Occupational Therapy and Older People

Second Edition

Edited by

Anita Atwal and Anne McIntyre

Division of Occupational Therapy
School of Health Sciences and Social Care
Brunel University
London
UK

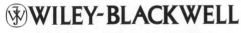

WILEY-BLACKWELL

A John Wiley & Sons, Ltd., Publication

This edition first published 2013 © 2013 Blackwell Publishing Ltd

Blackwell Publishing was acquired by John Wiley & Sons in February 2007. Blackwell's publishing program
has been merged with Wiley's global Scientific, Technical and Medical business to form Wiley-Blackwell.

Registered Office
John Wiley & Sons, Ltd, The Atrium, Southern Gate, Chichester, West Sussex, PO19 8SQ, UK

Editorial Offices
9600 Garsington Road, Oxford, OX4 2DQ, UK
The Atrium, Southern Gate, Chichester, West Sussex, PO19 8SQ, UK
111 River Street, Hoboken, NJ 07030-5774, USA

For details of our global editorial offices, for customer services and for information about how
to apply for permission to reuse the copyright material in this book please see our website at
www.wiley.com/wiley-blackwell.

Library of Congress Cataloging-in-Publication Data
Occupational therapy and older people / edited by Anita Atwal and Anne McIntyre. – 2nd ed.
    p. ; cm.
  Includes bibliographical references and index.
    ISBN 978-1-4443-3333-6 (pbk. : alk. paper) – ISBN 978-1-118-55612-2 (eMobi) –
ISBN 978-1-118-55613-9 (ePDF) – ISBN 978-1-118-55614-6 (ePub)
I. Atwal, Anita. II. McIntyre, Anne.
[DNLM: 1. Occupational Therapy. 2. Aged. 3. Aging. WB 555]
    615.8′5150846–dc23
                                                  2012043161

A catalogue record for this book is available from the British Library.

Wiley also publishes its books in a variety of electronic formats. Some content that appears in print may not
be available in electronic books.

Cover image: © iStock – sbayram
Cover design by Meaden Creative

Set in 10/12.5pt Times by SPi Publisher Services, Pondicherry, India
Printed in Singapore by Ho Printing Singapore Pte Ltd

1   2013

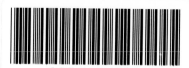

Occupational Therapy and Older People

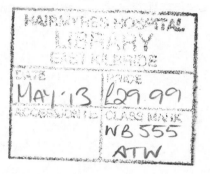

Acknowledgements

To our families, friends, colleagues and students. To our parents for being such inspirational role models.

Contents

List of Contributors

Stephen Ashford, PhD, MSc, BSc, MCSP, PGCE
Steve trained in Physiotherapy at Salford University and qualified in 1993. He undertook an MSc in Neuro-rehabilitation. Steve is a clinical specialist and gained teaching experience at Brunel University, being appointed course director for the Neuro-rehabilitation MSc course from 2001 until 2003. Steve has published a number of peer-reviewed papers in the rehabilitation literature as well as book chapters and clinical guideline contributions.

Anita Atwal, PhD, MSc, DipCOT, FHEA
After qualifying from the Derby School of Occupational Therapy in 1989, Anita gained a wide experience in acute medicine, older people and neurology. Anita has a particular interest in older adults in the acute care setting and has published over 30 articles in international and national peer-reviewed journals. She regularly presents at international and national conferences. Anita is the Director for Professional Practice Research at Brunel University, which aims to support and empower students, academics, clinicians and service users to promote high standards in clinical practice.

Rachel Bentley, MSc, BSc
Rachel worked as a junior and senior occupational therapist in medicine, surgery and oncology. She then spent five years in the community, working in intermediate care rehabilitating patients and supporting palliative care patients. She is currently working in a lung care team/specialist palliative care team.

Sarah Buchanan
Sarah is Research Director at Thomas Pocklington, a small UK charity that provides direct services for people with sight loss. Sarah has worked in the voluntary and public sectors for many years after being involved within academic research.

Margaret Gallagher, MA, DipCOT, FHEA
Margaret is an occupational therapy lecturer at Brunel University and manages the Practice Placement Educators course, preparing colleagues for practice education. She leads the OT programme for interprofessional learning. Her practice experience includes working with children with disabilities and their families. Her management experience was as a senior manager and spans mental health, learning disabilities,

community services and the acute sectors. Margaret's research interests are supervision in practice education and interprofessional working.

Linda Gnanasekaran, MSc, BSc(Hons), DipCOT, FHEA
Linda has worked in higher education for 23 years, teaching student occupational therapists and physiotherapists at undergraduate and postgraduate levels. Currently, she is the programme leader for the BSc Occupational Therapy course at Brunel University. Her teaching and scholarship focuses upon physiology, neurology, cognition, and neuro-rehabilitation. She has a particular interest in the physiology of ageing, and frailty. Prior to teaching, Linda worked in neuro-rehabilitation and community physical disability services.

Mary Grant, MSc, DipCOT
Mary qualified as an occupational therapist in 1984 and has worked in clinical practice, education and research. She has been a lecturer at Brunel University and Coventry University and is currently working as a research occupational therapist at the University of Nottingham.

Thérèse Jackson, MSc, DipCOT
Thérèse is the Consultant Occupational Therapist in Stroke for NHS Grampian and is the lead Allied Health Professions for the Stroke Management Clinical Network. She is the occupational therapy advisor to the National Advisory Committee for Stroke at the Scottish Government and has worked in the areas of stroke and neurosciences for most of her career. Thérèse has extensive teaching experience and runs courses nationally and internationally and has published several articles and written book chapters on topics related to stroke.

Jacqueline Lawson, MSc, BSc
Jacqueline is an occupational therapist who has a research interest in recovery and has been involved in several projects to promote recovery including the recovery arts and narrative project. She has spent many years working as a clinician and has presented at numerous conferences

Alison Lillywhite, MSc, BSc
Alison has mainly worked in community-based services for people with learning (intellectual) disabilities, Since 2009, she has worked as a Practitioner Researcher with the NIHR's CLAHRC for Cambridgeshire and Peterborough, supporting research into the design and delivery of community-based specialist learning disability services, particularly for people whose behaviour is 'challenging' or have unmet mental health needs. Alison continues to provide professional supervision to occupational therapists in clinical services.

Kee Hean Lim, MSc, DipCOT
Kee Hean is an occupational therapy lecturer at Brunel University. His research interests include occupational therapy in mental health, service users' involvement and empowerment,

cultural awareness and competency and the Kawa Model Framework. He is a co-author of the book *Advancing Occupational Therapy Practice in Mental Health Practice*.

Alice Mackenzie, MSc, PGCertHE, BSc OT (Can) DipCOT

Alice worked as an occupational therapist in mental health services and elderly care services for many years in London and Canada. In 2000, Alice came to Brunel University as an occupational therapy lecturer. She has had particular responsibility for practice placement education and teaching first-year undergraduates.

Melanie Manley, BSc (OT)

Melanie is an occupational therapist who has expertise in mental health, particularly in relation to older adults.

Anne McIntyre, PhD, MSc, PGCertTLHE, DipCOT

Anne is currently programme lead for the MSc (pre-reg) Occupational Therapy course at Brunel University, where she has been an OT lecturer since 1997. She teaches occupational therapy and physiotherapy students at undergraduate and postgraduate level. Anne has worked in acute health care, neurological rehabilitation, with children with motor disorders as well as community rehabilitation with older people. Her interests are successful ageing and the use of the ICF in practice. Her doctoral research explored the experience of falling for older people with dementia and their carers. She is a member of the Brunel Institute of Ageing Studies.

Anna L. Pratt, MSc, PGCert LTHE, DipCOT

Anna specialised in the area of hand therapy soon after qualifying as an occupational therapist. She has worked as a Clinical Specialist and Research Hand Therapist and has researched and published widely in the specialist area. She is currently the programme lead for the MSc Hand Therapy course at Brunel University.

Frances Reynolds, PhD, Dip. Psych. Couns, BSc, AFBPsS, FCOT

Frances is a Reader in Health Psychology at Brunel University and joined the Division of Occupational Therapy in 1992. She has a particular interest in supervising students' qualitative research projects, at MSc and PhD levels, and is a member of the Brunel Institute of Ageing Studies. She has particular research interests in the meanings of creative occupations, and their role in promoting positive identity, social networks and life satisfaction among people who are living with adversities associated with later life and/or disability. She has published articles in journals such as *Disability and Rehabilitation*, *Arts in Psychotherapy*, *The British Journal of Occupational Therapy*, and *Qualitative Health Research*.

Christina Richards, MSc, BSc(Hons)

Chris has worked in the physical health setting as both a junior and senior occupational therapist. This has encompassed specialist work with respiratory patients including setting up the occupational therapy component of a breathlessness clinic. She currently manages the therapy services within a general hospital.

Marcus Sivell-Muller, M.Phil, PG Dip OT, BA (Hons)

Marcus is a qualified occupational therapist and former Lecturer at Brunel University. He has been a Programme Manager supporting US Central Command and the International Security Assistance Force (ISAF) with numerous State-Building and Rule of Law projects in Afghanistan for almost a decade. Marcus has been at the forefront of pushing forward occupational therapy into the area of overseas development work. His expertise is focused in applying occupational theory and processes within a broader, empowerment: enabling a mentor/advisorship role amongst stability building and nation development projects in conflicted environments.

Anthony Slater

Anthony was Lighting Development Manager at Thomas Pocklington Trust where he was responsible for developing guidance on lighting for people with sight loss. Anthony has over 35 years' experience of lighting research and development and has published technical papers and served on international and UK technical and standards committees.

Kirsty Tattersall, BSc

Kirsty has worked as a junior and senior therapist within medicine, orthopaedics and neurology. She worked for five years as a clinical specialist at a tertiary cardiac and respiratory hospital, jointly setting up a rehabilitation programme for heart failure patients. She is currently working within critical care and surgery.

Sue Vernon, DipCOT DSA ADI (Car)

Sue qualified as a Driving Standards Agency Approved Driving Instructor (Car) in 1992 and becoming the first dual qualified OT/ADI in the UK. Sue established her own business and is currently running two specially equipped assessment vehicles and her expertise and wide experience enables her to work effectively with the high level of complex trauma at trauma centres.

Alison Warren, MSc, DipCOT, PGCertHE

Alison has many years' experience of working with older people with mental health problems. Alison completed her Masters on the use of COPM in mental health and, more recently, completed research related to dementia and interprofessional education. She is currently working at Limerick University, and is undertaking a PhD in the area of role emerging placements in occupational therapy. Alison is a Health Research Board (HRB) Fellow for 2012–2013.

Jennifer Wenborn, PhD, MSc, DipCOT

Jennifer is currently Clinical Research Fellow in Occupational Therapy, University College London, Dementia Research Unit. She has primarily worked with older people within many settings. Jennifer is involved in a randomised controlled trial of reminiscence therapy for people with dementia and their family caregivers. She is a past Chair of the College of Occupational Therapists Specialist Section – Older People.

Lesley Wilson, MSc, DipCOT
Lesley is an occupational therapy lecturer who was the programme lead for the MSc Occupational Therapy (pre-registration) which she developed in 2007, until 2012. Previously, she was the programme leader for the part-time BSc (Hons) Occupational Therapy from 1998 to 2005. Her clinical background is in physical and neurological disability, paediatrics, community work and senior management within the NHS and Social Services. Her research interests include occupational science, the mind–body interaction, spirituality and the connections between mental and physical health linked to occupation.

Chapter 1

Introduction

Anne McIntyre and Anita Atwal (with contributions from Jennifer Wenborn)

This introductory chapter provides a justification for why occupational therapists should be interested in working with older people and explains the structure of the book. The demands of occupational therapy practice with older people are considered, and a brief explanation is given for how the World Health Organization's [WHO] International Classification of Functioning, Disability and Health [ICF] (WHO 2001) can be used in occupational therapy practice. We also present our own reflections and that of an occupational therapy expert, Jennifer Wenborn, interspersed in boxes within the chapter, on why we work with older adults. We are not proud of our initial attitudes, but we hope that we do convey our enthusiasm for occupational therapy with older people.

Ageing is a process which occupational therapists cannot ignore, for globally there will be 1.2 billion people over the age of 60 by the year 2025 and by 2050 these figures will have doubled, with 80% of older people living in developing countries (WHO 2002). It is also worth considering why there is a global increase in the ageing population. There are three main factors – a decline in mortality, an increase in longevity and also a decline in fertility (Beard et al. 2012). It is also important to realise that the numbers of the oldest-old (or those people aged over 85 years) has doubled in the last 25 years and is predicted to more than double in the next 20 years (Wise 2010). Instead of regarding the growth in the ageing population and also the increasing life expectancy as success stories, these are often viewed with doom and gloom. This doom and gloom is often associated with the belief that old age equals indignity and dependency, as well as economic concerns of the need for more money to pay for additional health and social care. Yet healthy older people can be considered a precious resource, making important contributions to their families, communities and the economy at large, by either paid or voluntary employment (WHO 2002).

The type of service provided by occupational therapists for older people varies internationally, and it has to be acknowledged that the authors of this book speak from their own perspective. The services that occupational therapists provide to older people are not only determined by the needs of a growing older population, but also by government policy – either at a local or national level. As occupational therapists that work in England, we have seen many changes in the way that services are delivered to older people, in both the public and private sectors. Health and social care services for older people are not only provided by public services in the acute or rehabilitation in-patient settings for older people with physical or mental health care needs, but also by community health or social care services. Occupational therapists also provide services to older people in residential and nursing home care. Increasingly, older people are receiving services provided by the commercial and also the voluntary sectors. These are exciting and challenging times for occupational therapists working with older people.

Using this book

As in the first edition of this book, we discuss the biological, psychological and social elements of health and wellbeing for older people rather than having a bio-medical focus on health conditions. There are several reasons for this; many older people are referred to occupational therapy services with multiple difficulties in occupational performance and not all of these are caused by a health condition – some may be the result of the normal ageing process, or by environmental and contextual factors. There is also an increasing emphasis within health and social care on health promotion, and occupational therapists are becoming increasingly aware of their role with the 'well' older age group.

Once again, we have used the World Health Organization's [WHO] bio-psycho-social model of health, the International Classification of Functioning, Disability and Health [ICF] to provide a framework for the book, and the domains of the ICF have provided definitions for the content of each chapter (WHO 2001).

The motivation for writing a second edition of our book is our desire and wish for occupational therapists to continue to move towards an 'active ageing' approach (WHO 2002). Active ageing (Box 1.1) signifies an important paradigm shift: away from a 'needs based' approach to a 'right based' approach which support the rights and continued participation of older people both in the community and the political process (WHO 2002).

This chapter provides an introduction to the core issues that influence our practice as occupational therapists, including some personal reasons. Chapter 2 considers common concepts and theories of ageing, contextualising them within an occupational science perspective. Chapters 3, 4 and 9 consider other contextual factors such as social, cultural, environmental and economic factors. Chapter 5 does consider some of the more common health conditions that affect people in old age, but also directs the reader towards the evidence base for occupational therapy intervention as well as highlighting some

---

Box 1.1   What is active ageing?

It is the process of optimising opportunities for health, participation and security in order to enhance quality of life as people age. (WHO 2002: 12)

'Active' refers to continued participation in society and to realise their potential for physical, social, and mental wellbeing whilst ensuring adequate protection, security and care when assistance is needed. This includes continued participation in social, economic, cultural and spiritual, and civic affairs.

commonly- used outcome measures. Chapters 6 and 7 consider the ageing body in terms of body functions and structures. Chapter 8 presents how activity and participation changes in older age.

It is hoped that this book encourages the reader to view the strengths of older people during the ageing process, to consider old age as a time of celebration and to promote occupational justice for their older clients whilst still meeting all the demands of present-day practice.

The demands of occupational therapy practice

Although policies, demands and service provision vary from country to country, there is an increasing need for occupational therapists to clearly articulate the importance of their role and the evidence base of occupational therapy interventions to other professionals who might hold the power to commission services on behalf of older people, or to older people themselves and their families. Within the UK, public health and social care service provision is being increasingly determined by guidance provided by the National Institute for Health and Clinical Excellence [NICE] and the Social Care Institute for Excellence [SCIE]. What is encouraging is the inclusion of occupational therapy research within the UK NICE guidelines (NICE 2008). This guidance refers to occupational therapy and physical activity to promote the mental wellbeing of older people. These guidelines are extremely important for supporting and developing interventions within UK clinical practice.

Interestingly, where occupational therapy is well established, there is often little or no evidence for the service provided. Indeed, a systematic review of occupational therapy practice for older adults with lower limb amputations found that research evidence with this population is limited and scarce, and yet occupational therapists are key members of the multidisciplinary team for these older adults (Spiliotopoulou and Atwal 2011). However, complacency is dangerous, as one reason for occupational therapy posts being axed or services being contracted is a lack of evidence to support interventions or to provide evidence of its cost-effectiveness.

Box 1.2   Why work with older adults? – Jennifer Wenborn.

"I left occupational therapy college in 1979 very undecided about which speciality I wanted to work in – except I was clear I was NOT going to work in 'geriatrics' (as older people were then known). This was due to a very unsatisfactory first clinical placement at a (well-known) geriatric hospital, following which I seriously considered leaving the course as I didn't think OT was the right job for me. I started a rotational post in a central London hospital but almost immediately the unit was shut to save money and I was transferred to 'slow stream geriatric rehabilitation'. Not the most auspicious start to my brand-new career! However, I soon found that I enjoyed building relationships over time with the patients and working as part of a multidisciplinary team. Senior and Head OT posts followed, and I enjoyed and developed a broad range of experience, predominantly working with older people. After 15 years in the NHS I opted for redundancy when yet another reorganisation came along.

Eighteen months at the College of Occupational Therapists establishing their consultancy service followed before becoming self-employed. Over the next ten years I provided a wide range of services: individual assessments and interventions; setting up new services – occupational therapy within a private hospital; fast-track technician to facilitate NHS discharge; long-term care insurance assessment service for a reinsurance company; Commission for Health Improvement (CHI) reviews; Department of Health and Health Advisory Service project work; NHS management and supervision; education and training. I increasingly worked in care homes – with older people and adults with severe disability – learning more about people with dementia and acquiring specialist skills such as seating provision and multisensory stimulation.

I was then asked to provide some input to a new NHS Nursing Home until appointed to the 50:50 clinical/academic post. Having caught the research bug when I completed my Masters in Occupational Therapy ten years earlier I couldn't resist applying. I went on to complete my PhD, based on a randomised controlled trial of occupational therapy intervention for people with dementia in care homes. I now work full-time for University College London, using my OT skills to evaluate non-pharmacological interventions for people with dementia and their family caregivers. My next goal is to do more occupational therapy research to add to our profession's evidence base.

I definitely ended up in the right speciality! I love meeting older people, learning from their life experience and resilience. Those we meet in our work often have a complex mix of abilities and needs and I enjoy 'unpicking' these to achieve the best 'fit' solution – not least because it utilises my full range of occupational therapy skills creatively. I enjoy working within a team – the core members being the older person and their family. The range and diversity of what I have done has made it the best job ever!"

Jennifer Wenborn

Providing an evidence base

It is encouraging that there has increasingly been some high-quality research that does provide an evidence base for occupational therapy practice. Interestingly, studies by Clark et al. (1997, 2001, 2011), Steultjens et al. (2004), Graff et al. (2006), and Logan et al. (2010) have all involved older people (and are discussed in more detail in Chapter 2). Indeed, the amount of research involving older people has increased dramatically over the last 10 to 15 years, possibly because of global emphasis of user involvement and client-centred practice as part of health promotion policy (WHO 1986).

It would be naïve to say that research with older people is easy, and research by McMurdo et al. (2005, 2011) suggests that there is still a widespread exclusion of older people from research. There are many reasons given as to why older people are still excluded from research, such as:

- Obtaining consent is too time consuming (Bayer and Tadd 2000)
- Inclusion in research often deterred by others (Zermansky et al. 2005)
- Older people are perceived as too vulnerable or frail by researchers (Department of Health 2001, McMurdo et al. 2005)
- Older people are commonly excluded if they have cognitive impairment or dementia (Wilkinson 2002)
- Older people have multiple health conditions and medications, which increase likelihood of attrition, mortality rates and confounding variables within a study (McMurdo et al. 2005, Zermansky et al. 2005)

- They may require longer explanations about the study or more time to decide in consultation with family (Harris and Dyson 2001, Davies et al. 2010)
- Screening of oldest-old could take longer because of fatigue, mobility problems, social care or transportation issues (McMurdo et al. 2005, Zermansky et al. 2005, Davies et al. 2010).

However, it is suggested that the danger of not recruiting older people to health and social care research (and especially clinical and intervention trials) is a loss of autonomy and poor scientific outcome. There is also a paradox, with those people with the greater need and usage of services and interventions being excluded by ill health and social isolation (McMurdo et al. 2005, 2011).

It is acknowledged that researching with older people as participants requires more time, planning and expertise (Owen 2001, McMurdo et al. 2011) and an understanding of, and flexibility within, the consent process within both quantitative and qualitative research studies. Harris and Dyson (2001) and Davies et al. (2010) identified that the initial approach to older people by using 'gatekeepers' such as familiar and trusted health professionals, or by family members, enhanced recruitment. Recruitment to a study can also be enhanced by the personal contact with the researcher to gain information about the study, either face-to-face or by telephone (Harris and Dyson 2001, Davies et al. 2010).

The choice of design can often influence the reliability of the data collected from older people. Atwal and Caldwell (2005) identified that older people are often reluctant to express criticism of services during face-to-face interviews, and yet could have difficulty reading and completing potentially less-intrusive postal questionnaires because of small font size or language barriers. More frail older people mighty also have difficulty in sustaining their participation in interviews or questionnaire-based surveys because of fatigue (Davies et al. 2010). Cross-sectional and matched pair designs are often thwarted by the heterogeneity of an older sample population, but longitudinal cohort studies commonly suffer from participant attrition (Matthews et al. 2004, McMurdo et al. 2005). Indeed, in a review of randomised control trials, McMurdo et al. (2011) identified an attrition rate of up to 37% of older participants within the studies reviewed, often due to declining cognitive functioning, admission to long-term care or mortality.

The use of one-to-one or focus group interviews in qualitative research is said to be especially appropriate when involving older participants. The use of a semi- (or unstructured) interview process following a conversational style is also advocated to facilitate an older participant to reconstruct past experiences in a relatively free and unprompted way (Gearing and Dant 1990, Montazeri et al. 1996). Researching with older people with dementia is also said to be enhanced by the use of qualitative methodologies, a flexible interview schedule (i.e. finding the right time), allowing the participant to return to the topic, being supportive and alert to non-verbal signals, and being willing to accept the person's narrative as truth (Bond and Corner 2001, Wilkinson 2002, Hubbard et al. 2003).

Although there is increasing advice and guidance on methodological factors that need to be considered when researching with older people, there remains a disappointing lack of evidence to support occupational therapy practice in many areas. For example, there is still a lack of research evidence for occupational therapy for people with long-term health conditions and to support interventions within acute care settings for older adults and yet, in the UK, we have experienced a growth in the number of occupational therapists working within Accident and Emergency Departments. Whereas, in other more established areas of occupational therapy practice with older people (for example, dementia care, stroke, falls and Parkinson's disease), the interventions are highly rated by service users and clients, although the evidence base for intervention is ambiguous. It is important to explore both service user perspectives and the efficacy of interventions in the recently-expanding areas of occupational therapy with older adults such as those older people entering old age with disability, those with learning disability, older people using acute care and also intermediate care services.

As consumers of occupational therapy research, we need this evidence too. We also need the skills to critically appraise research articles so that we can determine the quality of the research, and to make a decision about how this research could impact upon our practice. In particular, therapists need to understand both qualitative and quantitative methods. Managers of services also have a part to play in building infrastructure to support evidence-based practice.

We write this chapter at a time of global economic recession, with public sector funding cuts and subsequent contraction and rationalisation of services. It is therefore even more important to consider the most appropriate and effective place (economically, socially, scientifically and professionally) for occupational therapists to work. As therapists, we need to start considering what our contribution is to our older clients. We have both practice experience and an interest in older people's acute care services, and the following are questions that we ask ourselves:

- What contribution do occupational therapists make to the quality of life and occupational justice of older adults in acute care settings?
- Is the role of occupational therapy in this setting simply to expedite hospital discharge or to prevent or delay a hospital admission?
- Are occupational therapy services in the acute care setting cost-effective?
- Could this service be offered by another member of the interprofessional and interagency team at a lower cost?
- Are occupational therapists working in the acute care setting carrying out their duties in an occupationally just and client-centred way?

These questions may be controversial, but we do believe that there is a role for occupational therapy for older adults in acute care settings. However, there appears to be a role dilemma for occupational therapists when working with older adults who are admitted into acute health care settings. Whilst discharge planning is an important process, perhaps it is more important for occupational therapists to focus on how they will contribute to this process rather than with the actual coordination of the discharge? Perhaps occupational therapists need to give a higher focus to preventive and rehabilitative interventions that promote optimal occupational performance and occupational justice? Likewise, community occupational therapists should also consider how rehabilitation can be integrated more into their practice, and ascertain further evidence to demonstrate how the provision of assistive technology and/or environmental adaption support this process. This will be explored further in Chapter 9. It is therefore important for occupational therapy practitioners to continually evaluate their service provision in a methodologically robust way to add to the evidence base for occupational therapy and older people.

Box 1.3   Why work with older adults – Anita Atwal.

"At the age of 21 I had absolutely no intention of working with older adults. I had just got my first job and real taste of independence in a large teaching hospital. I was going to focus on having fun and trying to avoid 'hard work'. On reflection, this was of course not the ideal attitude to have! Occupational therapy is more than work, it's a commitment to certain principles.

However, after completing a mental health rotation I started my first physical rotation, which was on an acute older persons' ward. I remember walking onto the ward and thinking that this was not for me! The ward was busy and full of commodes and people rushing by. However, I was then introduced to Rose. Rose was a dancing 70-year-old with flaming red hair who served the tea. The nurses, doctors and physiotherapists were dynamic and sociable. This was fun and, moreover, the two consultants were fantastic. On reflection, it was their attitude towards their management of the older person that changed the way I viewed older people. The older people were treated with respect and dignity. Their concerns were listened to and, more importantly, so were ours. We were given time to rehabilitate the person and given news about their progress in the day hospital. The consultants' attitude and leadership meant that the team adopted their ethos. Moreover, whilst working with older people was challenging and thought provoking, it was not 'hard work', it was fun. It meant that I really was utilising my skills and each day there was a new challenge.

My advice is to gather as much experience as possible and work in lots of physical areas such as neurology and orthopaedics. This will enhance your occupational therapy skills and shape your future development as an occupational therapist."

Anita Atwal

A new and exciting innovation has been the growth of knowledge transfer activity as there are often criticisms that academic researchers live and working in ivory towers with little application to everyday practice. Knowledge transfer (KT) describes the collaborative problem-solving and sharing of experiences, perspectives, and knowledge among caregivers, researchers and policy makers that arises through developing partnerships and exchanging information and ideas (ESCR 2010). This has the potential to prepare organisations and practitioners to receive the new knowledge resulting from research and implement it in practice. We have used this process successfully in partnership with members of the Specialist Section – Trauma and Orthopaedics of the College of Occupational Therapists, in formulating guidelines for occupational therapists working with people with lower limb amputations (Atwal et al. 2011). The success of the collaboration was the fusion of academic and expert skills in producing the guidelines. The expert clinicians received training in critical appraisal skills and on the process of producing guidelines. The academics faced the challenges of translating the research evidence into meaningful guidelines for practitioners (Atwal and Spiliotopoulou 2011).

ICF and Occupational Therapy

The International Classification of Functioning, Disability and Health (ICF; Box 1.4) is a member of the WHO's group of classifications devised to provide a global language. It can be linked with the ICD-10 which considers diagnosis and disease, whereas the ICF considers health and wellbeing in terms of the way we function in the context of our lives.

Box 1.4   The International Classification of Functioning, Disability and Health [ICF] (WHO 2001).

The World Health Organization's International Classification of Functioning, Disability and Health [ICF] (WHO 2001) can be accessed and explained in more detail at:
   http://www.who.int/classifications/icf/en/

The College of Occupational Therapists [COT] have also produced a guidance document on the ICF:

COT (2004) *Guidance for the Use of the International Classification of Functioning, Disability and Health and the Ottawa Charter for Health Promotion in Occupational Therapy Services.* London, COT.

The ICF has been adopted by occupational therapy associations and bodies in the UK, Canada, the US, Australia and Scandinavia, as well as the World Federation of Occupational Therapists (WFOT) as a model of health and disability because of its person–context interaction. It is not an occupational therapy-specific model but is a universally devised and accepted tool that involved many professions, organisations and user groups from around the world in its construction. It is not just a health and social care classification but for any agency including economic, education and transportation. Because of its universality, it is useful for interprofessional and interagency working as a 'common ground' or language for communication and intervention planning. Therefore, where occupational therapists work in interprofessional or interagency teams it allows for shared understanding of issues and concepts such as disability, impairment or participation (Tempest and McIntyre 2006).

   The ICF is considered as a bio-psycho-social model of functioning, because of its body-person-context interaction, applying to all people throughout the world. Even though it is used as a means of classifying and collecting data on functioning and disability of populations on a global scale, it also provides a framework to consider the occupational performance of individuals and how this is impacted by extrinsic factors. It therefore fits in with the ideals of client-centred practice.

   In the past, the consequences of health conditions for older people have been considered in terms of mortality rates; however, the ICF provides an opportunity to collect evidence of what older people can and cannot do. It enables us to consider the links between intrinsic factors from a health condition and also the contextual barriers or facilitators that impact upon their functioning. The ICF considers that the different elements within the classification can interact to a lesser or greater degree, rather than having a causal or hierarchical effect (see Figure 1.1). For example, an older person might not have any impairment or activity limitation but does have participation restriction because of the attitudes of their family or the society in which they live.

   The main components of the ICF are body functions and structures, activity, participation and the personal and environmental contextual factors. This fits easily with occupational therapy thinking of the person-environment-occupation interaction described in models of Occupational Performance (Christiansen and Baum 1997). Each component can be described and defined in a positive or negative way (e.g. impairment of body structure or function). Each of the body functions and structures are considered by systems rather than organs because of

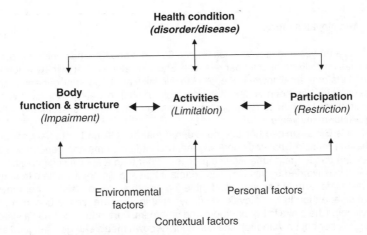

Figure 1.1 The World Health Organisation's International Classification of Functioning, Disability and Health [ICF] (*Source*: WHO 2001:18).

overlapping functions between many structures. Activity and participation can be considered in terms of activity limitation and participation restriction, with personal and environmental contextual factors described in terms of potential facilitators or barriers for the client's activity or participation. An example of this could be that the cessation of the local bus service acts as a barrier to an older person being able to do their food shopping independently, but the acquisition of a home computer and easy internet access can facilitate the older person to order their weekly food shopping online and have it delivered by their supermarket of choice.

Each of the components is subdivided into separate domains and these are defined within the ICF, providing much-needed universal definitions of self care and mobility, for example. The reader is advised to explore these on the ICF website mentioned in Box 1.4.

Use of the ICF as a framework

In the following chapters in this book, it will hopefully become clearer how the normal ageing process and pathological change of body functions and structures and contextual factors can interact to create activity limitations or participation restrictions for an older person. It is worthwhile considering Mrs Nowak's story in Box 1.5 and then explore how the occupational therapist has extracted relevant issues from this story using the ICF (WHO 2001) as a framework, to inform intervention (Figure 1.2). The ICF codes have also been included so that the reader can consult the classification and definitions on the ICF website.

The ICF framework is a useful tool to identify Mrs Novak's problems and potential issues. By considering these as differing concepts, it allows the therapist to consider whether the limitation in activity or participation restriction ares caused by an impairment of body function or structure, or by an environmental barrier. Therefore, the occupational therapist can consider if the outcome measure of choice will focus on impairment or on contextual factors; or, indeed, necessitate the need for both types of outcome measure to be used. The most appropriate intervention can then be determined. However, the choice

---

Box 1.5   Mrs Novak's story.

Mrs Novak is a 96-year-old lady who left Poland 60 years ago. She has been a widow for 30 years and has no children or any near relatives. She lives alone in her own two-storey house on the outskirts of a small town in the UK. Mrs Novak went to see her general practitioner [GP] because she has been finding it increasingly difficult to walk to her local shops and becomes tired easily when carrying out her housework. She has been suffering with osteo-arthritis [OA] for many years.

Mrs Novak's GP examined her and considered that her OA had not changed, and suggested that her muscle weakness and wasting, mobility problems and generalised feelings of fatigue were due to the normal ageing process rather than a specific diagnosis.

Mrs Novak was worried by this and was adamant that she did not want help from her local social services department as she was frightened that they would insist on her moving into residential care. Although Mrs Novak is independent in self-care, she is beginning to have difficulty climbing the stairs to her bedroom and bathroom. Fortunately, she has a toilet on the ground floor of her house. Although she can cook her own meals she gets fatigued standing for long periods. Her only social contact is from attending a daily service at her local church, which she is struggling to attend. This upsets her, as her observance of her beliefs is very important to her.

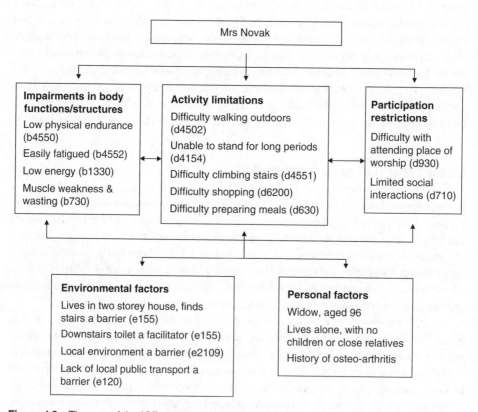

Figure 1.2   The use of the ICF as a framework for practice.

of intervention will also be determined by the beliefs, philosophy and theoretical model of the occupational therapist and the organisation.

One could suggest that, in the absence of any identifiable health condition, Mrs Novak is becoming frailer and less able to cope with her everyday tasks. As an occupational therapist, it is perhaps pertinent to consider that Mrs Novak is now 96 years of age, and that her physiological capacity is probably reduced. Therefore, it might be appropriate to consider a compensatory approach to address Mrs Novak's occupational performance difficulties. This approach may be the best option for Mrs Novak to preserve her current level of body functioning, to conserve her energy and capacity for her most valued occupations. Hence Mrs Novak's activity limitations or participation restrictions could be considered in terms of environmental facilitators and barriers to improve performance, and therefore these will be the focus of assessment and intervention. For example, the OT could discuss with Mrs Novak whether her kitchen could be organised in such a way to reduce unnecessary energy consumption, and that perhaps the provision of a perching/high stool could assist her in carrying out kitchen activities. The OT could carry out an assessment of Mrs Novak's stairs to consider if provision of extra rails would reduce the amount of effort required and improve Mrs Novak's ability to safely ascend and descend her stairs. Mrs Novak's local place of worship might also have a rota to collect and transport parishioners so they could attend services and events, and perhaps have a local community organisation that helps more frail or disabled parishioners with everyday activities such as shopping, so perhaps enabling Mrs Novak in such a way that she feels supported and empowered rather than threatened and monitored so that her sense of autonomy remains intact.

Using the ICF as a framework not only highlights the areas of importance for the client but also the type of services that could be involved. Mrs Novak's story highlights how the interagency team often involves local community services, such as voluntary organisations or places of worship, as well as the public sector. The ICF can also clarify roles and identify areas of overlap and discrepancies in service provision when working in interprofessional and interagency teams where roles seem to be blurred. Using the ICF can also assist in clinical reasoning – of the choice of intervention approach and focus of assessment. Such clarification can avoid two services working at odds with each other – one with a rehabilitative approach (working on activity capacity) and another with a compensatory one (working on activity performance) with the same client.

Why work with older people?

It is interesting that all three of our stories given in Boxes 1.2, 1.3 and 1.6 show that we all have had similar experiences. None of us wanted to work with older people initially, and fell into this area of practice by accident. What also comes across is that we all enjoy the interdisciplinary team working that is necessary when working with older people, because of the many needs and problems an older person normally faces when they are referred to healthcare services.

It is perhaps fair to say that our own early attitudes were not unusual and mirrored those explicitly expressed in health and social care at the time, with older people being excluded

---

Box 1.6   Why work with older people – Anne McIntyre.

"I would like to say that I had always wanted to work with older people, but this was not the case. I qualified as an occupational therapist in 1980, and, like Jennifer, was determined never to work with older people. I was ambitious and knew that if I wanted to 'get on' in OT, then working with older people was not the right career path to take. I hadn't been able to decide whether I wanted to work in a physical or a mental health care setting, and for many years I specialised in neurological rehabilitation as I felt it gave me the best of both worlds. It was not until my last clinical post before becoming an academic OT that I started working in an older people's service. The post was, I am afraid, chosen because of its proximity to my children's school and not because of the client group. However, here my love for older people's practice began. I worked in a community day hospital for older people with 'physical' health problems. I helped set up the service and worked in a very enthusiastic and supportive interdisciplinary team. Until this time, I had worked within a medical model of practice, but soon learnt that a bio-psycho-social model was more appropriate here.

I found working with older people a challenge and very stimulating, as my interventions had to be client-centred and multifaceted. No two clients (or, indeed, interventions) were alike, because of the differing personal and environmental contextual factors. I listened to people's stories of their past lives – of their struggles and losses during WWII, and the hardships faced during their childhood in the 1920 and 1930s. I realised that these past experiences influenced the older person that they had become. I became aware that even the most affluent client suffered deprivation of some kind – as they were often socially isolated and looked after by a succession of paid carers, with little opportunity for developing any kind of relationship. Unfortunately, we also had to address incidences of physical, emotional or financial abuse, and co-existing mental health problems, so I was fully aware of the vulnerability of our older clients. I became interested in falls prevention whilst at the day hospital, and this interest has continued until today. My PhD research explored the experiences of older people with dementia and their carers of falling. Once again, I listened to peoples' stories and realised how these participants were struggling to maintain their autonomy and identity whilst dealing with the consequences of falls, dementia and ageing.

So what do I enjoy about working with older people? I enjoy the challenge of enabling each individual, to maintain their optimal health and wellbeing in a holistic way. I relish that my clinical reasoning skills are continually challenged, my 'tool box' of interventions is constantly added to, and my negotiation skills are honed. I have a hatred of being bored, and one thing I have never been, when working with older people, is bored."

Anne McIntyre

---

from services and interventions because of their age. These beliefs are no longer explicitly expressed; however, it is worth reflecting whether these attitudes still prevail but are implicit in current practice.

One of the reasons why we are so passionate about working with older adults is because we believe occupation can enhance the lives of everyone in society. What all three of us enjoy is the challenge and complexity of practice with older people. We have developed skills and a greater awareness of the need to manage interrelated health, social, environmental and political factors to ensure occupational justice for our older clients.

Summary

This chapter has introduced the structure of this book and the concept of active ageing. Current challenges to the occupational therapy profession and the need for evidence base practice have been discussed. An understanding of the underlying issues and potential solutions to researching with older people have also been presented. The WHO (2001) ICF has also been presented, along with a suggestion for its use in occupational therapy to assist clinical reasoning and service provision. We have also presented our own stories of how we came to work with older people, how our initial prejudices were changed and why we find working with older people enjoyable, challenging and stimulating. This chapter provides a background to the chapters that now follow. We hope that this book with inspire you to adopt an active ageing approach to older adults and for you to reflect on current and future practice. We also hope you enjoy our colleagues' contributions.

References

Atwal, A. and Caldwell, K. (2005) The enigma of satisfaction surveys. *Australian Occupational Therapy Journal* **52**(**1**), 10–16.

Atwal, A., McLaughlin, J. and Spiliotopoulou, G. (2011) Occupational therapy with people who have had lower limb amputation: Evidence-based guidelines. College of Occupational Therapists: London.

Atwal, A. and Spiliotopoulou, G. (2011) Knowledge transfer: Developing guidelines for occupational therapists working with people with lower limb amputations. (Editorial), *British Journal of Occupational Therapy* **74**(**3**), 109–109.

Bayer, A. and Tadd, W. (2000) Unjustified exclusion of elderly people from studies submitted to research ethics committee for approval: Descriptive study. *BMJ* **321**, 992–993.

Beard, J.R., Biggs, S., Bloom, D.E., Fried, L.P., Hogan, P., Kalache, A. and Olshansky, S.J. (2012) Introduction. In World Economic Forum (ed.) *Global Population Ageing: Peril or promise?* Global Agenda Council on Ageing Society, pp. 4–13.

Bond, J. and Corner, L. (2001) Researching dementia: Are there unique methodological challenges for health services research? *Ageing and Society* **21**, 95–116.

Christiansen, C.H., and Baum, C.M. (1997) *Occupational Therapy: Enabling function and well-being*, 2nd edition. Thorofare, NJ: SLACK.

Clark, F., Azen, S.P., Zemke, R., Jackson, J., Carlson, M., Mandel, D., Hay, J., Josephson, K., Cherry, B., Hessel, C., Palmer, J. and Lipson, L. (1997) Occupational therapy for independent-living older adults: A randomised controlled trial. *Journal of the American Medical Association* **278**(**16**), 1321–1326.

Clark, F., Azen, S.P., Carlson, M., Mandel, D., LaBree, L., Hay, J., Zemke, R., Jackson, J. and Lipson, L. (2001) Embedding health-promoting changes into the daily lives of independent-living older adults: Long-term follow-up of occupational therapy intervention. *Journals of Gerontology Series B Psychological and Social Sciences* **56**(**1**), 60–63.

Clark, F., Jackson, J., Carlson, M., Chou, C.P., Cherry, B.J., Jordan-Marsh, M., Knight, B.G., Mandel, D., Blanchard, J., Granger, D.A., Wilcox, R.R., Lai, M.Y., White, B., Hay, J., Lam, C., Marterella, A. and Azen, S.P. (2011) Effectiveness of a lifestyle intervention in promoting the well-being of independently living older people: Results of the Well Elderly 2 Randomised Controlled Trial. *J Epidemiological Community Health*, doi:10.1136/jech.2009099754

Davies, K., Collerton, J.C., Jagger, C., Bond, J., Barker, S.A.H., Edwards, J., Hughes, J., Hunt, J.M. and Robinson, L. (2010) Engaging the oldest old in research: Lessons learnt from the Newcastle 85+ study. *BMC Geriatrics* **10**, 64; doi:10.1186/1471-2318-10-64

Department of Health (2001) *National Service Framework for Older People*. London. HMSO.

ESCR (2010) Society Today. Introduction to Knowledge Transfer. Available at http://www.esrc.ac.uk/ESRCInfoCentre/Support/knowledge_transfer/index.aspx

Gearing, B. and Dan, T. (1990) Doing biographical research. In: Peace, S.M. (ed.) *Researching Social Gerontology*. London: Sage Publications, pp. 143–159.

Graff, M.J.L., Vernooij-Dassen, M.J.M., Thijssen, M., Dekker, J., Hoefnagels, W.H.L. and Olde Rikkert, G.M. (2006) Community based occupational therapy for patients with dementia and their care givers: Randomised controlled trial. *BMJ* **333(7580)**, 1196–1199.

Harris, R. and Dyson, E. (2001) Recruitment of frail older people to research: Lessons learnt through experience. *Journal of Advanced Nursing* **36(5)**, 643–651.

Hubbard, G., Downs, M.G. and Tester, S. (2003) Including older people with dementia in research: Challenges and strategies. *Aging and Mental Health* **7(5)**, 351–362.

Logan, P.A., Coupland, C.A., Gladman, J.R.F., Sahota, O., Stoner-Hobbs, V., Robertson, K., Tomlinson, V., Ward, M., Sach, T. and Avery, A.J. (2010) Community falls prevention for people who call an emergency ambulance after a fall: Randomised controlled trial. *BMJ* **340**, c2101, doi:10.1136/bmj.c2102

Matthews, F.E., Chatfield, M., Freeman, C., McCracken, C., Brayne, C. and MRC CFAS (2004) Attrition and bias in the MRC cognitive function and ageing study: An epidemiological investigation. *BMC Public Health* **4**, 12, doi:10.1186/1471-2458-4-12

McMurdo, M.E.T., Witham, M.D. and Gillespie, N.D. (2005) Including older people in clinical research. *BMJ* **331**, 1036–1037.

McMurdo, M., Roberts, H., Parker, S., Wyatt, N., May, H., Goodman, C., Jackson, S., Gladman, J., O'Mahony, S., Ali, K., Dickinson, E., Edison, P. and Dyer, C. (2011) Improving recruitment of older people to research through good practice. *Age and Ageing* **40**, 659–665, doi:10.1093/ageing/afr115

Montazeri, A., Milroy, R., Gillis, C.R. and McEwen, J. (1996) Interviewing cancer patients in a research setting: The role of effective communication. *Supportive Care in Cancer* **4**, 447–454.

National Institute for Health and Clinical Excellence (NICE) (2008) Occupational Therapy Interventions and Physical Activity Interventions to Promote the Mental Wellbeing of Older People in Pprimary Care and Residential Care. London: National Institute for Health and Clinical Excellence. Available at http://www.nice.org.uk/nicemedia/pdf/PH16Guidance.pdf

Owen, S. (2001) The practical, methodological and ethical dilemmas of conducting focus groups with vulnerable clients. *Methodological Issues in Nursing Research* **36(5)**, 652–658.

Spiliotopoulou, G. and Atwal, A. (2011) Is occupational therapy practice for older adults with lower limb amputations evidence-based? A systematic review. *Prosthetics and Orthotics International* **36(1)**, 7–14.

Steultjens, E.M.J., Dekker, J., Bouter, L.M., Jellema, S., Bakker, E.B. and van den Ende, C.H.M. (2004) Occupational therapy for community dwelling elderly people: A systematic review. *Age & Ageing* **33(5)**, 453.

Tempest, S. and McIntyre, A. (2006) Using the ICF to clarify team roles and demonstrate clinical reasoning in stroke rehabilitation. *Disability and Rehabilitation* **28(10)**, 663–667.

Wilkinson, H. (2002) Including people with dementia in research: Methods and motivations. In Wilkinson, H. (ed.) *The Perspectives of People with Dementia: Research methods and motivations*. London: Jessica Kingsley, pp. 9–24.

Wise, J. (2010) Number of "oldest old" has doubled in the past 25 years. *BMJ* **340**, c3057.

World Health Organization (1986) *Ottawa Charter for Health Promotion*. Ottawa, Canada, First International Conference on Health Promotion. Geneva: World Health Organization.

World Health Organization (2001) *The International Classification of Functioning Disability and Health*. Geneva: World Health Organization.

World Health Organization (2002) *Active Ageing. A policy framework*. Geneva: World Health Organization.

Zermansky, A.G., Petty, D.R., Raynor, D.K. and Alldred, D.P. (2005) Including care home residents in clinical research. *BMJ* **331**, 1036–1037.

Chapter 2

Perspectives of ageing

Anne McIntyre

Our understanding and perception of old age influences our therapeutic approach and service provision as occupational therapists. Our practice is also influenced by our professional philosophical belief that health and wellbeing is enabled through occupation. This chapter discusses concepts and theories of ageing, how personal factors (such as those considered in the ICF (WHO 2001) influence the ageing process, and also how those transitions more apparent in older age such as retirement, frailty and end of life occur within an occupationally just framework.

What is old age?

Old age is commonly perceived as the later stage of life, or the last stage within the life cycle. In 'As You Like It', by Shakespeare, Jacques gives a monologue on the seven ages of man. It is perhaps the last two stages described within the monologue that could be said to relate to older age:

> "...The sixth age shifts
> Into the lean and slipper'd pantaloon,
> With spectacles on nose and pouch on side,
> His youthful hose, well saved, a world too wide
> For his shrunk shank; and his big manly voice,
> Turning again toward childish treble, pipes
> And whistles in his sound. Last scene of all,
> That ends this strange eventful history,
> Is second childishness and mere oblivion,
> Sans teeth, sans eyes, sans taste, sans everything."
> ('As You Like It' Act 2, Scene 7,
> William Shakespeare)

In many societies, when an individual enters old age is socially constructed; either determined by cultural assumptions or, more often, by policy or legislation. Most international and national policy-making organisations determine older adulthood by

Occupational Therapy and Older People, Second Edition. Edited by Anita Atwal and Anne McIntyre.
© 2013 Blackwell Publishing Ltd. Published 2013 by Blackwell Publishing Ltd.

chronological age. Indeed, the United Nations suggests that an older person is 60+ years of age (WHO 2002), although many industrialised countries, such as the UK, the USA and Australia, have used 65 years of age to determine older age and provision of older adult services. In the past this age has related to retirement and eligibility for state pension or benefit; however, pensionable age is now being extended over the next few decades to 66 and 67 years of age for both men and women in England. The use of the term 'old age' is also debated, with Higgs and Gilleard (2006) preferring the term 'later life'.

Personal factors and old age

The ICF (WHO 2001) identifies that personal factors such as age, gender, personal beliefs, coping styles and attitudes, education, social background and life experience (past and present) all contribute to how an individual functions. These factors are addressed in subsequent chapters; chronological age, personal beliefs and gender differences are specifically considered here.

Using chronological age to determine the boundary between old age and middle age, and as the determinant of service provision, is increasingly challenged as being overly simplistic. Our own experiences indicate discrepancies between chronological and biological ageing. These discrepancies are increasingly acknowledged within research, policy and service provision, alongside the homogeneity of older people being also challenged (Freude et al. 2010). The heterogeneity of old age was considered by Baltes and Baltes (1990) who suggested that the great interpersonal variations in rate and type of ageing for older individuals are determined by genetics, environment and onset of disease.

From our own observation we are also aware of the differences in occupational performance and expectations of people aged 65 and 85. Therefore, researchers and service providers are increasingly differentiating between groups of older people by means other than chronological age. However, how this is determined or defined is not uniform. Baltes and Smith (2003), Cartensen and Fried (2012) and the UK Office for National Statistics (2012) consider older people as belonging to two distinct groups – the young-old and oldest-old, with the suggestion that those in the latter group would be aged 85+. Others consider older people as belonging to three groups, with the UK Department of Health (2001) describing these as those people entering old age, those in transition between healthy old age and frailty and frail older people. In the USA the three groups are often termed the young-old (60–74 years), old-old (75–89) or oldest-old (90+) (Salthouse 2009). It is perhaps useful to be aware of these differences when reading research literature to inform practice.

Old age is also determined not only by the beliefs of governments and organisations, but also by society and individuals themselves. In Chapter 3 of this book, the negative beliefs of others are discussed in terms of ageism and age discrimination, but it is also worth considering how the personal beliefs of the older individual impact upon their attitude to old age. In Chapter 4, Isabel, a retired headmistress, describes becoming older as 'a shock'. Clarke (2005) suggests that older people can internalise ageist attitudes of society and others, believing that decline is inevitable. Thompson (1992) considers that ageing is a lifelong process and therefore one's attitude to old age is based upon experience of previous life events rather than one single event (i.e. such as becoming 65).

There is a widespread belief that the baby boomers, born after World War II (between the years 1949 and 1961) and just entering old age, have greater expectations of themselves and society. In many industrialised countries around the world, the generation of baby boomers was born into a time of great social change, with the emergence of the youth culture. The baby boomers were better educated than their predecessors, are now entering old age in better health and are used to a greater disposable income than their predecessors (Cartensen and Fried 2012, Ehnes 2012). Many of them wish to preserve their quality of life, continue their employment, more youthful physical and social activities and expect to take up new challenges, voluntary work, or care for older frail parents or grandchildren. From a societal perspective, it is important that these young-old people retain their positive self-belief, their health, independence and contribution to society for as long as possible, delaying the frailty that tends to be associated with poor health and older age (Dillaway and Byrnes 2009, Cartensen and Fried 2012). Studies have also identified that positive self-belief amongst older people enables them to cope better with serious health events (Wurm et al. 2008) and increases their longevity (Levy et al. 2002). A study of centenarians identified that they had been highly motivated and self-disciplined in their activities and maintained their physical and mental health throughout their lives. They could adapt and change their interests with enthusiasm and curiosity, remaining goal-driven with all new challenges until their death (Antonini et al. 2008).

Those older people with more negative self image and poorer expectations of ageing are said to attribute any new disability to old age rather than a treatable health condition and are therefore less likely to seek health care or intervention (Sarkisian et al. 2001). It has also been observed that older people's attitudes to their social and occupational engagement influence their response to, and motivation for, rehabilitation, more than their health condition or limitations in occupational performance (Lilja et al. 2003). Cousins (2003) presents similar findings in relation to the participation in physical activity, suggesting that older people's reticence or lack of motivation to take physical activity is influenced by negative past experiences or lack of opportunity. It can therefore be seen that the lifelong interrelationship between personal beliefs about old age, self-belief and functioning is an important issue for occupational therapists to consider, especially when older people can internalise the ageist attitudes of others (be they family members, friends or health professionals), believing that decline is an inevitable part of ageing.

It is acknowledged that there are gender differences in older people's experiences of ageing, with the WHO (2003) reporting differences in the incidence of various health conditions between older men and women such as cardiovascular disease, cancer, osteoporosis and mental health conditions. Although these gender differences occur, it is difficult to know if they occur because of differences in ageing of body functions and structures, or because of environmental factors (Kryspin-Exner et al. 2011).

Differences in activity and participation also occur between men and women, and especially the types of activities that men and women benefit from. Although both men and women benefit from participating in leisure activities, women seem to benefit more from these. Whereas older women benefit from leisure activities involving social engagement, men benefit more from solitary interests and hobbies (Agahi and Parker 2008). Therefore, it is important to consider the individual preferences of older people when providing them with interventions, especially group-based sessions.

There are also contrasting socio-cultural expectations and opportunities for men and women around the world. Women may have had more restrictions in education, employment, access to healthcare, legal, financial and social support during their lifespan which would impact on their experiences of older age (WHO 2003).

Theories of ageing

From the previous sections in this chapter, it is evident that as a practising occupational therapist, one needs to be aware of differing perceptions and definitions of old age as well as individual beliefs and attitudes. It is also important to consider different theories of how and why we age, so that our practice promotes occupational justice, and optimal health and wellbeing. Although many people would like to deny that ageing occurs, it is necessary to remind ourselves that ageing is inevitable and a lifelong process. Indeed, our health and social behaviours in early life will often predetermine how well or successful our old age becomes. Whereas some theories of ageing focus on the concept of longevity, others promote living longer with better health, wellbeing and quality of life. It is also important to understand how and why we age so that we can distinguish between normal ageing and pathological processes caused by a health condition; these are considered more fully in Chapters 6 and 7 where ageing of body functions and structures is discussed. In this section we will consider biological, psycho-social and bio-psycho-social theories of ageing.

Biological theories of ageing

Even though the maximum lifespan for humans has not changed radically over the centuries, the average life expectancy has increased in the industrialised world. There are many biological theories of ageing which seek to explore the rationale for both the maximum and average lifespan; however, no single theory fully explains the ageing process in humans. Biological ageing has its basis in cellular and sub-cellular change with many researchers hypothesising how and why cells die and whether cell death can be prevented or slowed.

Hayflick limit theory (Hayflick and Moorhead 1961) suggests that there is a finite limit on the number of cell divisions and replications, with different types of cells (e.g. muscle, nerve or skin) having differing limits of replication. Cell replication and consequent death can be accelerated or slowed by extrinsic factors such as calorie intake and lifestyle, as the DNA in cells which is crucial to cell division can be easily damaged by diet, toxins, pollution and trauma (Hayflick 2000).

Free radical theory (Harman 1956) considers that ageing occurs because of production of free radicals within cells as a result of energy production from mitochondria. Production of free radicals occurs as a result of normal behaviours such as eating, drinking and breathing, but diet, lifestyle, drugs (e.g. tobacco, alcohol), radiation and pollution all accelerate the production of free radicals within cells. These free radicals create metabolic waste products, which disrupt cell membranes, cause mitochondrial damage and the eventual death of the cell.

Genetic and evolutionary theories: Early theories advocated an ageing gene that programmed when an organism died to prevent overcrowding and overpopulation of a species, but existed for long enough to produce the next generation (Weismann 1891, cited by Kirkwood 2002, p. 738). Later evolutionary theories advocate that there is a physiological allocation of resources between growth, maintenance and reproduction, with a trade-off between reproduction and life expectancy (Kirkwood 2002). Kirkwood and Austad (2000) also suggest that there are multiple genes that influence ageing and longevity, as there are lifespan differences between species, and similarities within families and monozygotic twins.

It is also hypothesised that genetics influence ageing by approximately 25%, whereas environment and lifestyle have a 75% impact on ageing (Kirkwood 2003). Perls and Terry (2003) suggest that centenarians and other very old people have genetic variations that can impact upon the ageing process and the ability to withstand age-associated diseases such as Alzheimer's disease. However, they also identified that genetic make-up was only one factor in the centenarian's longevity.

All of these biological theories of ageing identify extrinsic influences on cellular activity. For example, if our environment causes high metabolic activity within cells to maintain body functions and structures then the rate of cellular ageing and subsequent death will increase. Conversely, good nutrition, physical activity, healthy environments, and freedom from disease and trauma minimise metabolic activity within cells and cell death. Such theories identify that ageing can be partly manipulated and under the control of the individual or of society, with Hayflick (1998) suggesting that ageing is a construct of civilisation, in that where there are more comforts of modern life there is a greater life expectancy.

Compression of morbidity theory (Fries 1980)

Current healthy life expectancy (i.e. freedom from disability and disease) differs from the average life expectancy by several years and some of the global differences for men and women are apparent in Table 2.1. Therefore, any increase in life expectancy should be accompanied by freedom from disease and disability to enhance the quality of life in older age, as discussed further in Chapter 4.

Table 2.1   Global differences between actual and healthy life expactancy.

	Actual life expectancy	**Healthy life expectancy**
Sierre Leone	40	29
Japan	83	75
Australia	82	73
UK	79	71
USA	78	69
Canada	81	72

(Source: WHO 2008)

Fries (1980) advocated that morbidity (i.e. ill health and disability) should be compressed into fewer and later years before death. This compression of morbidity theory has been validated by the increase in healthy years as a result of health promotion programmes such as immunisation, smoking cessation, health checks and screening (Fries 2003, Lupien and Wan 2004). It forms the basis for the WHO's Active Ageing programme and policy (Kalache et al. 2002) and, indeed, all lifelong health promotion policies. The reader is signposted to Chapter 4, where health promotion and social policy are discussed. It is interesting to note that the centenarians in the retrospective study by Hitt et al. (1999) also demonstrated that these oldest-old participants tended to live with good health and independence in everyday activity for most of their lives, with a rapid deterioration in health and activity at the very end of life.

Psycho-social theories of ageing

Even though biological theories of ageing explain how our bodies age, psycho-social ageing theories encompass both the attitudes of the self and others to occupational performance as well as the social and physical environments that either facilitate or act as barriers to occupation. These theories are highly relevant when exploring occupations or encouraging older people in their participation in occupations, as they inform clinical reasoning and planning of intervention. It is worth reflecting on whether these theories allow for the heterogeneity of older people and are relevant to one or all of the broad groups of older people identified earlier in this chapter.

Activity theory (Havighurst and Albrecht 1953): This theory suggests that greater life satisfaction is achieved through increased activity which is meaningful and creative. It reinforces the importance of the maintenance of active roles and relationships. However, this theory assumes that we all wish to be active and perhaps denies biological, psychological and social changes.

Continuity theory (Atchley 1989): This theory suggests that there is a continuous thread that runs through our lives but that how we carry out occupations adapts and changes in response to intrinsic and extrinsic changes of ageing. These adjustments in people's behaviours and activities are made according to their lifestyle and interests. This theory addresses how we can engage in the same activity or occupation throughout our lives but in different ways. For example, whereas we may have played tennis in our youth, we can still be engaged in tennis as we age but as an umpire or club committee member, not as a player.

Disengagement theory (Cumming and Henry 1961): This theory suggests that old age is the time to reap the benefits of life and allow older people to disengage from roles, activities and relationships. It is suggested that this a biologically-driven natural reduction in social involvement and responsibility, with a corresponding decrease in activity and is supported and needed by society to cope with loss and death. This theory has been accused of being very negative, perceiving older people as passive members of society and encouraging an expulsion of older people from society. More recent interpretations of this theory focus on the needs of the individual to disengage from everyday worries rather than to fulfil the needs of society, and is best described by Tornstam (1989) below.

Gerotranscendence theory (Tornstam 1989): This theory suggests that there is a stage where older people 'cross over' to another, higher stage, where they have a disappearing fear of death and connect to earlier generations. Older people will be more concerned with the self by confronting themselves with a shift from egoism to altruism and rediscovering the child within. The meaning and importance of relationships changes with people demonstrating everyday wisdom and emancipated innocence (Wadenstein 2005).

Theory of psycho-social development (Erikson 1950): This theory considers an individual's life in eight stages, from birth to old age. The eighth stage – old age – is represented by the theme of integrity and despair. Erikson et al. (1986) identify that whether an individual enters old age positively with integrity and wellbeing or in despair and discontent is dependent upon their positive and or negative past experiences and, more importantly, their ability to reflect on these experiences. Erikson et al. (1986) advocate that wisdom and integrity emerge from reflection, understanding and acceptance of past experience.

Bio-psycho-social theories of ageing

More recent theories acknowledge that ageing is not just a biological or social phenomenon but also a combination of many factors. These are perhaps more relevant to modern industrialised society, as baby boomers entering old age are less likely to suffer from pathological changes and disability in later years. It is thought that this new and current generation of older people will therefore avoid institutionalisation because of advances in medicine, public health, education and financial resources. However, there is concern for the much younger generations where there are increasing trends of obesity, tobacco use and reduction in physical activity, which will impact upon future disease and disability rates.

The two most commonly-used terms to encompass these bio-psycho-social theories of ageing are 'active ageing' and 'successful ageing'. Since the previous edition of this book, both of these terms are increasingly used within international, national and local policies as well as in the literature. However, both terms are hotly debated within the literature, because of the possible interpretations and definitions.

As already stated in the introduction to this book, the WHO (2002) considers active ageing to be a multifaceted and lifelong concept. Active ageing as defined by the WHO (2002) involves involvement and maintenance in physical activity, paid employment, participation in social, economic, spiritual and civic activities. In Chapter 4, these concepts are related to social policy and occupational therapy practice.

This concept has been strongly influenced by activity theory (Havighurst and Albrecht 1953) and compression of morbidity theory (Fries 1980), because of the strong evidence that an active lifestyle can delay the onset of first disability. However, this concept identifies that early and lifelong prevention is required so that people enter old age maintaining their activity and participation for as long as possible, and is not specifically targeting older people (Kalache et al. 2002). The WHO (2002) identifies that active ageing is not only determined by personal and lifestyle factors but also by contextual factors such as economic resources, and the physical, social, legislative and political environment.

Interestingly, the European Union (EU) declared 2012 as the 'European Year for Active Ageing and Solidarity Between Generations' (Europa 2012). The EU considers active ageing to encourage older people to grow old, contributing to society through staying in paid employment for longer, contributing to civic life as carers and volunteers, and staying as healthy and independent as possible. Whereas the WHO (2002) definition of active ageing could be seen to be empowering and aspirational in promoting human rights and security for older people worldwide, the EU and national government concepts of active ageing seemingly focus on the economic contribution of older people to society (Bowling 2009, Stenner et al. 2011).

Lay concepts of active ageing are multifaceted. Two studies by Bowling (2009) and Stenner et al. (2011) identified that older people in the UK consider active ageing to incorporate physical activity and good health, keeping mentally and socially active (volunteering, caring, participating in hobbies and interests), maintaining autonomy and agency as well as independence in everyday activities. Many participants associated being old with a reduction in activity, loss of autonomy and control, development of health conditions, bereavement and entering residential care. Interestingly, although volunteering was perceived as important, none of the participants identified staying in paid employment as an integral part of active ageing. It is also interesting to note that in the study by Bowling (2009), those participants from ethnic minority groups were less likely to consider that they had aged well, according to the criteria used in the study.

There are many theories and definitions of successful ageing, with this term proposed by Havighurst (1961) in relation to activity theory (Havighurst and Albrecht 1953) as a way of 'adding life to years' (p. 8), and also by Rowe and Kahn (1987). The bio-medical theory proposed by Rowe and Kahn (1987) was the first to gain popularity. This initial theory differentiated between usual ageing and successful ageing, suggesting that loss of function and independence associated with ageing is actually associated with lifestyle, and that an older person could be considered to have aged successfully if they had managed to avoid disease or disability (Rowe and Kahn 1987). The definition was further developed to also include physical and cognitive functioning, and engagement in social and productive activities (Rowe and Kahn 1997).

Baltes and Baltes (1990) considered that successful ageing is an adaptive process of selection, optimisation and compensation (SOC) of activity and participation. Successful ageing is seen as multifaceted and demonstrated through longevity, physical and mental health, cognitive functioning, social participation, productivity, autonomy and life satisfaction (Baltes and Baltes 1990). These researchers suggested that there are three ways to age – normally (without disease or disability), optimally (in a facilitatory physical and social environment) or pathologically (with disease, such as dementia).

Autonomy, agency, dignity and a positive sense of self have also been advocated as important elements in successful ageing (Glass 2003, Bowling and Illiffe 2006). Over the last 10 years, more user-focused definitions of successful ageing have developed. Older people's definitions include being in good health, independence in everyday activity, personal resilience, autonomy and agency, financial and environmental security, maintenance of social roles, activities and relationships, and a productive lifestyle (Phelan et al. 2004, Bowling and Illiffe 2006).

Glass (2003) suggested that concepts of successful ageing should also include quality of life, dignity and absence of suffering. Moreover, Baltes and Smith (2003) considered that the concept of successful ageing relates more to those young-old people but not the oldest-old who are more frail. To this purpose, more recent research has explored the concepts of successful ageing held by the oldest-old (those people aged 85+) and frail older people living in residential care. These older participants highlighted a sense of wellbeing, a positive attitude, social functioning and being able to adapt and change to circumstances as being the most important determinants of successful ageing (Guse and Masesar 1999, von Faber et al. 2001). Research in South Korea of older people with low income also identified that relationships with others and a positive outlook on life were considered crucial elements of successful ageing (Chung and Park 2008).

The current concepts of active and successful ageing are being increasingly debated and accused of being discriminatory, oppressive and ageist (Dillaway and Byrnes 2009, Stenner et al. 2011). Indeed, it could be argued that anyone entering old age with, or acquiring a disease or disability during old age, has already failed to age successfully. Liang and Luo (2012) also suggest that successful ageing is a discriminatory concept because it encourages expectations of agelessness and denial of normal ageing. These authors suggest that the concept has become consumer driven to encourage the consumption of anti-ageing products in western society. Moreover, Liang and Luo (2012) discuss that activity and productivity (as advocated in theories of activity and continuity by Havighurst and Albrecht 1953, Atchley 1989) are valued in Western successful and active ageing theories but overlook other more reflective and spiritual experiences that are prized in eastern societies and philosophy. Liang and Lu (2012) propose an alternative concept of harmonious ageing, where an older person is encouraged to maintain a dynamic balance in mind and body, social and intergenerational relationships.

Glass (2003) states that interventions at both a governmental and service provider level should maximise the potential of successful and active ageing, but that this might need new approaches to health and social care provision. Successful and active ageing theories advocate an obvious role for occupational therapy with this age group. The importance of maintenance of functioning, independence, social relationships and the environment to promote health and wellbeing reflects the philosophical basis of occupational science and occupational therapy practice. The concept of successful ageing by Baltes and Baltes (1990) of selection, optimisation and compensation (SOC) also fits with many occupational therapy intervention approaches involving adaptation, maximisation or compensation.

It can therefore be seen that bio-psycho-social theories of ageing are still debated in terms of their conceptual focus and also their terminology. Although these theories promote a more positive approach to ageing, their inclusivity and interpretation still need global discussion.

Entering old age with disability

There is an increasing number of people entering old age already with disability, such as those with learning disability, respiratory conditions or arthritis (as discussed in Chapter 5) or those with cerebral palsy, spinal cord injury, multiple sclerosis or post-polio syndrome, for example. It is because of improvement in medical technology, rehabilitation and assistive devices that many people with lifelong disability or long-term chronic illness now live into older age (Zarb and Oliver 1993).

Studies of older people with multiple sclerosis (MS) have identified that many experience the transition into retirement at earlier ages because of their disability arising from MS (Fong et al. 2006) and also experience age-related or acceleration of ageing changes and difficulties in occupational performance (Finlayson et al. 2009). McColl et al. (1999) also report early or accelerated onset of ageing in people with spinal cord injury. Those people with post-polio syndrome (PPS) have a different experience. This syndrome has only been recognised within the last 20–30 years, and seems to appear 20–40 years after the initial contraction of polio (Bridgens et al. 2010). As the last epidemic of polio in the UK and USA occurred in the 1950s some of these people are now entering old age with PPS. These people experience muscle weakness and atrophy, fatigue, muscle and joint pain, sleep and respiratory problems and cold intolerance, which requires management (Bridgens et al. 2010, British Polio Fellowship [accessed 20.06.2012]).

It is important to appreciate that people entering old age with disability will have different experiences than those who have newly- acquired disability and health conditions. They will have already accessed health and social care services, but may experience greater activity limitations and participation restrictions because of their disability (Fong et al. 2006). It is also important to consider that not only might their existing condition accelerate the ageing process but also new symptoms and issues could arise from their condition (Bridgens et al. 2010). For occupational therapists working with older people, it is important to be aware that this client group will increase in numbers and may require different interventions or have different expectations of services.

Older people and occupational justice

For occupational therapists, the concept of meaningful activity is seen as essential to health and wellbeing (Wilcock 1999, Yerxa, et al. 1990). Wilcock (1999) first described occupation as a synthesis of 'doing, being and becoming', with 'doing' and 'being' essential for 'becoming' (i.e. an expression of autonomy or self-actualisation). For many people, as they become frailer the opportunity to remain autonomous and carry out their occupations of choice diminishes, because of the attitudes of their families, carers or service providers, and/or because of risk management or organisational restrictions. Wilcock (2006) terms this 'occupational deprivation', and advocates that if we wish to practise in an occupationally just way we should consider how, as part of intervention, we can facilitate an older person to have a meaningful lifestyle that allows them to 'do' or 'be' to meet their unique 'becoming' needs (Wilcock 2005, 2006).

Indeed, an important part of successful ageing and active ageing concepts and policies is the promotion of good health, autonomy and self-actualisation and prevention of inequalities and deprivation (WHO 2002). Client-centred practice is an integral part of these policies and also a crucial underpinning of occupational justice. It is important that occupational therapists provide every opportunity for older people to participate in their chosen occupations, to exercise choice and control in their daily routines and are supported in their decision making, thus maintaining occupational justice – even when this is perceived as taking risk. This is especially pertinent for those occupational therapists working with older people in acute healthcare settings and planning discharge home, or when working with the oldest-old.

Taking risks

Occupational therapists need to balance older people's opportunities in risk taking, their rights, autonomy and empowerment and also the potential harm that might come to the older person as a result of their risk-taking behaviour (Taylor 2005, Moats 2006). It is important for occupational therapists to examine their own values and perceptions of risk, as it would seem that health professionals are more likely to base their opinion of risk on their own beliefs and those of their colleagues, rather than on research evidence or protocols (Richard et al. 2005). In Chapter 9, risks are discussed in relation to home and home visits and the reader is referred to Table 9.4.

Where risk is associated with conflict, uncertainty or refusal of services or recommendations by an older person, it is not uncommon that their capacity to make decisions is questioned (Huby et al. 2004), thus creating occupational deprivation. Findings from our own research suggest that therapists are willing to take risks in intervention and recommendations with older people, as long as they feel that the individual has the mental capacity and insight to fully understand the possible outcome. But our research also indicates that risk causes uncertainty and anxiety among professionals and this is particularly evident within the discharge process (Atwal et al. 2011).

Sumsion (2006) identifies that therapists' concepts of risk, capacity and levels of insight can all act as barriers to client-centred practice and, therefore, occupational justice. It is important for occupational therapists to move away from being risk managers or being perceived as risk averse, to become risk activators or enablers to maintain the rights, autonomy and dignity of older people. It is acknowledged that the management of risk could be problematic, therefore frameworks have been published in the UK (DH 2007, 2010) to guide how clinicians manage risk in practice. These frameworks, however, do not provide clinical solutions and therefore occupational therapists must reflect upon their own values, use their clinical reasoning skills and the expertise of other team members to manage risk in a client-centred way.

Research by Wicks (2006) and Hocking et al. (2011) identified that older people themselves develop strategies that not only enable them to carry out their chosen occupations but also address and reduce risk. These strategies still ensure that the older person's needs are adequately met, either by obtaining help or by making different occupational choices. It is also important that older people do not become bogged down in self-care activities if these activities preclude them from carrying out the occupations that are more meaningful and challenging for them (Jackson et al. 1998, Wicks 2006). It is therefore crucial to ascertain what the occupational priorities of our older clients are. It is also essential to explore how the older person carries out their occupations and the strategies they use to reduce risk, to facilitate a sense of autonomy and self-efficacy, thus ensuring that occupational justice prevails.

Occupational transitions

It is important to consider how successful ageing can be maintained during periods of transition during old age. The majority of older people experience transition where the choice of occupation or the way in which they 'do' the occupation alter because of intrinsic or extrinsic factors. Perhaps the most symbolic of these is retirement, as this could be perceived to be the transition from adulthood to old age.

Retirement

For some older people, retirement is a positive experience with relief from obligations of work allowing an increased involvement in other occupations (either new or continued) such as volunteering, caring, grandparenting or part-time working. It would seem that men and women have different experiences of retirement and that these experiences change post-retirement (Barnes and Perry 2004). Retirement can also be experienced as a time of loss – of routine, role, purpose, social contacts, relationships, income and of meaningful occupations (Jonsson et al. 2000a). For some older people, retirement also means loss of their home and loss of place where these are tied to their place of work – especially in farming or rural communities (Wythes and Lyons 2006).

Not all changes to occupations are negative; some older people engage in occupations that are related to their previous work, or long-term hobbies, or interests carried out with family members. For many retirees, these occupations are meaningful because they are reaffirming of the individual's identity, require commitment or responsibility, have a community attachment where activities/occupations are the focus, or are the by-product of community membership (Jonsson et al. 2000b).

Many older people find that, on retirement, there are many changes to their occupations, in terms of their routine being altered by the freedom from work demands or a change in daily rhythm so that occupations reserved for weekends or holidays can occur anytime. For some, these changes are positive and for others these devalue the meaning of the occupation (Jonsson et al. 2000b). Indeed, Pettican and Prior (2011) suggest that the establishment of a satisfying routine in retirement is more important than filling their time, so that the individual has some flexibility in what they choose to do when. More successful transition to retirement occurs when there is opportunity of social engagement, a carryover of meaningful occupations into retirement, a positive outlook and a gradual adaptation to environmental changes (Wythes and Lyons 2006) as well as choosing occupations that challenge and develop existing abilities (Pettican and Prior 2011).

The oldest-old

Another transition is into oldest-old age. The oldest-old are also the fastest growing group in the global population. This time in life is frequently associated with frailty, ill health and declining independence. Although it is important to realise that not all very old people are dependent on others or live in residential care, it is also relevant to remember that this age group is most likely to experience biological ageing and reduced physical reserve. For these older people, it is essential to ascertain their body functioning as well as contextual barriers so that they can maintain their treasured occupations for as long as they wish in order to enhance their health and wellbeing.

Increasingly, more research is carried out with the oldest-old population, including that which considers their views of successful ageing and their subjective experiences of occupations. von Faber et al. (2001) describe a 'disability paradox' (p. 2699) in their study of successful ageing and those aged 85+, where more older participants consider themselves to have aged successfully, even though they have limitations in functioning (as defined within the ICF by WHO (2001)). These older participants equate successful ageing with personal factors such as being able to adapt and integrate losses and change (including loss in functioning) that come with ageing, as well as having social contacts (von Faber et al. 2001). These findings are reinforced by studies of older people aged 90+ who relate successful ageing, health and quality of life to their opportunity to not only adapt to change, but also to find meaning and enjoyment in their everyday lives (Antonini et al. 2008, Lapid et al. 2011) and their engagement with their chosen occupations (Häggblom-Kronlöf et al. 2007). In particular, the 99-year-old participants in the study by Häggblom-Kronlöf et al. (2007) found satisfactory involvement in their occupations either through actively 'doing', by being an active spectator or by recalling previously-satisfying experiences. Being an active spectator involved being included in decisions and drawing on personal themes of meaning to still engage in and validate the occupation (Jackson 1996, Wicks 2006, Craig and Mountain 2007).

These oldest-old also described how they found challenge in their everyday occupations, by pushing themselves and testing the limits of their abilities to gain mastery of occupations that would seem to be beyond their capabilities. Mastery of occupations included problem solving, planning how to deal with difficulties in body functions or structures, or environmental barriers, and also learning new skills or new ways of carrying out valued occupations. The 99-year-old participants valued having a pattern and rhythm to the day as this provided them with a reference point, control and autonomy over their occupations, whereas a pattern disrupted by visitors or an imposed change in routine caused irritation, stress and anxiety (Häggblom-Kronlöf et al. 2007). The need for a supportive environment also emerged as important to enable the oldest-old to engage in their occupations in a meaningful way. Both physical barriers, such as bad lighting, heavy doors, uneven pavements, and social or attitudinal barriers of those who were caring for them made it more difficult for the oldest-old to participate in their chosen occupations and often caused them to withdraw from these (Hovbrandt et al. 2007).

It is important to consider that such a retreat from occupations because of life events, failing capacity (i.e. body versus environment), dominance in self-care tasks, a reliance on or a lack of recognition by others of the meaningful nature of occupations can be a cause of occupational injustice (Jackson 1996, Wicks 2006, Hovbrandt et al. 2007). However, it is worth considering that not all older people wish to be engaged in occupation and it is important to differentiate between a conscious decision to disengage from occupations and a lack of opportunity to participate in them (Borell et al. 2001).

Frailty

An insidious withdrawal from valued occupations can be a time of the transition from healthy old age to frailty. Although the prevalence of frailty increases as people age, it is

---

Box 2.1   Definition of frailty.

Frailty is a clinical syndrome diagnosed by the presence of three of the following criteria:

- Unintentional weight loss (10 lbs in previous year)
- Self-reported exhaustion
- Weakness (grip strength)
- Slow walking speed
- Low physical activity

(*Source*: Fried et al. 2001)

---

no longer considered synonymous with being very old (Fried et al. 2001, Lang et al. 2009). There are many definitions of frailty, but the one most commonly accepted within biomedical studies is that by Fried et al. (2001) (see Box 2.1).

However, this is increasingly perceived as being a multidimensional construct (Syddall et al. 2010, Roland et al. 2011). Lang et al. (2009) define frailty as:

> "… an extended process of increasing vulnerability, predisposing to functional decline and ultimately leading to death." (p. 540)

Lang et al. (2009) suggest that age, gender, lifestyle, and socio-economic background all contribute to frailty, along with co-morbidities, affective, cognitive and sensory impairments. Frailty is not just observed in the oldest-old, with Syddall et al. (2010) identifying frailty in a population of 64–74-year-old participants in the UK, and especially women and those from lower socio-economic groups.

Lang et al. (2009) have suggested that frailty can be prevented, by encouraging those identifiable as being in a 'pre-frail' group (by using the criteria of Fried et al. 2001) to eat an adequate diet, take physical exercise, prevent infection, and prevent of stressful events. Although occupational therapists provide interventions for frail older people this often involves 'crisis management'. However, the occupational therapy and physiotherapy participants in the study by Roland et al. (2011) suggested that pre-frailty is 'a time bomb waiting for a catastrophic event' (p. 279). They perceived that an event such as a fall, hospital admission or loss of social contacts could tip an individual over the edge into frailty. Therefore, a successful ageing approach and maintenance of occupational balance for older people could be crucial to prevent or delay frailty for as long as possible.

End of life

It could be argued whether dying is an integral part of successful ageing. Some could consider that dying means that a successful ageing approach has failed. However, it is important to consider successful ageing as a lifespan approach and therefore dying is as fundamental a part of life as birth. It is perhaps easier to consider having a good death or dying well as part of successful ageing or active ageing approaches and policies. It is argued whether dying is an occupation, with Pollard (2006) suggesting that this is an event; however, preparing for death could be considered an occupation (Box 2.2).

Box 2.2   End of life care strategies.

The following end of life strategies can be accessed:

DH (2008) The End of Life Care strategy for England. http://www.endoflifecareforadults.nhs.
uk/assets/downloads/pubs_EoLC_Strategy_1.pdf

Australian Government (2011) Guidelines for a palliative approach for aged care in the community setting. http://www.health.gov.au/internet/main/publishing.nsf/Content/400BE269B
92A6D73CA2578BF00010BB0/$File/COMPAC-30Jun11.pdf

WHO European Region (2011) Palliative care for older people: Better practices. http://www.
euro.who.int/__data/assets/pdf_file/0017/143153/e95052.pdf

Two-thirds of all people who die each year in the UK and Australia are over 65 years of age, with nearly a half of all deaths occurring in the over-80 age group (Australian Government 2011, UK National End of Life Intelligence Network [NEoLIN], 2012). End of life care policies have been developed by various countries to ensure that people are suitably cared for towards the end of life, in their place of choice, with effective and appro-priate pain relief and with their wishes taken into account (Department of Health 2008, Australian Government 2011). Unfortunately, many deaths are sudden, and the incidence of unexpected death increases with age. Whereas older people would prefer to die in a hospice, they are more likely to die in hospital, and unfortunately it would seem that the quality of care for people dying in hospital is perceived as poor (NEoLIN 2012). The need to provide appropriate care at the end of life for people with dementia, for example, is also important, especially as 25% of people with dementia die in hospital (NEoLIN 2012).

Where death is expected and can be planned, it is easier to maintain a successful ageing approach. Within the English End of Life care strategy (DH 2008), advance care planning is advocated, so that the individual's wishes can be heard and followed and that the carers' needs are assessed in order that a good death can be experienced. Jacques and Hasselkus (2004) discuss that people at the end of life tend to disengage from the every-day occupations and focus more on getting their life in order – financially, legally, emotionally and spiritually and interpersonal relationships. Jacques and Hasselkus (2004) and Pollard (2006) advocate that, for occupational justice to prevail, an individual requires help to live meaningfully at the end of life. It is therefore important for people at the end of life to successfully carry out their valued occupations, rather than getting overwhelmed by medical interventions or poor personal care.

Successful ageing and occupational justice

The previous sections in this chapter have highlighted theories of ageing and the transitions that people go through in later life. The threats to occupational justice have also been discussed, especially in relation to the transitions that take place in older age. What, hopefully, is obvious is that occupational therapists need to have a pro-active approach to work within a successful or active ageing framework. As already stated in Chapter 1, few high-quality studies that provide the evidence base for occupational therapy interventions were carried out with older people. Two of these studies are discussed here, as they are good examples of how occupational therapy interventions fit within a successful ageing framework.

The Lifestyle Redesign programme published by Mandel et al. (1999) and reported as the Well Elderly study by Clark et al. (1997) is one of the few randomised control trial studies of occupational therapy interventions. What makes this particularly pertinent is that it aimed to address lifestyle rather than specific activities for independently-living older people by explicitly linking everyday activity to health and wellbeing. The 6–9 month individualised programme encouraged and promoted participation in a range of occupations and is described by Jackson et al. (1998). This programme has also been carried out and evaluated in the UK but renamed Lifestyle Matters (Craig and Mountain 2007, Mountain et al. 2008). The occupation-focused programme fits perfectly with concepts of successful ageing and compression of morbidity, complementing the recent evidence for physical, leisure and creative activities in the promotion of health and wellbeing discussed in Chapter 4.

Older participants were involved in individual sessions where specific goals, concerns and issues could be addressed and in group sessions where didactic teaching, peer exchange of ideas, experiences and reflections were based on chosen themes (i.e. transportation, finances, physical and mental activity). Group outings were also carried out where members could test their new knowledge and skills and challenge them in a safe and supported way. What is of particular interest is that older participants were encouraged to carry out their own occupational analyses so they could understand the components of their occupations, their significance, and their contribution to their health and wellbeing. The older people gained an overview of their occupational balance by exploring the frequency and duration of their activities and their relevance to their roles, habits and routines. Using narratives (or occupational story-telling) the older people were able to discuss, share and reflect upon the importance, value and meaning of their occupations and to share the personal experiences with others which they could then draw upon when challenged by future activities and occupations. The participants were creative in their ability to think laterally and problem solve as well as in their self-expression through media such as art and photography.

In subsequent studies Clark et al. (2001, 2011) (with Clark et al. 2011, being a repeated and a much larger study), established that long-term benefits to health and wellbeing for a group of older adults are possible. Clark et al. (2011) were able to demonstrate that these positive effects were still apparent at six months post intervention for their ethnically diverse group of participants. Participants benefitted from improved mental functioning, social engagement, self-rated physical health and reduction in bodily pain. All of these factors can be seen to contribute to concepts of successful ageing, in an occupationally just way.

The role of occupational therapy for persons with dementia is discussed in Chapter 5. One study that has given additional evidence about occupational therapy intervention is a study by Graff et al. (2006). This study examined the effectiveness of community-based occupational therapy on the daily functioning of patients with dementia and the sense of competence of their care givers. This study concluded that occupational therapy improved patients' daily functioning and reduced the burden on the care giver, despite the patients' limited learning ability. Longer-term effects for both members of the dyad were still being experienced at 12 weeks after the intervention had been provided. In this study, older people with dementia and their carers received 10 sessions of occupational therapy over five weeks, during which time the participants were encouraged to define their problems and prioritise those meaningful everyday activities that they wanted to improve. In the study, a compensatory approach and environmental modification were used and the participants shown how to improve their performance in their chosen activities by utilising the compensatory strategies and environmental modifications appropriately. Carers were shown how to use appropriate and effective supervisory, problem-solving and coping strategies for themselves and the person with dementia.

Summary

This chapter has discussed differing theories of ageing, including the bio-psycho-social theories of successful and active ageing. How occupational justice for older people can be challenged or maintained has also been discussed. The varying transitions that take place during later life, such as retirement, becoming very old, becoming frail and at the end of life have also been discussed.

References

Agahi, N. and Parker, M.G. (2008) Leisure activities and mortality: Does gender matter? *Journal of Aging and Health* **20**, 855–871.

Antonini, F.M., Magnolfi, S.U., Petruzzi, E., Pinzani, P., Malentacchi, F., Petruzzi, I. and Masotti, G. (2008) Physical performance and creative activities of centenarians. *Archives of Gerontology and Geriatrics* **46**, 252–261.

Atchley, R.C. (1989) A continuity theory of normal aging. *Gerontologist* **29**, 183–190.

Atwal, A., Wiggett, C. and McIntyre, A. (2011) Risks with older adults in acute care settings: Occupational therapists and physiotherapists' perceptions. *British Journal of Occupational Therapy* **74**:9, 412–418.

Australian Government (2011) *Guidelines for a Palliative Approach for Aged Care in the Community Setting*. Canberra: Department of Health and Ageing.

Baltes, P.B. and Baltes, M.M. (1990) Psychological perspectives in successful ageing: The model of selective optimisation with compensation. In: Baltes, P.B. and Baltes, M.M. (eds) *Successful Ageing: Perspectives from the behavioural sciences*. Cambridge: Cambridge University Press, pp. 1–36.

Baltes, P.B. and Smith, J. (2003) New frontiers in the future of aging: From successful aging of the young old to the dilemmas of the Fourth Age. *Gerontology*, **49**, 123–135.

Barnes, H. and Perry, J. (2004) Renegotiating identity and relationships: Men and women's adjustments to retirement. *Ageing and Society* **24**(2), 213–233.

Borell, L., Lilja, M., Sviden, G.A. and Sadlo, G. (2001) Involvement in occupations among older adults with physical and functional impairments is influenced by positive belief and a sense of hope. *American Journal of Occupational Therapy* **53**, 311–316.

Bowling, A. (2009) Perceptions of active ageing in Britain: Divergences between minority ethnic and whole population samples. *Age and Ageing*, London, doi: 10.1093/ageing/afp175

Bowling, A. and Iliffe, S. (2006) Which model of successful ageing should be used? Baseline findings from a British longitudinal survey of ageing. *Age and Ageing* **35**, 607–614.

Bridgens, R., Sturman, S. and Davidson, C. (2010) Post-polio syndrome – polio's legacy. *Clinical Medicine* **10**(3), 213–214.

Cartensen, L.L. and Fried, L.P. (2012) The meaning of old age. In: World Economic Forum (ed.) *Global Population Ageing: Peril or promise?* Global Agenda Council on Ageing Society, pp. 15–17.

Chung, S. and Park, S.-J. (2008) Successful ageing among low-income older people in South Korea. *Ageing and Society*, **28(8)**, 1061–1074.

Clark, F., Azen, S.P., Zemke, R., Jackson, J., Carlson, M., Mandel, D., Hay, J., Josephson, K., Cherry, B., Hessel, C., Palmer, J. and Lipson, L. (1997) Occupational therapy for independent-living older adults: A randomised controlled trial. *Journal of the American Medical Association* **278(16)**, 1321–1326.

Clark, F., Azen, S.P., Carlson, M., Mandel, D., LaBree, L., Hay, J., Zemke, R., Jackson, J. and Lipson, L. (2001) Embedding health-promoting changes into the daily lives of independent-living older adults: Long-term follow-up of occupational therapy intervention. *Journals of Gerontology Series B Psychological and Social Sciences* **56(1)**, 60–63.

Clark, F., Jackson, J., Carlson, M., Chou, C.P., Cherry, B.J., Jordan-Marsh, M., Knight, B.G., Mandel, D., Blanchard, J., Grander, D.A., Wilcox, R.R., Lai, M.Y., White, B., Ha,y J., Lam, C., Marterell,a A. and Azen, S.P. (2011) Effectiveness of a lifestyle intervention in promoting the well-being of independently living older people: Results of the Well Elderly 2 Randomised Controlled Trial. *J Epidemiol Community Health*, USA, doi: 10.1136/jech.2009.099754

Clarke, J. (2005) Adverse factors and the mental health of older people: Implications for social policy and professional practice. *Journal of Psychiatric and Mental Health Nursing* **12**, 290–296.

Cousins, S.O. (2003) A self-referent thinking model: How older adults may talk themselves out of being physically active. *Health Promotion Practice* **4(4)**, 439–448, doi: 10.1177/15248399903255417

Craig, C. and Mountain, G. (2007) *Lifestyle Matters*. Brackley: Speechmark Publishing Ltd.

Cumming, E. and Henry, W.E. (1961) *Growing Old: The process of disengagement*. New York: Basic Books.

Department of Health (DH) (2001) *National Service Framework for Older People*. London: Department of Health.

Department of Health (DH) (2007) *Cancer Reform Strategy*. London: Department of Health.

Department of Health (DH) (2008) *End of Life Care Strategy – Promoting high quality care for all adults at the end of life*. London: Department of Health.

Department of Health (DH) (2010) *Quality Outcomes for People with Dementia: Building on the work of the National Dementia Strategy*. London: Department of Health.

Dillaway, H.E. and Byrnes, M. (2009) Reconsidering successful aging: A call for renewed and expanded academic critiques and conceptualizations. *Journal of Applied Geronotology* **28**:6, 702–722.

Ehnes, J. (2012) Ageing and financial (in)security. In: Beard, J., Biggs, S., Bloom, D., Fried, L., Hogan, P., Kalache, A. and Olshanky, J. (eds.) (on behalf of the World Economic Forum) *Global Population Ageing: Peril or promise?* Geneva: World Economic Forum Global Agenda Council on Ageing Society, pp. 18–20.

Erikson, E.H. (1950) *Childhood and Society*. New York: WW Norton & Co. Inc.

Erikson, J., Erikson, E.H. and Kivinick, H.Q. (1986) *Vital Involvement in Old Age*. New York. London: Norton & Co.

Europa (2012) European Year for Active Ageing and solidarity between generations 2012. Accessed 20.06.2012, http://europa.eu/ey2012/

Finlayson, M., Preissner, K. and Garcia, J. (2009) Pilot study of an educational programme for caregivers of people ageing with multiple sclerosis. *British Journal of Occupational Therapy* **72(1)**, 11–20.

Fong, T., Finlayson, M. and Peacock, N. (2006) The social experience of aging with a chronic illness: Perspectives of older adults with multiple sclerosis. *Disability and Rehabilitation* **28(11)**, 695–705.

Freude, G., Jakob, O., Martus, P., Rose, U. and Seibt, R. (2010) Predictors of the discrepancy between calendar and biological age. *Occupational Medicine* **60**, 21–28.

Fried. L.P., Tangen. C.M., Walston. J., Newman. A.B., Hirsch. C., Gottdiener. J., Seeman. T., Tracy. R., Kop. W.J., Burke. G. and McBurnie. M.A. (2001) Frailty in older adults: Evidence for a phenotype. *Journal of Gerontology* **56A(3)**, M146–M156.

Fries, J.F. (1980) Aging, natural death and the compression of morbidity. *New England Journal of Medicine* **303(3)**, 130–135.

Fries, J. (2003) Measuring and monitoring success in compressing morbidity. *Annals of Internal Medicine* **139**, 455–459.

Glass, T.A. (2003) Assessing the success of successful aging. *Annals of Internal Medicine* **139(5)**, 382–383.

Graff, M.J.L, Vernooij-Dassen, M.J.M., Thijssen, M., Dekker, J., Hoefnagels, W.H.L. and Rokkert, M.G.M.O. (2006) Community based occupational therapy for patients with dementia and their care givers: Randomised controlled trial. *BMJ*, doi: 10.1136/bmj.39001.688843.BE

Guse, L.W. and Masesar, M.A. (1999) Quality of life and successful ageing in long term care: Perceptions of residents. *Mental Health Nursing* **20(6)**, 527–539.

Häggblom-Kronlöf, G., Hultberg, J., Eriksson, B.G. and Sonn, U. (2007) Experiences of daily occupations at 99 years of age. *Scandinavian Journal of Occupational Therapy* **14(3)**, 192–200.

Harman, D. (1956) Aging: A theory based on free radical and radiation chemistry. *Journal of Gerontology* **11**, 298–300.

Havighurst, R.J. (1961) Successful aging. *The Gerontologist* **1**, 8–13.

Havighurst, R.J. and Albrecht, R. (1953) *Older People*. New York: Longmans, Green.

Hayflick, L. (1998) How and why we age. *Experimental Gerontology* **33(7/8)**, 639–653.

Hayflick, L. (2000) The future of ageing. *Nature Insight* **408**, 267–269.

Hayflick, L. and Moorhead, P.S. (1961) The serial cultivation of human diploid cell strains. *Experimental Cell Research* **25**, 585–621.

Higgs, P. and Gilleard, C. (2006) Departing the margins: Social class and later life in a second modernity. *Journal of Sociology* **42(3)**, 219–241.

Hitt, R., Young-Xu, Y., Silver, M. and Perls, T. (1999) Centenarians: The older you get the healthier you have been. *Lancet* **354(9179)**, 652.

Hocking, C., Murphy, J. and Reed, K. (2011) Strategies older New Zealanders use to participate in day-to-day occupations. *British Journal of Occupational Therapy* **74**:11, 509–516.

Hovbrandt, P., Fridlund, B. and Carlsson, G (2007) Very old people's experiences of occupational performance outside the home: Possibilities and limitations. *Scandinavian Journal of Occupational Therapy* **14(2)**, 77–85.

Huby, G., Stewart, J., Tierney, A. and Rogers, W. (2004) Planning older people's discharge from acute hospital care: Linking risk management and patient participation. *Health, Risk & Society* **6**, 115–132.

Jackson, J. (1996) Living a meaningful existence in old age. In: Zemke, R. and Clark, F. (eds) *Occupational Science: The evolving discipline*. Philadelphia: FA Davis, pp. 339–362.

Jackson, J., Carlson, M., Mandel, D., Zemke, R. and Clark, F. (1998) Occupation in Lifestyle Redesign: The Well Elderly Study Occupational Therapy Program. *The American Journal of Occupational Therapy* **52(5)**, 326–336.

Jacques, N.D. and Hasselkus, B.R. (2004) The nature of occupation surrounding dying and death. *Occupation, Participation and Health* **24(2)**, 44–53.

Jonsson, H., Josephsson, S. and Kielhofner, G. (2000a) Evolving narratives in the course of retirement:A longitudinal study. *American Journal of Occupational Therapy* **54**, 463–470.

Jonsson, H., Josephsson, S. and Kielhofner, G. (2000b) Narratives and experience in an occupational transition: A longitudinal study of the retirement process. *American Journal of Occupational Therapy* **55**, 424–432.

Kalache, A., Aboderin, I. and Hoskins, I. (2002) Compression of morbidity and active ageing: Key priorities for public health policy in the 21st century. *Bulletin of the World Health Organization* **80(3)**, 243–244.

Kirkwood, T.B.L. (2002) Evolution of ageing. *Mechanisms of Ageing and Development* **123(7)**, 737–745.

Kirkwood, T.B.L. (2003) The most pressing problem of our age. *British Medical Journal* **326**, 1297–1299.

Kirkwood, T.B.L. and Austad, S.N. (2000) Why do we age? *Nature Insight* **408**, 233–237.

Kryspin-Exner, I., Lamplmayr, E. and Felnhofer, A. (2011) Geropsychology: The gender gap in human aging – A mini-review. *Gerontology, Germany* **57**, 539–548, doi: 10.1159/000323154

Lang, P.O., Micheal, J.P. and Zekry, D. (2009) Frailty Syndrome: A transitional state in a dynamic process. *Gerontology, France* **55**, 539–549, doi: 10.1159/000211949

Lapid, M.I., Rummans, T.A., Boeve, B.F., McCormick, J.K., Pankratz, V.S., Cha, R.H., Smith, G.E., Ivnik, R.J., Tangalos, E.G. and Petersen, R.C. (2011) What is the quality of life in the oldest-old?*International Psychogeriatrics* **23**:6, 1003–1010.

Levy, B.R., Slade, M.D. and Kasl, S.V. (2002) Longitudinal benefit of positive self-perceptions of aging on functional health. *Journal of Gerontology, Series B, Psychological Sciences and Social Sciences* **57(5)**, 409–417.

Liang, J. and Luo, B. (2012) Toward a discourse shift in social gerontology: From successful aging to harmonious aging. *Journal of Aging Studies, USA* **26**:3, 327–334, doi: 10.1016/j.jaging.2012.03.001

Lilja, M., Bergh, A., Johansson, L. and Nygard, L. (2003) Attitudes towards the rehabilitation needs and support from assistive technology and the social environment among elderly people with disability. *Occupational Therapy International* **10(1)**, 75–93.

Lupien, S.J. and Wan, N. (2004) Successful ageing: From cell to self. *Philosophical Transactions of the Royal Society B, Biological Sciences* **359(1449)**, 1413–1426.

Mandel, D.R., Jackson, J.M., Zemke, R., Nelson, L. and Clark, F.A. (1999) *Lifestyle redesign: Implementing the Well Elderly programme.* Bethesda, MD: American Occupational Therapy Association.

McColl, M.A., Stirling, P., Walker, J., Corey, P. and Wilkins, R. (1999) Expectations of independence and life satisfaction among ageing spinal cord injured adults. *Disability and Rehabilitation, Canada* **21(5/6)**, 231–240.

Moats, G. (2006) Discharge decision-making with older people: The influence of the institutional environment. *Australian Occupational Therapy Journal* **53**, 107–116.

Mountain, G., Mozley, C., Craig, C. and Ball, L. (2008) Occupational therapy led health promotion for older people: Feasibility of the Lifestyle Matters Programme. *British Journal of Occupational Therapy* **71(10)**, 406–413.

National End of Life Care Intelligence Network (2012) What do we know now that we didn't know a year ago? New intelligence on end of life care in England. Accessed 20.05.2012, http://www.endoflifecare-intelligence.org.uk/resources/publications/what_we_know_now.aspx

Office for National Statistics (2012) Population ageing in the United Kingdom, its constituent countries and the European Union. Accessed 20.06.2012. http://www.ons.gov.uk/ons/dcp171776_258607.pdf

Pettican, A. and Prior, S. (2011) "It's a new way of life": An exploration of the occupational transition of retirement. *British Journal of Occupational Therapy* **74(1)**, 12–19.

Perls, T. and Terry, D. (2003) Understanding the determinants of exceptional longevity. *Annals of Internal Medicine*, suppl **139**, 445–449.

Phelan, E.A., Anderson, L.A., LaCroix, A.Z. and Larson, E.B. (2004) Older adults' views of "successful ageing". How do they compare with researchers' definitions? *Journal of the American Geriatrics Society* **52(2)**, 211–216.

Pollard, N. (2006) Is dying an occupation? *Journal of Occupational Science* **13(2)**, 144–152.

Richard, S., Donovan, S., Victor, C. and Hunt, J. (2005) Standing secure amidst a falling world? Practitioner understandings of old age in response to a case vignette. *Journal of Interprofessional Care* **21**, 335–349.

Roland, K.P., Theou, O.. Jakobi, J.M., Swan, L. and Jones, G.R. (2011) Exploring frailty: Community physical and occupation therapists' perspectives. *Physical & Occupational Therapy in Geriatrics, USA* **29(4)**, 270–286, doi: 10.3109/02703181.2011.616986

Rowe, J.W. and Kahn, R.L. (1987) Human aging: Usual and successful. *Science* **237**, 143–149.

Rowe, J.W. and Kahn, R.L. (1997) Successful aging. *The Gerontologist* **37(4)**, 433–440.

Salthouse, T.A. (2009) When does age-related cognitive decline begin? *Neurobiology of Aging, University of Virginia* **30**, 507–514.

Sarkisian, C.A., Liu, H., Ensrud, K., Stone, K.L. and Mangione, C.M. (2001) Correlates of attributing new disability to old age. *Journal of the American Geriatrics Society* **49(2)**, 134–141.

Stenner, P., McFarquhar, T. and Bowling, A. (2011) Older people and "active ageing": Subjective aspects of ageing actively. *Journal of Health Psychology* **16(3)**, 467–477,

Sumsion, T. (2006) Overview of client centred practice. In: Sumsion, T. (ed.) *Client Centred Practice in Occupational Therapy*, 2nd ed. Edinburgh: Churchill Livingstone Elsevier, pp. 1–18.

Syddall, H., Roberts, H.C., Evandrou, M., Cooper, C., Bergman, H. and Sayer, A.A. (2010) Prevalence and correlates of frailty among community-dwelling older men and women: Findings from the Hertfordshire Cohort Study. *Age and Ageing* **39**, 197–203, doi: 10.1093/ageing/afp204

Taylor, J. (2005) Risk management paradigms in health and social services for professional decision making in the long term care of older people. *British Journal of Social Work* **36**, 1411–1429.

Thompson, P. (1992) 'I don't feel old: Subjective ageing and the search for meaning in later life. *Ageing and Society* **12**, 23–47.

Tornstam, L. (1989) Gerotranscendence: A metaphysical reformulation of the disengagement theory. *Aging: Clinical and Experimental Research* **1(1)**, 55–63.

von Faber, M., Bootsma-van der Wiwl, A., van Exel, E., Gussekloo, J., Lagaay, A.M., van Dongen, E., Knook, D.L., van der Geest, S. and Westendorp, R.G.J. (2001) Successful ageing in the oldest old. *Archives of Internal Medicine* **161(22)**, 2694.

Wadenstein, B. (2005) Introducing older people to the theory of gerotranscendence. *Journal of Advanced Nursing* **52(4)**, 381–388.

Wicks, A. (2006) Older women's "ways of doing": Strategies for successful ageing. *Ageing International* **31(4)**, 263–275.

Wilcock, A.A. (1999) Reflections on doing, being, becoming. *Australian Journal of Occupational Therapy* **46**, 1–11.

Wilcock, A.A. (2005) Older people and occupational justice. In: McIntyre, A. and Atwal, A. (eds) *Occupational Therapy and Older People*. Oxford: Blackwell Publishing, pp. 14–26.

Wilcock, A.A. (2006) *An Occupational Perspective of Health*. 2nd edition. Thorofare NJ: Slack Inc.

World Health Organization (2001) *The International Classification of Functioning Disability and Health*. Geneva: World Health Organization.

World Health Organization (2002) *Active Ageing. A Policy Framework*. Geneva: World Health Organization.

World Health Organization (2003) *Gender, Health and Ageing*. Geneva: World Health Organization.

World Health Organization (2008) *World Health Statistics*. Geneva: World Health Organization..

World Health Organization European Region (2011) *Palliative care for older people: Better practices*. Accessed 20/05/2012 at: http://www.euro.who.int/__data/assets/pdf_file/0017/143153/e95052.pdf

Wurm, S., Tomasik, M.J. and Tesch-Romer, C. (2008) Serious health events and their impact on changes in subjective health and life satisfaction: The role of age and a positive view on ageing. *European Journal of Ageing, Germany*, doi: 10.1007/s10433-008-0077-5

Wythes, A.J. and Lyons, M. (2006) Leaving the land: An exploratory study of retirement for a small group of Australian men. *Rural and Remote Health* **6**, 531 (online). Retrieved 11/08/2008.

Yerxa, E.J., Clark, F., Frank, G., Jackson, J., Parham, D., Pierce, D., Stein, C. and Zemke, R. (1990) An introduction to Occupational Science, a foundation for Occupational Therapy in the 21st century. *Occupational Therapy in Health Care* **6(4)**, 1–17.

Zarb, G. and Oliver, M. (1993) *Ageing with a Disability: What do they expect after all these years?* London: University of Greenwich.

Chapter 3

The social context of older people

Frances Reynolds and Kee Hean Lim

Older people are as different in their skills, needs, resources and interests as younger people, and are a far from homogeneous group. Whilst negative social attitudes continue to exist, over the past 10 years or so there has been increasing awareness that many of the accepted challenges of later life, such as ill-health and shrinkage of social networks, disproportionately affect people over 80 years of age, and that many people expect to be active players in their social context and to retain valued occupations for at least 15 years after statutory retirement age (Gergen and Gergen 2001).

We begin this chapter by firstly addressing ageism and discrimination within the health and social care system. As well as examining personal attitudes, occupational therapists need to be sensitive to the cultural dimensions of ageing. We do not live in a homogeneous culture, so it is important for occupational therapists to be attuned to the various patterns of social support and prevalent attitudes towards ageing that are commonly found in different ethnic and cultural groups. Such cultural sensitivity enhances the therapists' capacity to form effective partnerships with older people from diverse social groups.

We will also explore the immediate social context of older people, including family, friends, pets, health professionals and local communities. We will show how older people live within a variety of social support networks, and that these have an enormous influence over the individual's quality of life, identity/self-esteem, and strategies of coping with ill-health. There are also profound links between older people's engagement in valued occupations and their social support networks. Moreover, the size and functioning of the social network could even influence physical health and longevity, and we will consider the mechanisms that may be involved. Far from presenting older people as passively dependent upon care, the chapter will explore the complex *reciprocal* social relationships that form part of the majority of older people's everyday experiences.

Some of the challenges inherent in residential settings will also be highlighted. Sadly, this social context can, at its worst, completely undermine the older person's wellbeing, and some of the psycho-social factors associated with neglect and abuse are mentioned. The chapter ends by considering certain strategies that occupational therapists could adopt to improve partnership-working with older people, and to help older clients strengthen and extend their social networks. Such strategies help clients to gain better health and

Occupational Therapy and Older People, Second Edition. Edited by Anita Atwal and Anne McIntyre.
© 2013 Blackwell Publishing Ltd. Published 2013 by Blackwell Publishing Ltd.

quality of life. To illustrate the points made and to encourage personal reflection, the chapter includes not only published research, but also two case studies, and a collection of quotations and recounted incidents.

Ageist attitudes, values, assumptions and stereotypes

Henley and Schott (1999, p. 51) define 'attitude' as 'A settled opinion or way of thinking'. Such 'settled' opinions are often resistant to empirical evidence and, furthermore, influence behaviour, leading to discriminatory practices. Ageism reflects both a categorisation of people solely on the basis of age, and an attribution of shared characteristics to all who are placed in this category. Williams and Giles (1998) suggest that some stereotypes present older people as 'frail' and 'useless', whereas others are equally condescending in presenting this age group as especially 'worthy' and 'deserving'. Both forms of stereotype neglect the individuality of each older person, and place older people in a special social 'ghetto'. Ageist attitudes are widespread in Western societies (Cuddy et al. 2005). One illustration is provided by a recent review of research into advertising. The authors report that people aged over 65 years are underrepresented in advertisements, compared with their proportion of the general population, and also that when they do appear, they tend to be negatively portrayed as weak, helpless, comic, or requiring special aids and adaptations (Zhang et al. 2006). Other research has found that older people are readily categorised as worthless, inflexible, and declining in cognitive and other abilities (Henley and Schott 1999), although recently there seems to be a welcome increase in public initiatives to combat such assumptions (Featherstone and Hepworth 2009). Older people are aware of negative stereotyping and report feeling patronised, and limited by it in many aspects of their lives (Cuddy et al. 2005).

Ageist attitudes may be held unconsciously, even when people believe they hold positive views (Levy and Banaji 2002). Health and social care professionals are not immune to the stereotypes that prevail in the wider culture (Cuddy et al. 2005; Davys 2008; Duthie and Donaghy 2009), and may discriminate against older clients, even if unintentionally (Carruthers and Ormondroyd 2009). To form non-judgemental, empowering relationships with older clients, there is a need for occupational therapists to be aware of the prejudices to which they have been exposed through their own socialisation, and to confront discriminatory policies and practices in their local social contexts.

Cross cultural perspectives on ageing and older people

Differences exist in how older people are perceived and treated within different cultures. In the West, growing old is often viewed negatively, being linked with images of disease, illness, dependence on others, loss of status and diminished autonomy. This depressing image is not found in more traditional and Eastern societies, where being old is synonymous with attaining greater wisdom and knowledge. In less individualistic societies, the extended family confers high status and respect on its older members, as well as involving them in its patterns of *reciprocal* care-giving (Henley and Schott 1999, Helman 2000).

Chiu and Yu (2001, p. 683), reporting on their study of immigrant Chinese families, explain: 'older people in the traditional Chinese family are more than cared-for persons: they are senior family members with authority and status to guide the direction of the family. Hence, they receive not only care but also respect.'

Within 'traditional' or non-Western families and communities, older people tend to have a culturally recognised role in offering advice, guidance and sharing experiences. They also contribute actively to caring for other family members. For example, the older person could play an active and culturally valued role as grandparent, cook and house-keeper in extended families. These roles and responsibilities promote the health, self-worth and wellbeing of older persons, as they provide real purpose and opportunities to keep active and involved (see Box 3.1). We must, however, as health professionals be aware of culturally bound stereotypes. To immediately assume that all 'non-Western' families are willing to care for their elderly relatives, without seeking any form of professional help or support, is too presumptuous, and risks disenfranchising older people (especially those who are immigrants) from statutory services (Chiu and Yu 2001, Chau and Yu 2009). It is also important to realise that different ethnic/cultural groups and communities may have different ideas and understandings of what contributes to an individual's health and wellbeing, They may, for example, reinforce dependent behaviour (by taking over the everyday self-care activities of older members recovering from stroke or other illness). Immigrant families might find it difficult to reconcile their traditional values with the pressures of the host society (for example, to work long hours

---

Box 3.1   Consider the strengths and limitations of Mrs Gopal's social context

Mrs Rena Gopal is a 78-year-old woman of Indian origin who lives in an extended family of three generations, in the UK. She is widowed and lives with her eldest son, Rajendra, and daughter-in-law, Meena, and four grandchildren. Mrs Gopal had a stroke four months ago and was in hospital for three months. She suffered a right CVA, with a left side neglect and has been discharged back home. She now attends the Community Rehabilitation Unit where she receives occupational therapy input twice weekly. Although Mrs Gopal appears keen to get better and has engaged in the rehabilitation programme on offer, her recovery is being hampered to a certain extent by her immediate family's commitment to do every-thing for her. This has proven to be a disincentive for her to participate fully in rehabilitation as she does not have the opportunity to undertake and practise any of the tasks at home. Mrs Gopal has two other daughters who live nearby with their families and together they feel that it is their responsibility to care for her. The extended family have been reluctant to accept any assistance from social services as they feel it is their duty to care and provide for her needs. Mrs Gopal is only able to speak basic English and her main interests prior to suffering the stroke included cooking for the family, attending family gatherings, participating in Hindu religious events and attending a women's social group in her local community centre for two hours each week. She was also responsible for looking after her grandchildren, which is a role that she has not been able to continue with after the stroke. Since returning home, she has been mainly cared for by her eldest granddaughter, Amar, who is 17. Mrs Gopal has not been encouraged to do any 'hands on' cooking at home but she has been given a supervisory role, instructing what needs to be done. So far, she has not attended the women's social gathering as her family are concerned for her safety out-side of the home. Mrs Gopal has two close female friends who visit her daily. Although she is keen to be mobile and independent again, and to be able to go out with her friends, she is also fearful that she may not be able to manage this.

away from home), leading to less shared care of older members than might be assumed (Chiu and Yu 2001). Not only attitudes, but also changing patterns of behaviour in the wider culture (such as increasing levels of divorce, reduced fertility rates, and dual career families) limit the resources which are available for the informal care of older people regardless of whether the family originates within minority or majority ethnic groups (Tomassini et al. 2007).

Whilst remaining mindful of broad cultural differences in family structures and values, we need to treat each client as an individual, with specific needs and requirements. Only in this way can we effectively provide culturally sensitive and appropriate care (Lim 2001). In the UK, the College of Occupational Therapists' revised Code of Ethics and Professional Conduct (2010; p. 14) suggests that occupational therapists shall ensure that they are sensitive to 'factors that affect service users' cultural and lifestyle choices, incorporating this into any service planning, individual assessment and/or intervention where possible'. Standard 2 of the National Service Framework for Older People (DH 2001) in England, similarly supports the need to be person-centred (see Chapter 4).

Exploring the social networks of older people

There are two fairly widespread, somewhat contradictory, stereotypes about the social context of older people. The first is that older people are much more likely than younger people to be living alone, feeling isolated and lonely. The second unwarranted assumption is that older people have a child-like status, passively dependent upon the care of their families, especially daughters. Research is showing that neither pattern of living is widespread and that the social networks of large numbers of older people are rich and complex. We need to recognise that older people who live alone may find this choice agreeable, and that they may retain regular contacts with a variety of relatives and friends, rather than being socially isolated. Loneliness is distinct from living alone or social isolation, and refers to the experience of having fewer social ties or confidantes than a person expects, desires, or feels is admissible (Victor and Scharf 2005). It is an experience that is highly associated with depression (Victor et al. 2005).

According to a review of four surveys carried out between 1945 and 1999, on average about 5–9% of older people regard themselves as 'often lonely' (rising to 14% of those who live alone), a pattern that showed little change during that follow-up period (Victor et al. 2002). It is unclear whether loneliness is now affecting greater numbers of older people. A similar percentage of English participants report being 'severely lonely' in a more recent study, as in previous research, although a large minority (43%) described themselves as moderately lonely (Scharf and de Jong Gierveld 2008). Golden et al. (2009) report in their study of over 1000 older people that about one-third described themselves as lonely, 'with 9% describing it as painful and 6% as intrusive' (p. 694). Loneliness is more likely to affect the 'oldest old' who are most vulnerable to loss of partner and other relationships through bereavement, and also disproportionately affects those who are in poor health and in poverty. It could be the experience that best explains the elevated risk of depression amongst those who are widowed (Golden et al. 2009). Social isolation and loneliness are also associated with neighbourhood variables, such as a deprived physical and social urban environment, poor transport and other services, and insecurity/threats of crime. These factors limit older people's engagement in community activities and sense of belonging (Scharf and de Jong Gierveld 2008).

A social network comprises all of the interlinked relationships of a person. Networks vary in 'size, composition and density, and the geographical dispersion of the members' (Keating et al. 2003, p. 117). Kahn and Antonucci (1980) proposed the more dynamic concept of the social network 'convoy', comprising the numerous relationships – some stable, some changing – that accompany people over the course of their lives. As years pass, some relationships continue, some come to an end, and some people enter the convoy (e.g. new friends, or grandchildren). The social network is overall likely to shrink, especially amongst the over-80s. There is increasing recognition that broad social changes which have increased rates of divorce and geographical mobility in younger people, threaten older people's family relationships. For example, break-up in the families of adult children can result in older people losing contact with their children's partners and with their grandchildren, to the detriment of their health and psychological wellbeing (Drew and Smith 1999, Drew and Silverstein 2007). Older people are also vulnerable to losing relationships through bereavement and relocation (including friends leaving the local district to live near their own adult children or to enter residential homes). The evolving social network of an older man is illustrated in Box 3.2.

No health professional appears in this network, as Mr Jameson has been fiercely independent and has made minimal use of any health or social service until recently. But for some clients, health and social professionals might play an important supportive role.

Box 3.2   Read the case study, identify the members of Mr Jameson's social network, and the exchange of social support within this network

Mr Edward Jameson is 81 years old. He is in fair health, but experiences chronic pain from osteoarthritis, particularly in his knees and back. He came to the attention of occupational therapists recently, after a knee replacement operation. It emerges that he cares for his wife, Dorothy, who is 78 years old. She had a stroke two years ago. His wife requires considerable help with transfers and personal care, but is cognitively bright and usually cheerful. Mr Jameson does most of the housework, although his daughter, Anne, who lives nearby, brings in shopping. There is a close bond between Anne and her parents. The Jamesons see much less of their son-in-law, Paul, but they enjoy quite a positive relationship with him. Mr Jameson sometimes helps his daughter with jobs such as checking that her rather ancient car has sufficient oil, and taking it to the garage for servicing. As well as having a daughter, the Jamesons have a 12-year old granddaughter, Claire, whom they sometimes care for during half-term holidays. The Jamesons have a mutual friend, Emily, whom they met shortly after their wedding. They now keep in touch by letter, but they rarely see her since she moved into a residential home about 50 miles away. Mrs Jameson's closest friend died about a year ago, leaving a void in her life. Because it is difficult for her to get out of the house, she sees few other people apart from her immediate family. Mr Jameson has recently become friends with one of the next-door neighbours, Jim, who is a widower, and they often chat over the garden fence. The neighbour is diabetic and Mr Jameson keeps a watchful eye to make sure that he is not becoming ill. The neighbour often has to attend hospital appointments, and Mr Jameson always takes him there in his car, and brings him home. Mr Jameson himself is wary of doctors and hospitals, regarding himself as 'strong' and 'uncomplaining'. Only severe pain some months ago made him attend for a medical consultation about his knee.

Types of social support

Several large social surveys have shown not only that most older people are satisfied with their social context, but that the relationships of older people – except among the oldest or most frail – are usually characterised by *reciprocity*, that is, mutual support rather than 'one-way' caring. This is shown in both case studies (Box 3.1, Box 3.2). In line with theories of friendship which propose that stable relationships are founded on an equitable basis of give-and-take, the networks of older people seem generally to both give help to the older person and to receive help from this person. Older people, for example, take great satisfaction from being able to give help to their adult children as well as receiving support (Lowenstein et al. 2007). Many older people also offer considerable child care in their roles as grandparents, through which they gain a sense of purpose and value (Thiele and Whelan 2008).

Various types of social support have been identified, such as emotional, informational and practical support. Krause (2007, p. 458) argues that these various forms of support are not only directly helpful but that they convey 'subtle messages' to the older person, helping 'recipients feel they are esteemed and valued, and this helps them see they have a set place in the wider social order…[into which] they belong'. Close family members tend to provide most of the long-term instrumental/practical support that is available to older people, although neighbours may offer short-term help (e.g. information, or help with fairly straightforward practical tasks, such as moving a heavy dustbin). Older people tend to prefer receiving practical support from family than friends or neighbours. However, close friends offer welcome emotional support, and have a large impact on morale (Henley and Schott 1999, Keating et al. 2003, Litwin 2001). Friends mighty offer practical assistance when family members are not available for whatever reason, but there is some evidence that friendship relationships can become more quickly strained by non-reciprocal helping (Crohan and Antonucci 1989). The sense of obligation plus the presence of long-standing emotional attachments may encourage close family members, especially daughters, to continue in practical caring for long periods, sometimes even at the expense of their own health and wellbeing.

The emotional support and affirmation offered by friends – as well as close family members – tend to play an important role in helping the older person to maintain a familiar identity and self-esteem, as well as offering opportunities to share stressful experiences, and perhaps to gain advice. Frequency of contact with friends is associated with life satisfaction among older women (Sener et al. 2008), and may even confer some protection against mortality according to a longitudinal study by Harris and Thoresen (2005). Friends of similar ages may help to 'normalise' difficulties (such as bereavement or disability), encouraging the person to feel more accepting of the challenges that later life can present. On the other hand, loss of peers can leave the older person without confidantes, especially among those aged over 80, increasing the risk of depression (Askham et al. 2007, Wenger & Jerrome 1999). Women seem particularly likely to be devastated by loss of a confidante, even when they have a spouse (Crohan & Antonucci 1989, Wenger and Jerrome 1999). Any loss of close friends from the social network can also create strains for other family members who mightattempt to plug the gaps by, for example, making more visits or inviting the older person to stay. These adaptive changes can work well for some families, but increase strain or conflict for others, for a number of reasons. Some older people do not like to feel 'indebted'; some feel awkward because they never had close emotional ties with their adult children in previous years; some family members feel overwhelmed by conflicting role obligations (to their own families, to their work and to the older person).

Although loss of peers is an inevitable part of growing older, not all social networks shrink dramatically with increasing age. Some older people – particularly women – seem able to maintain their support 'convoys' through, for example, joining new organisations, doing voluntary work, remaining active within religious organisations, and making new friends (Wright 1989). Even weak social ties, when they exist in some numbers, make a difference to older people's wellbeing (Haines and Henderson 2002).

Older men appear particularly vulnerable to losing work-mates on retirement, and many come to depend on a few female relatives for social support, especially their spouse. Not surprisingly, they therefore seem especially vulnerable to loneliness, if widowed or caring for a disabled spouse (de Jong Gierveld et al. 2009). Widowers face particular difficulties in maintaining their support networks, perhaps because there are fewer men in this situation than women (as women tend to live longer than men, outlasting their husbands). This can result in greater loneliness for men who have lost their wives (who were often their sole confidantes), than for women. It appears more difficult for them to meet other widowed men who share their social situation. Maintaining involvement in hobby or recreational groups seems to protect the wellbeing of older men suffering from declining health, more so than for women who may have more alternative sources of support (Greenfield and Marks 2007). Network losses seem to create increased risks, particularly for older men's ill-health (Davidson and Arber 2004). Peer support appears to be as important to the wellbeing of older people living in residential settings as for those in the community (Carpenter 2002), suggesting that staff in such settings need to ensure that opportunities exist for social contact and friendship, for example by making available a wide range of sociable leisure activities (Silverstein and Parker 2002, Atwal et al. 2003).

Older people also value providing support *to* others in their social networks (such as adult children and grandchildren). In one study, 90% of older people reported being satisfied with the amount of tangible support that they received, whereas 39% wished they could provide more support to others (Krause and Markides 1990). Those who are involved in caring for grandchildren tend to report taking great pleasure in their new roles and activities (Clarke and Roberts 2004). Even in residential homes, a considerable exchange of social support has been observed, such as buddy systems where individuals look out for each other (Lawrence and Schigelone 2002). These supportive alliances increase feelings of solidarity and wellbeing.

Some older people extend their social networks by volunteering. Warburton et al. (2001) found that older volunteers appreciated the opportunity to gain social contacts in roles recognised as useful to the community. Volunteering not only enhances morale and decreases the risk of depression, but seems to extend life, according to two longitudinal studies (Harris and Thoresen 2005, Lum and Lightfoot 2005). The findings challenge traditional stereotypes of the 'needy' older person, who is simply in receipt of care. Certain occupations apart from volunteering help to extend social networks – as they do for all people regardless of age. Some older people take up new activities during retirement that successfully extend their social networks. For example, most of the participants in a study of creative art-making in later life highly valued the social aspects of their art-making, having made new friends since retirement age (Reynolds, 2010). A 75-year-old woman with health problems illustrated the social context of art-making by describing how she had joined a spinning group after retiring, and how these new friends had then decided to engage in further creative occupations together:

> "Several people from the spinning group, there are about four of us … we get together and just sit and draw in the garden once a week. So it's quite a sociable activity really. You know that you're very much doing it in the company … of friends. Well you have to when you retire, you have to make an effort to do something. At least it's a way of getting out and meeting people. … Everyone focusing on something together is sort of pleasant." (Reynolds, 2010 p. 141)

Types of support network

As well as documenting the size of social networks and their various supportive functions, some researchers have attempted to categorise different types of social network, exploring their relative strengths and vulnerabilities for supporting the older person. Wenger (1994) has put forward a fivefold classification based on a longitudinal study of older people in North Wales. Firstly, let us consider aspects of the research method.

Focus on research: The social networks of older people in North Wales

The Bangor Longitudinal Study consists of a number of surveys carried out since 1978, in which a cohort of older people have been followed up every few years to document stability and change in their social support networks, in relation to factors such as illness, bereavement and migration (Wenger & Jerome 1999). In one analysis, carried out in the 1990s, the social networks of people in rural North Wales were compared with those in Liverpool (Wenger 1995). Wenger's analysis uncovered five main types of family network among older people in North Wales. These should not be regarded as totally fixed, because changes in a person's network can occur over time, as friends, offspring and siblings die, move away, or move nearer to the older person. The birth of grandchildren can have positive effects on the network, but changes in the health of the older person can have negative effects. Also, the increasing prevalence of divorce, remarriage and step-families complicates the social networks of older people in ways that require much greater attention from researchers. According to Wenger (1994), the five main types of network are as follows:

- *Local family dependent*: In these networks, the older person has close ties with at least some family members who live close at hand – at least within five miles. Such family members – typically one or more daughters – are in regular contact, offering assistance and emotional support. The older person tends to have few ties outside the family (e.g. with friends or neighbours). This network type is more common among widowed older people, and among those in poorer health.

- *Locally integrated*: Such networks are characterised by the presence of friends and neighbours as well as family members living locally. The person may have close ties with church and voluntary bodies, and the social network, developed over a long period, may be large. Older people in these networks tend to be in better health.
- *Local self-contained*: These networks tend to be small, and consist of only a few relatives, sometimes emotionally as well as geographically distant. The older person is unlikely to know many people in the local community, but may be reliant on neighbours in times of emergency.
- *Wider community-focused*: Older people in this type of network tend to have a large number of ties with the local community, including membership of local clubs, societies, charitable organisations and so on. They are often involved in helping others, and have relatively little need for assistance, at least when in good or fair health.
- *Private restricted*: These networks are tiny, and might reflect only minimal contacts with a few friends – who may in reality be more like acquaintances. Wenger argues that, in many cases, it represents a life-long pattern of extreme independence or, indeed, aloofness.

More recent studies confirm the influence of social network type on the wellbeing of older people. For example, Golden et al. (2009) administered a number of quantitative scales face-to-face with 1299 older people living in the community. About two-thirds lived in a locally integrated social network and most of the remainder lived in a family-dependent network. Participants living in the locally integrated networks tended to report greater levels of happiness and life satisfaction. Those living in a non-integrated network were nearly twice as likely to report depression and more than twice as likely to report loneliness or hopelessness. Field et al. (2002) studied older people living in sheltered accommodation and found that those with a more locally integrated network participated in more activities and were less lonely. However, unlike Golden et al. (2009), they found no association between network type and depression (or dementia). There will be further exploration of relationships between social context and valued occupations in a subsequent section.

Pets as members of the older person's social context

In recent years, there has been increasing recognition that pets may be much-loved members of the older person's social context (McColgan and Schofield 2007). However, not all studies show any psychological health benefits from pet ownership (Parslow et al. 2005). The latter study illustrates that it is not easy to measure the distinctive effects of having a pet on the wellbeing of older people, as other variables (which can themselves be associated with pet ownership) such as loneliness and widowhood, also play a powerful role in shaping wellbeing. For some people, though, caring for a pet seems to satisfy the human need to nurture and care for another living being, and the pet's loyalty and affection could be perceived as a form of unconditional emotional support. Pets also provide a valued sense of continuity and identity (Cookman 1996), and may encourage better self-care and more active daily routines. Raina et al. (1999) noted that older people who owned a dog or cat seemed to maintain their engagement in activities of daily living over the course of a year to a greater extent than those who lacked a companion animal, even when other factors such as age had been taken into account. Having a dog could be particularly health-promoting. A small-scale study of 10 older people living in a residential setting observed that those with a dog walked further than those without (Herbert and Greene 2001). As pets are important members of the social context of many older people, their death can be as distressing as the loss of a friend or relative, and yet this distress may not be socially recognised or accepted.

Health professionals as sources of social support

It is difficult to generalise about the contribution that health professionals make to the social support systems of older people. Wenger (1994) argues that the formal support provided by social and healthcare professionals can offer a valuable supplement, in particular to the smaller family-based social networks. However, a qualitative study by Tanner (2001) reveals that seeking and accepting professional help can be a source of discomfort and stigma, as it may be experienced as threatening the older person's view of self as independent.

Some older people do not perceive their rehabilitation specialists to be emotionally supportive or holistic, but rather to operate within the medical discourse that treats patients primarily as objects of treatment (Lund and Tamm 2001). Some older men treated for coronary artery disease saw their healthcare professionals as offering limited tangible or emotional support, and instead regarded their relatives as their main source of comfort (Yates 1995). A recent study of older people's families reported similar concerns, with perceptions that professionals lacked skills for communicating about depression (Mellor et al. 2008). Yet healthcare professionals can potentially play an important role in older people's support networks. A review of research suggests that professionals who establish continuities in their relationships with older people, and who listen effectively and invite the older person to be a collaborative partner in decision-making are likely to achieve the most satisfactory outcomes (Stewart et al. 2000). The importance of communication and written information is discussed further in Chapter 9.

Dysfunctional social contexts

Sadly, in some cases, the social context has deleterious effects on the physical and psychological wellbeing of the older person. For example, the family can behave in disempowering and infantilising ways, even whilst intending to act in the older person's 'best interests'. A UK survey by Biggs et al. (2007) of older people living in private households found that 2.6% reported overt maltreatment, including physical abuse, financial abuse and neglect. Even more alarming figures were reported by an Israeli survey of hospitalised older people, which contrasted the 5.9% of older patients who disclosed abuse when in hospital with the 21.4% who showed evident signs (Cohen et al. 2007). Clearly all forms of abuse and neglect demean and frighten the older person, and contribute to feelings of worthlessness and depression, as well as resulting in physical harm.

Which network types are most prone to neglect and abuse? Clearly the more private networks, in which the older person is supported with minimal outside contact, are most capable of hiding abuse. Whilst some research suggests that highly neglectful or abusive family members are likely to have mental health or alcohol problems (Pillemer and Finkelhor 1989), some findings encourage us to look at the functioning of the network as a whole. Clinicians and researchers adopting the systemic perspective do not seek to condone abuse, but argue that effective intervention depends upon identifying all the factors that contribute to dysfunctional social contexts. Neglect and abuse are likely to occur when support systems are shrinking and under heavy strain (Bradley 1996, Shugarman et al. 2003), when care-givers have a history of conflictual relationships with the older person (who may also have been abusive as a parent), and/or when carers are experiencing prolonged stress associated with poverty or looking after other family members. Victims of mistreatment tend to be highly vulnerable, for example, suffering from depression or dementia, possibly as a result making increased demands upon care-givers (Dyer et al. 2000, Shugarman et al. 2003). However, we must also acknowledge the influence of the social and physical environment, as well as wider social attitudes that devalue older people. Even though many people feel frustrated from time to time when caring for family members, most do not act out these feelings. Enclosure within the home, and family withdrawal from external social contacts, heighten the risk for the vulnerable older person.

The social context, health and longevity

The chapter so far has suggested that the older person's social context exerts a powerful influence over morale and wellbeing. Through emotional intimacy, affirmation, advice and practical assistance, the older person could be supported in living independently and with dignity. The social context may also offer the older person a strong sense of continuity with past identity, and self-esteem. Rather than being in passive receipt of care, the social context for most older people is a place where equitable relationships and reciprocal support occur. Such relationships affirm beliefs in one's usefulness. Social contacts can also offer stimulation, fun and challenge, and they could empower collective action. These experiences all help to reduce the individual's risk of depression and helplessness. As a result, the older person may be better able to cope with chronic pain and functional limitations. Such effects have been shown in a study of older people with osteoarthritis (Blixen and Kippes 1999). Perceived health appears to be greater among older people who belong to groups and associations, which have a community-oriented purpose, perhaps because of the validation offered by others (Young and Glasgow 1998).

In addition to the psychological and perceived health benefits, some evidence exists that social support confers greater objective physical health and longevity. In a classic study, Berkman and Syme (1979) surveyed a large representative sample of the general community-dwelling population in California to establish whether those with fewer social ties were more susceptible to death over a period of nine years. They obtained a questionnaire return rate of 86%, and a fairly complete number of death certificates, ensuring valid data. The authors reported that people aged 30–69 years old who had a large number of social ties (including married partners, friends, family, church

---

Box 3.3   How may social support affect physical health?

Consider the person whose social network was represented in Box 3.2.
 If Mr Jameson's daughter moved much further away, what effects might this have on his physical, as well as psychological, health?

---

membership and membership of community groups) had significantly lower mortality rates over the nine-year period. The most isolated men were 2.3 times more likely to die than the men with extensive social contacts. The risk for isolated women was even greater. These findings were not confined to a single survey. Seeman et al. (1987) continued the survey for 17 years. They found that people aged 70 and over with the most limited social networks had a 50% greater risk of mortality, even when many other relevant variables were controlled in the analysis. House et al. (1982, 1988), reported similar findings. Lyyra and Heikkinen (2006) in a 10-year longitudinal study found that emotional support (in the form of reassurance of worth, sense of belonging, opportunities for nurturing others, and emotional closeness) predicted longevity among women. These various findings have important implications for occupational therapists as they suggest that social networks are an important resource for health and that engagement in social activities promotes health.

The mechanisms linking social support to physical health are hotly debated (Bath and Deeg 2005). Some have questioned whether cause and effect are being confused in these research studies, and whether the apparent link exists simply because the healthier, more mobile person is better able to sustain social relationships over time (Vaillant et al. 1998). Alternatively, it may be questioned whether other factors, such as poverty, are influencing both social context and mortality. However, Berkman and Syme (1979), and other researchers, have considered these issues carefully, and showed through their statistical analysis that the people with fewer social ties had a greater risk of premature death, even when other health-jeopardising factors such as smoking status, obesity, alcohol use, and physical activity were taken into account. There may be several processes linking social context to physical health:

- Supportive friends and family in the local vicinity may alert the older person to the need to consult medical practitioners, or to take medication, in times of illness. Early action might then result in more effective treatment for health problems, and/or better adherence to treatment. The unsupported older person may neglect to act so promptly when physical symptoms of ill-health appear, and might forget to take medication. Berkman and Syme (1979) showed that people with more extensive social networks tended to use preventive health services more often.
- The older person may engage in more health-promoting activities when part of a social network. For example, it has been found that having supportive friends to walk with encourages older people to take more exercise (Booth et al. 2000). People living alone may get by on snacks rather than making the effort to prepare nutritious meals. Berkman and Syme (1979) showed that people with more numerous social ties adopted healthier lifestyle behaviours, such as eating breakfast, exercising and having sufficient sleep.

More recently, Burnett et al. (2006) found that limited social contact was associated with self-neglect among older people (even when other relevant factors such as age and poverty were taken into account).

- The social context may affect health through the buffering effects of support against stress. Older people who have less support (for example, when providing care to a partner with chronic illness or dementia) suffer prolonged physiological stress responses. Such changes eventually lead to the down-regulation of the immune system, leaving the body more vulnerable to infection. Chronically stressed people who lack support also experience slower healing (e.g. of wounds). Any long-term down-regulation of the immune system may also elevate the risk of cancer. These links are subject to much current investigation (Evans et al. 2000).

- Social contact may support participation in a greater range of activities, alleviating depression and promoting a meaningful quality of life. Such experiences might encourage self-esteem, self-care, and self-efficacy for managing the challenges of later life (Jorm 2005). Relationships between social network characteristics and activity participation will be further considered in the final section.

The evidence linking social networks and health is considered so strong that Jorm (2005) suggested that intervention studies were called for, including evaluations of befriending initiatives.

Social context and valued occupations

The social context appears to influence the quality and quantity of older people's leisure occupations which, in turn, affects their life satisfaction and wellbeing. An early study by House et al. (1982) found that mortality among older people was not only linked with the quality of their social networks but with their engagement in active social and organisational activities. Beneficial associations between the survival of older people and their social, productive and physical activities have also been demonstrated by Glass et al. (1999). Whilst relationships between good health and physical activities might be considered unsurprising, their analysis showed that those who engaged in more social activities (requiring no substantial exertion) typically enjoyed longer lives. A review of additional evidence on this topic can be found in Bath and Deeg (2005).

Having a rich social network seems to offer older people more opportunities to stay active and engaged. In turn, engagement in valued leisure occupations offers older people a buffer against stress, especially among those who have been bereaved (Silverstein and Parker 2002). Paillard-Borg et al. (2009) conducted a large survey in one area of Sweden of people aged 75 years and over. They documented a wide range of leisure occupations, and linked these to the older people's social network, which was rated on a four-point scale. Those with a richer social network (reflecting, for example, the number of social ties, frequency of interaction and older person's satisfaction with their social relationships) reported more numerous leisure activities, even when other contextual influences such as age, gender and health were taken into account statistically.

Implications for Occupational Therapists

This chapter has shown that the social context of the older person has profound effects on wellbeing, identity, capacity to cope with functional impairments, and physical and psychological health. Whilst some older people experience loneliness, we need to avoid stereotyping all older people as lonely and needing care. Many studies emphasise that large numbers of older people are involved in giving care to others, and that relatively few are passive recipients of care. Older people, even when living with chronic ill-health, provide a great deal of reciprocal support within their social contexts, affirming their adult status, identity and self-esteem. Older clients may therefore benefit psychologically and physically within the therapy process from identifying the support that they already make to others in their social network (whether emotional, informational, or practical), and by exploring, if they so wish, how they can make further contributions to their families, friends and communities – for example, in volunteering or charity work if they feel physically able to do so, or through providing emotional support to others. Explicit recognition that older people make an enormous difference to the people they serve may help to enhance self-esteem (Kincade et al. 1996, Wheeler et al. 1998).

Occupations that provide opportunities to forge new social contacts (e.g. through joining a support group or adult education class) could enhance the quality of life and self-confidence of older people. The internet is making such contacts more accessible and there is interest among researchers regarding how older people are making use of its social potential (Dickinson and Hill 2007, Russell et al. 2008). The richer and more community-integrated the social network, the more likely it is that the older person will preserve valued leisure activities and remain healthier. Nevertheless, it is important for therapists to avoid an over-romantic ideal of social support. Some older people, by reason of their upbringing and personality, have always been socially quite isolated, and for some, meeting new people is an anxiety-provoking experience. Therapists also need to be mindful that some older people dislike age-segregated activities. Yet engagement in meaningful occupations within a social context can help older people to develop new relationships, and to break out of a highly family-focused, restricted network. These are important goals, as similar aged friends make a distinctive contribution to morale (Litwin 2001). Some older people may benefit from interventions specifically designed to help them to extend their social networks. Stevens (2001) described working with older people to help them analyse their social networks, and to identify their friendship goals and strategies. This was a helpful intervention as, one year later, the participants reported being less lonely and having more friends.

For relatively isolated older people, group-based therapy or support groups can offer empowerment and assistance. Groups that share common experiences and coping strategies help to achieve collective action, and challenge helplessness and depression. Routasalo et al. (2009) reported a randomised controlled trial in which they evaluated a group support intervention for older people who reported loneliness. Whilst the intervention did not improve measures of loneliness, participants did report developing more new friendships, greater wellbeing and feeling needed. Thus a relatively modest social support intervention achieved significant outcomes, and further initiatives evaluated by occupational therapists would be helpful.

Occupational therapists need to be mindful of the older person's social network type. Each type has distinct strengths and vulnerabilities. When it functions well, the smaller, more integrated network types can offer high levels of emotional and practical assistance, but they are liable to place more strain on care-givers. The wider community-focused type can provide excellent practical help, over fairly short time-scales, but may leave an older person who is in failing health with very limited emotional support. The more intense, private networks may hide abuse in a minority of cases, and health professionals need to be vigilant about this. Family structures and attitudes towards older people in different ethnic and cultural groups also differ and result in varying levels and sources of support. It is important for occupational therapists to refrain from making assumptions and to be well-informed about such variations.

Intergenerational projects may be worthwhile for enhancing social integration. As noted previously, Granville (2001) described a project involving older people working success-fully on equal terms with children in a school setting to improve the local environment. Both groups found that the experience dismantled their prejudices and were surprised at finding so many shared concerns and goals. The collaborative project provided purpose and promoted self-worth. Occupational therapists can do much to assist older clients to gain quality of life through helping them to consider and extend their social support networks which, in turn, may help them to expand their repertoire of activities and occupations.

Occupational therapists need to work more extensively with older people in residential settings, as meaningful occupations can facilitate social contacts and friendship (which in turn facilitate more shared activities). Residents commonly value both social relation-ships and absorbing occupations, but often find that neither is facilitated. Instead, they are left to sit in large common rooms with other residents with little common purpose (Atwal et al. 2003). This practice continues even though there is evidence that increased partici-pation in leisure activities makes an important contribution to quality of life, especially among people in their 80s with few relatives (Silverstein and Parker 2002). Better consul-tation with residents to establish their needs and preferences is a first step towards assist-ing them to engage in meaningful and rewarding occupations (Squire 2001).

Sensitivity is required by all therapists offering or setting in place formal supports, as some older people may regard external help as demeaning and threatening to their famil-iar identity (Tanner 2001). Client-centred practice, in which therapists really listen to their clients' preferences in relation to therapy and social support, is vital. Furthermore, it is crucial that occupational therapists and other health and social care professionals do not impose their own value system or ageist stereotypes on others but instead focus on nego-tiating acceptable goals with each individual client. Such an imposition of an intervention on an older client is illustrated in the case of Barbara in Box 3.4.

In the case of Barbara, the health and social care professionals, together with the family, all believed that they were acting in her best interest. Yet they had in fact failed to take into account her wishes. As occupational therapists, we must ensure we do not make the error of imposing our own values, or prejudices, on our older clients. Rather, we need to work in partnership with the client and their carers to arrive at mutually acceptable solutions.

Sensitivity to the cultural and ethnic needs and preferences of older clients must also be paramount. Diversity and difference should be celebrated rather than frowned upon. Therapists need to find ways of resolving conflicts between personal and

---

Box 3.4   Why can't Barbara make herself heard?

When reading the case study, reflect on why the health professionals ignored Barbara's views. To what extent might ageist stereotypes – or other factors – have played a part?

- In what ways might the social context have enabled or disempowered Barbara?
- What ethical (and emotional) conflicts do therapists and families face when the older client rejects assistance that they regard as promoting safety and security?

Barbara, a 76-year-old woman, was admitted to hospital following a fall, which resulted in a fracture of her tibia. After a period of six weeks in hospital, Barbara was discharged home where she lived on her own. She has only two friends who live close by, both of whom are in rather poor health. Her two sons live about 30 miles away and she sees them about once a month. Social Services were requested to conduct a needs assessment and to provide her with a care package. They decided to look into adapting her bathroom which was too small to allow Barbara the required space to get in and out of her bath safely. On the assessment visit, both the occupational therapist and social worker agreed with Barbara that having a shower installed in place of her bath would allow her to manoeuvre around her bathroom more freely.

Unknown to Barbara, an additional assessment was made during the visit. This concerned the possibility of having central heating installed. Although the professional team appeared to have Barbara's best interest in mind when deciding that having central heating would be beneficial to her, they did not directly consult with her about her needs and preferences. Barbara was therefore surprised to discover on the second visit that this additional project had been planned and agreed upon. She was also upset at the prospect of vacating her home for at least three months whilst the additional work was carried out, and she did not know where she could live during that time.

Barbara objected that she had lived in the same house contentedly for over 50 years, with only a gas fire in her lounge and electric blankets. In addition to feeling anxious about the temporary living arrangements that the project required, she did not see any need for central heating, and disliked what she called 'stuffy' environments. Her views were, however, disregarded by her family, Social Services and health professionals alike. All were adamant that her quality of life and comfort would be greatly improved.

This case example, taken from recent clinical practice, highlights a professional failure to consult fully with the older client and the imposition instead of personal values and judgements. Barbara's encounter with the occupational therapist and social worker was clearly disempowering and upsetting.

---

professional viewpoints and older clients' preferences. Identifying our own ageist and culturally blinkered views and stereotypes through self-examination is the first step to dismantling them.

In conclusion, the challenge for occupational therapists working with older people is, firstly, to counter any ageist attitudes that may guide their thinking and practice. Secondly, they need to avoid infantilising or patronising older clients and engage with them instead as equal partners in every stage of the process of treatment and care. Thirdly, although the focus of occupational therapists is often on functional assessments and rehabilitation, it is crucially important that therapists are also involved in enhancing the quality of life of the older person through health promotion, meaningful occupation, providing autonomy and choice, and by assisting the client to enlarge their social support networks. Finally, therapists need to be mindful of the various strengths and vulnerabilities of the different network types that older people inhabit, and adapt their interventions accordingly.

References

Askham, J., Ferring, D. and Lamura, G. (2007) Personal relationships in later life. In: Bond, J., Peace, S., Dittmann-Kohli, F., and Westerhof, Gerben J. (eds) *Ageing in Society: European perspectives on gerontology*, 3rd edition. Thousand Oaks, CA: Sage Publications Ltd, pp. 186–208.

Atwal, A., Owen, S. and Davies, R. (2003) Struggling for occupational satisfaction: Older people in care homes. *British Journal of Occupational Therapy* **66(3)**, 118–124.

Bath, P. and Deeg, D. (2005) Social engagement and health outcomes among older people: Introduction to a special section. *European Journal of Ageing* **2(1)**, 24–30.

Berkman, L. and Syme, S. (1979) Social networks, host resistance, and mortality: A nine-year follow-up study of Alameda County residents. *American Journal of Epidemiology* **109**, 186–204.

Biggs, S., Manthorpe, J., Tinker, A., Doyle, M. and Erens, B. (2007) Mistreatment of older people in the United Kingdom: Findings from the First National Prevalence Study. *Journal of Elder Abuse & Neglect* **21(1)**, 1–14.

Blixen, C. and Kippes, C. (1999) Depression, social support, and quality of life in older adults with osteoarthritis. *The Journal of Nursing Scholarship* **31(3)**, 221–226.

Booth, M., Owen, N., Bauman, A., Clavisi, O. and Leslie, E. (2000) Social-cognitive and perceived environment influences associated with physical activity in older Australians. *Preventive Medicine* **31(1)**, 15–22.

Bradley, M. (1996) Caring for older people: Elder abuse. *British Medical Journal* **313**, 548–550.

Burnett, J., Regev, T., Pickens, S., Prati, L., Aung, K., Moore, J. and Dyer, C. (2006) Social networks: A profile of the elderly who self-neglect. *Journal of Elder Abuse and Neglect* **18(4)**, 35–49.

Carpenter, B. (2002) Family, peer and staff social support in nursing home patients: Contributions to psychological well-being. *Journal of Applied Gerontology* **21(3)**, 275–293.

Carruthers, I. and Ormondroyd, J. (2009) Achieving Age Equality in Health and Social Care: A report to the Secretary of State for Health. http://www.dh.gov.uk/dr_consum_dh/groups/dh_digitalassets/documents/digitalasset/dh_107398.pdf (Accessed 3.2.10)

Chau, R. and Yu, S. (2009) Culturally sensitive approaches to health and social care: Uniformity and diversity in the Chinese community in the UK. *International Social Work* **52(6)**, 773–784.

Chiu, S. and Yu, S. (2001) An excess of culture: The myth of shared care in the Chinese community in Britain. *Ageing & Society* **21(6)**, 681–699.

Clarke, L. and Roberts, C. (2004) The meaning of grandparenthood and its contribution to the quality of life of older people. In: Walker, A. and Hagan Hennessy. C. (eds), *Growing Older: Quality of life in old age*. Maidenhead: Open University Press, pp. 188–208.

Cohen, M., Levin, S., Gagin, R. and Friedman, G. (2007) Elder abuse: Disparities between older people's disclosure of abuse, evident signs of abuse, and high risk of abuse. *Journal of the American Geriatrics Society* **55(8)**, 1224–1230.

College of Occupational Therapists (2010) *Code of Ethics and Professional Conduct*. London: College of Occupational Therapists.

Cookman, C. (1996) Older people and attachment to things, places, pets and ideas. *Image: The Journal of Nursing Scholarship* **28(3)**, 227–231.

Crohan, S. and Antonucci, T. (1989) Friends as a source of social support in old age. In: Adams, R. and Blieszner, R. (eds) *Older Adult Friendship: Structure and process*. Newbury Park, CA: Sage Publications, pp. 129–146.

Cuddy, A., Norton, M. and Fiske, S. (2005) This old stereotype: The pervasiveness and persistence of the elderly stereotype. *Journal of Social Issues* **61(2)**, 267–285.

Davidson, K. and Arber, S. (2004) Older men: Their health behaviours and partnership status. In: Walker A. and Hagan Hennessy, C. (eds), *Growing Older: Quality of life in old age*. Maidenhead: Open University Press, pp. 127–148.

Davys, D. (2008) Ageism with occupational therapy? *British Journal of Occupational Therapy* **71(2)**, 72–74.

de Jong Gierveld, J., Broese Van Groenou, M., Hoogendoorn, A. and Smit, J. (2009) Quality of marriages in later life and emotional and social loneliness. *The Journals of Gerontology: Series B: Psychological Sciences and Social Sciences* **64B(4)**, 497–506.

Department of Health (2001) *National Service Framework for Older People*. London: HMSO.

Dickinson, A. and Hill, R. (2007) Keeping in touch: Talking to older people about computers and communication. *Educational Gerontology* **33(8)**, 613–630.

Drew, L. and Silverstein, M. (2007) Grandparents' psychological well-being after loss of contact with their grandchildren. *Journal of Family Psychology* **21(3)**, 372–379.

Drew, L. and Smith, P. (1999) The impact of parental separation/divorce on grandparent–grandchild relationships. *International Journal of Aging and Human Development* **48**, 191–215.

Duthie, J. and Donaghy, M. (2009) The beliefs and attitudes of physiotherapy students in Scotland toward older people. *Physical & Occupational Therapy in Geriatrics* **27(3)**, 245–266.

Dyer, C., Pavlik, V., Murphy, K. and Hyman, D. (2000) The high prevalence of depression and dementia in elder abuse or neglect. *Journal of the American Geriatrics Society* **48(2)**, 205–208.

Evans, P., Hucklebridge, F. and Clow, A. (2000) *Mind, Immunity and Health: The science of psychoneuroimmunology*. London: Free Association Books.

Featherstone, M. and Hepworth, M. (2009) Images of aging: Cultural representations of later life. In: Sokolovsky, J. (ed.) *The Cultural Context of Aging: Worldwide perspectives*, 3rd ed. Westport, CT: Praeger Publishers/Greenwood Publishing Group, pp. 124–144.

Field, E., Walker, M. and Orrell, M. (2002) Social networks and health of older people living in sheltered housing. *Aging & Mental Health* **6(4)**, 372–386.

Gergen, M. and Gergen, K. (2001) Positive aging: New images for a new age. *Ageing International* **27(1)**, 3–23.

Glass, T., Mendes de Leon, C., Marottoli, R. and Berkman, L. (1999) Population based study of social and productive activities as predictors of survival among elderly Americans. *BMJ* **319**, 478–483.

Golden, J., Conroy, R., Bruce, I., Denihan, A., Greene, E., Kirby, M. and Lawlor, B. (2009) Loneliness, social support networks, mood and wellbeing in community-dwelling elderly. *International Journal of Geriatric Psychiatry* **24(7)**, 694–700.

Granville, G. (2001) Intergenerational health promotion and active citizenship. In: Chiva, A. and Stears, D. (eds) *Promoting the Health of Older People*. Buckingham: Open University Press, pp. 40–50.

Greenfield, E. and Marks, N. (2007) Continuous participation in voluntary groups as a protective factor for the psychological well-being of adults who develop functional limitations: Evidence from the national survey of families and households. *The Journals of Gerontology: Series B: Psychological Sciences and Social Sciences* **62B(1)**, S60–S68.

Haines, V. and Henderson, L. (2002) Targeting social support: A network assessment of the convoy model of social support. *Canadian Journal on Aging* **21(2)**, 243–256.

Harris, A. and Thoresen, C. (2005) Volunteering is associated with delayed mortality in older people: Analysis of the Longitudinal Study of Aging. *Journal of Health Psychology* **10(6)**, 739–735.

Helman, C.G. (2000) *Culture, Difference and Healthcare*. Oxford: Butterworth Scientific.

Henley, A. and Schott, J. (1999) *Culture, Religion and Patient Care in Multi-ethnic Society*. London: Age Concern Books.

Herbert, J. and Greene, D. (2001) Effects of preference on distance walked by assisted living residents. *Physical and Occupational Therapy in Geriatrics* **19(4)**, 1–15.

House, J., Robbins, C. and Metzner, H. (1982) The associations of social relationships and activities with mortality: Prospective evidence from the Tecumseh community health study. *American Journal of Epidemiology* **116(1)**, 123–140.

House, J., Landis, K. and Umberson, D. (1988) Social relationships and health. *Science* **241**, 540–545.

Jorm, A. (2005) Social networks and health: It's time for an intervention trial. *Journal of Epidemiology and Community Health* **59(7)**, 537–538.

Kahn, R. and Antonucci, T. (1980) Convoys over the life course: Attachment, roles and social support. In: Baltes, P. and Brim, O. (eds) *Life-span Development and Behavior*, Vol **3**. New York: Academic Press, pp. 253–286.

Keating, N., Otfinowski, P., Wenger, C., Fast, J. and Derksen, L. (2003) Understanding the caring capacity of informal networks of frail seniors: A case for care networks. *Ageing and Society* **23**, 115–127.

Kincade, J., Rabiner, D., Bernard, S. and Woomert, A. (1996) Older adults as a community resource: Results from the National Survey of Self-Care and Aging. *Gerontologist* **36(4)**, 474–482.

Krause, N. (2007) Longitudinal study of social support and meaning in life. *Psychology and Aging* **22(3)**, 456–469.

Krause, N. and Markides, K. (1990) Measuring social support among older adults. *International Journal of Aging and Human Development* **30(1)**, 37–53.

Lawrence, A. and Schigelone, A. (2002) Reciprocity beyond dyadic relationships. *Research on Aging* **24(6)**, 684–704.

Levy, B. and Banaji, M. (2002) Implicit ageism. In Nelson, T. (ed.) *Ageism: Stereotypes and prejudice against older persons*. Cambridge, Mass: MIT Press, pp. 49–75.

Lim, K.H. (2001) A guide to providing culturally sensitive and appropriate occupational therapy assessments and interventions. *Mental Health Occupational Therapy Magazine* **6(2)**, 26–29.

Litwin, H. (2001) Social network type and morale in old age. *Gerontologist* **41(4)**, 516–524.

Lowenstein, A., Katz, R. and Gur-Yaishm N, (2007) Reciprocity in parent-child exchange and life satisfaction among the elderly: A cross-national perspective. *Journal of Social Issues* **63(4)**, 865–883.

Lum, T. and Lightfoot, E. (2005) The effects of volunteering on the physical and mental health of older people. *Research on Aging* **27(1)**, 31–55.

Lund, M. and Tamm, M. (2001) How a group of disabled persons experience rehabilitation over a period of time. *Scandinavian Journal of Occupational Therapy* **8(2)**, 96–104.

Lyyra, T. and Heikkinen, R. (2006) Perceived social support and mortality in older people. *The Journals of Gerontology: Series B: Psychological Sciences and Social Sciences* **61B(3)**, S147–S152.

McColgan, G. and Schofield, I. (2007) The importance of companion animal relationships in the lives of older people. *Nursing Older People* **19(1)**, 21–23.

Mellor, D., Davison, T., McCabe, M. and George, K. (2008) Professional carers' knowledge and response to depression among their aged-care clients: The care recipients' perspective. *Aging & Mental Health* **12(3)**, 389–399.

Paillard-Borg, S., Wang, H., Winblad, B. and Fratiglioni, L. (2009) Pattern of participation in leisure activities among older people in relation to their health conditions and contextual factors: A survey in a Swedish urban area. *Ageing and Society* **29(5)**, 803–821.

Parslow, R., Jorm, A., Christensen, H., Rodgers, B. and Jacomb, P. (2005) Pet ownership and health in older adults: Findings from a survey of 2,551 community-based Australians aged 60–64. *Gerontology* **51(1)**, 40–47.

Pillemer, K. and Finkelhor, D. (1989) Causes of elder abuse: Caregiver stress versus problem relatives. *American Journal of Orthopsychiatry* **59(2)**, 179–187.

Raina, P., Waltner-Toews, D., Bonnett, B., Woodward, C. and Abernathy, T. (1999) Influence of companion animals on the physical and psychological health of older people: An analysis of a one-year longitudinal study. *Journal of the American Geriatrics Society* **47(3)**, 323–329.

Reynolds, F. (2010) 'Colour and communion': Exploring the influences of visual art-making as a leisure activity on older women's subjective well-being. *Journal of Aging Studies* **24(2)**, 135–143.

Routasalo, P., Tilvis, R., Kautiainen, H. and Pitkala, K. (2009) Effects of psychosocial group rehabilitation on social functioning, loneliness and well-being of lonely, older people: Randomized controlled trial. *Journal of Advanced Nursing* **65(2)**, 297–305.

Russell, C., Campbell, A. and Hughes, I. (2008) Ageing, social capital and the internet: Findings from an exploratory study of Australian 'silver surfers'. *Australasian Journal on Ageing* **27(2)**, 78–82.

Scharf, T. and de Jong Gierveld, J. (2008) Loneliness in urban neighbourhoods: An Anglo-Dutch comparison. *European Journal of Ageing* **5(2)**, 103–115.

Seeman, T.A., Kaplan, G.A., Knudsen, L., Cohen, R. and Guralink, J. (1987) Social network ties and mortality among the elderly in the Alameda County Study. *American Journal of Epidemiology* **126(4)**, 714–723.

Sener, A., Oztop, H. and Dogan, N. (2008) Family, close relatives, friends: Life satisfaction among older people. *Educational Gerontology* **34(10)**, 890–906.

Shugarman, L., Fries, B., Wolf, R. and Morris, J. (2003) Identifying older people at risk of abuse during routine screening practices. *Journal of the American Geriatrics Society* **51(1)**, 24–31.

Silverstein, M. and Parker, M. (2002) Leisure activities and quality of life among the oldest old in Sweden. *Research on Aging* **24(5)**, 528–547.

Squire, A. (2001) Health-promoting residential settings. In: Chiva, A. and Stears, D. (eds) *Promoting the Health of Older People*. Buckingham: Open University Press, pp. 120–131.

Stevens, N. (2001) Combating loneliness: A friendship enrichment programme for older women. *Ageing and Society*, **21(2)**, 183–202.

Stewart, M., Meredith, L., Brown, J. and Galajda, J. (2000) The influence of older patient-physician communication on health and health-related outcomes. *Clinics in Geriatric Medicine* **16(1)**, 25–36.

Tanner, D. (2001) Sustaining the self in later life: Supporting older people in the community. *Ageing and Society* **21(3)**, 255–278.

Thiele, D. and Whelan, T. (2008) The relationship between grandparent satisfaction, meaning, and generativity. *The International Journal of Aging & Human Development* **66(1)**, 21–48.

Tomassini, C., Glaser, K. and Stuchbury, R. (2007) Family disruption and support in later life: A comparative study between the United Kingdom and Italy. *Journal of Social Issues* **63(4)**, 845–863.

Vaillant, G., Meyer, S., Mukamai, K. and Soldz, S. (1998) Are social supports in late mid-life a cause or result of successful ageing? *Psychological Medicine* **28(5)**, 1159–1168.

Victor, C. and Scharf, T. (2005) Social isolation and loneliness: In: Walker, A. (ed.) *Understanding Quality of Life in Old Age*. Buckingham: Open University Press, pp.100–116.

Victor, C., Scambler, S., Shah, S., Cook, D., Harris, T., Rink, E. and de Wilde, S. (2002) Has loneliness amongst older people increased? An investigation into variations between cohorts. *Ageing and Society* **22(5)**, 585–597.

Victor, C., Grenade, L. and Boldy, D. (2005) Measuring loneliness in later life: A comparison of differing measures. *Reviews in Clinical Gerontology* **15(1)**, 63–70.

Warburton, J., Terry, D., Rosenman, L. and Shapiro, M. (2001) Differences between older volunteers and nonvolunteers: Attitudinal, normative and control beliefs. *Research on Aging* **23(5)**, 586–605.

Wenger, G.C. (1994) *Support Networks of Older People: A guide for practitioners*. Bangor. Centre for Social Policy Research and Development, University of Wales.

Wenger, G.C. (1995) A comparison of urban with rural support networks: Liverpool and North Wales. *Ageing and Society* **15(1)**, 59–82.

Wenger, G.C. and Jerome, D. (1999) Change and stability in confidante relationships: Findings from the Bangor Longitudinal Study of Ageing. *Journal of Aging Studies* **13(3)**, 269–294.

Wheeler, J., Gorey, K. and Greenblatt, B. (1998) The beneficial effects of volunteering for older volunteers and the people they serve: A meta-analysis. *International Journal of Aging and Human Development* **47(1)**, 69–79.

Williams, A. and Giles, H. (1998) Communication of ageism. In: Hecht, M. (ed.) *Communicating Prejudice*. Thousand Oaks, CA: Sage Publishing, pp. 136–160.

Wright, P. (1989) Gender differences in adults' same and cross-gender friendships. In: Adams, R. and Blieszner, R. (eds) *Older Adult Friendship: Structure and process*. Newbury Park, CA: Sage Publishing, pp. 197–221.

Yates, B. (1995) The relation among social support and short- and long-term recovery outcomes in men with coronary heart disease. *Research in Nursing and Health* **18(3)**, 193–203.

Young, R.F. and Glasgow, N. (1998) Voluntary social participation and health. *Research on Aging* **20(3)**, 339–362.

Zhang, Y., Harwood, J., Williams, A., Ylanne-McEwen, V., Wadleigh, P. and Thimm, C. (2006) The portrayal of older adults in advertising: A cross-national review. *Journal of Language and Social Psychology* **25(3)**, 264–282.

Chapter 4

Policy development and implications for occupational therapy practice

Margaret Gallagher

This chapter explores the contemporary context of policy development and service delivery for older people through global and national policy. It examines how this affects the development of services for older people and occupational therapy practice, in a time of major financial and population challenges, through the consideration of current trends in policy development with an emphasis on interprofessional working and developments in England. The College of Occupational Therapists (COT) has highlighted the need for occupational therapists to change the way in which they operate so that the profession remains valued and relevant to the society (COT 2009). We want, and believe, that occupational therapists take a more active role within health and social care policy making and decision making. In order to do this, we need to be able to promote the core values of occupational therapy to politicians, commissioners, members of the multidisciplinary team and the general public. Only then can we make a real difference.

The global view

In the developed world, life expectancy has significantly increased but there are countries where there have not been similar improvements in life expectancy. This has been discussed in Chapter 2 within the compression of morbidity theory.

These inequalities in life expectancy can be considered in terms of the political and economic context, and the approach adopted by the country to health care provision, both in health promotion and condition management. The quality of life for individuals is another matter and this also depends on a variety of factors, many of them culturally driven and is defined by the World Health Organization (WHO) as the:

> "individuals' perceptions of their position in life in the context of the culture and value systems in which they live and in relation to their goals, expectations, standards and concerns." (WHO 1996, p. 5)

The progress that has been made through economic development, clean water, improved environments and healthcare systems means that, by 2050, the world's population aged 60 and over will more than triple and will present challenges for all health and social care

Occupational Therapy and Older People, Second Edition. Edited by Anita Atwal and Anne McIntyre.
© 2013 Blackwell Publishing Ltd. Published 2013 by Blackwell Publishing Ltd.

systems. What are the public health implications of global ageing? The key components of a well-functioning health system include equitable provision through people-centred care, including the opportunity to participate in decisions affecting their health and the health system, and the Perth framework for age-friendly, community-based primary healthcare (WHO 2010(a)). This framework recognised that there are particular concerns in delivering primary healthcare for older people.

In the European Union, The Healthy Life Years (European Union 2005) examines both longevity and the quality of life experienced by older people. This could broadly be expressed in the quality versus quantity debate. Life expectancy in the UK (European Union 2005), at age 65 was 19.5 years for women and 17.0 years for men. The concept of positive healthy life years is important in the public policy of supporting healthy lifestyles and planning for the management of declining capacity and participation in old age. Healthy life years (HLY) also includes acknowledgement of life with moderate and severe activity limitations. Differences between the genders are evident, with women living longer but with a longer period of ill health. Many of the health issues that are faced in the industrialised and post-industrial societies are connected to affluence, such as heart disease and obesity. Poverty is also an important factor as 18% of people over state pension age are judged to live below the government poverty line (Age UK 2010) and this has a significant effect on an individual's quality of life. A further discussion about retirement occurs in Chapter 2.

Health promotion is an integral aspect of health and social care policy (Department of Health (DH) 2011). Much of what determines successful or active ageing fits perfectly within the occupational therapy philosophy of Occupation. However, the role of occupational therapy within health promotion still needs to be further developed. In the UK, this role has been directly influenced by Wilcock (1998, 2002) who sets out strong arguments for the role of occupational therapists as health promoters in the public health arena. Her main proposition is that occupational therapy must extend beyond the amelioration of illness and become directly involved with the promotion of optimal states of health in line with health-promoting philosophies. Occupational therapists can be involved in primary, secondary or tertiary health promotion (Box 4.1). Guidance is available so that occupational therapists can enhance the quality of health promotion projects (see Lis et al. 2008).

It is evident that occupational therapists are already involved in different types of health promotion with older people. However, a recent study by Flannery and Barry (2003) concluded that the greatest perceived barrier to occupational therapists making a praxis shift to becoming health promoters was limited resources, including time, staffing levels and funds. The study by Clark et al. (1997) 'Occupational therapy for independent-living older people' demonstrated the benefit of occupational therapy in preventative intervention treatment groups and is discussed in Chapter 2. This seminal study provided evidence of the efficacy of occupational therapy and informed the National Institute for Health and Clinical Excellence (2008) guidelines 'Mental well being and older people', where the benefits of occupational therapy intervention are identified. This study demonstrated benefits and savings through: reduced risk of depression and anxiety, enhanced mood and self-esteem, improvement of physical and general health, mobility and independence, improved wellbeing and quality of life. Occupational therapy can

---

Box 4.1   Health promotion: Primary, secondary or tertiary

Primary health promotion (upstream activity) – targeting the well population and aiming at preventing ill health and disability. For occupational therapists this means working with well older people. (See Clark et al. 1997 in Chapter 2.)

Secondary health promotion (midstream activity) – directed at individuals or groups to change health-damaging habits and/or to prevent ill health moving to a chronic or irreversible stage, For example, teaching accident prevention techniques in falls prevention programmes. In addition, where possible, to restore people to their former state of health

Tertiary health promotion (downstream) – takes place with individuals who have chronic conditions and/or are disabled, to make the most of their potential. With older people, occupational therapists are already actively involved in health promotion through adaptation, compensation and equipment provision.

---

deliver evidence of efficacy, not just via the gold standard of randomised control trials but also through qualitative practice-based approaches (Reagon et al. 2010). The use of the Model of Human Occupation in the promotion of wellness for older people has produced beneficial results (Yamada et al. 2010).

There is an important recognition of the ageing population in Europe with projections that, by 2050, the number of people in the EU aged 65+ will grow by 70% and that the 80+ age group will grow by 170% (European Union 2007). The European Commission's (2009) initiative on Alzheimer's disease and other dementias estimated that, in 2006, 7.3 million Europeans between 30 and 99 years of age had a dementia. This report found almost twice as many women as men were living with the diagnosis. The proposed actions include: early diagnosis and the promotion of well being; sharing and coordination of knowledge and research of dementias across Europe in the promotion of best practice; and respecting the rights of people with dementia.

When planning for the future, governments have to consider a variety of options and WHO (2002b) developed a Long-Term Care Tool Kit for policy makers. This identifies four scenarios – steady progress, crisis and turmoil, civic connections and global transformation – through which a country's needs with regard to long-term care (which includes older people) can be assessed. The questions posed by the approach aim to shape policy and service delivery:

- What will families be expected to do, and for whom?
- Which members of the family are expected to shoulder these obligations, and why does the task fall to them?
- What supports can be provided to make the tasks easier?
- What limits should be set on the burdens imposed on the family?
- What is the responsibility of the community (and who in the community is expected to shoulder these responsibilities)?
- What is the responsibility of the State?

These questions are central to the current debate regarding the funding of long-term care for older people in the UK. The key issue is about who pays for the care needs of older people: the individual and the family, a mixed economy of the individual/family and

---

Box 4.2   Isobel: 'Older Age as a Shock'

My thoughts focus on my friend Isobel, a retired headmistress, who is currently managing the journey into old age with grace but has not made a friend of the process. She has described becoming older as 'a shock when it comes, as you never think becoming old will apply to you.'

- How do you prepare individuals for something that they don't think will apply to them?
- How can we understand a process we have not yet experienced?
- What do you, as a student or a novice practitioner, need to know about the policy context of services for older people?
- Can you answer this using any evidence from the literature?

---

the State, or the State? There has been consistent prevarication by UK governments as to how this could or should be funded.

International context

The World Health Organization, which operates within the United Nations, provides international leadership and is responsible for the direction and coordination of health policy and for shaping research. These initiatives have had a significant impact on the development of policies for older people. The four key concepts of Active Aging were articulated through 'Active Aging, A Policy Framework' (WHO 2002(a)) as are autonomy, independence, quality of life and healthy life expectancy (discussed in Chapter 2). While life expectancy at birth remains an important measure of population ageing, how long people can expect to live without disabilities is especially important to an ageing population.

Autonomy is a key aspect within the concept of Active Ageing and occupational therapists need to ensure that users are better informed and more empowered to make decisions by allowing persons to become key decision-makers in the treatment process (Department of Health 2010(a, b), 2012). Allowing service users to make their own assessment will allow service users to manage and take control of their life. (See Chapter 5 for a discussion of standardised assessment and outcome measures.) The Universal Declaration of Human Rights (1948) stated the right to 'medical care and necessary social services, and the right to security in the event of unemployment, sickness, disability, widowhood, old age' (article 25). It is important to note that this seminal document specifically cites old age and disability as requiring protection. This was also the year that the National Health Service (NHS) was founded in the UK. Both these developments should be seen in the context of the desire to create a better world following World War ll. The UK Government committed to the European Convention on Human Rights in 1951 and these rights were subsequently enshrined in the Human Rights Act (1998). This provides individuals with the opportunity to challenge health and social care legislation and service providers, for example, through the respect for private and family life and the right to life. The UN Madrid International Plan of Action on Ageing (United Nations 2002) 'Provision of health care, support and social protection for older persons, including preventive and rehabilitative health care'

(Objective 12 (h)), continues to maintain the focus on integrating the aspirations and needs of older people into mainstream international agendas.

Social policy in the United Kingdom

The themes from the international research and guidance reflected within our contemporary discourse are about human rights, individualism, consumerism, the impact this has on the cost of health and social care policies and how these services are delivered. The UK now has a devolved structure, so arrangements in England, Scotland, Wales and Northern Ireland differ in how services are funded and delivered, especially with regard to the payments for continuing care for older people. There has been a different settlement in Scotland after devolution as older people are eligible for free personal care. Currently, there is no agreed way forward in England. However, the key Act that will change health and social care is the Health and Social Care Act (2012), which aims to cut administration in the health service by a third. In addition, whilst care remains free (one of the founding principles of the NHS in 1948), the Health and Social Care Act (2012) allows General Practioners (GPs) to commission services on behalf of their patients, which could be from the private, public or voluntary sectors. GPs, however, might not wish to commission occupational therapy if there is no evidence to support its effectiveness. Therefore occupational therapists will have to require development entrepreneurship within the core skills of occupational therapy (Holmes and Scaffa 2009). Both the British Medical Association and the Royal College of Nurses opposed the Bill. The College of Occupational Therapists also sought to influence the policy agenda during the 2010 general election in the UK (COT 2010). Two key requests for older people were:

* Enabling older people to live independently: Government must provide sufficient resources for rehabilitation, re-enablement, adaptations and equipment.
* Supporting people with dementia: Government must use occupational therapists' expertise to address physical needs and behavioural challenges to optimise quality of life.

The National Quality Board (Department of Health 2010(c)) recognises that the move to GP commissioning could be problematic and suggests ways of managing this through targets. Social enterprise, which could include the voluntary and independent sectors, is highlighted as a way of delivering services. These plans open the way for multiplicity of providers in health and social care, which could also lead to further fragmentation of services and potential difficulties in maintaining appropriate standards of service. This presents significant challenges for occupational therapists in maintaining a professional identity and leadership with the current focus on delayering of management. Additionally, occupational therapists provide services across a variety of organisations where integration between the agencies is often an issue. A priority for the profession is to provide evidence of efficacy for occupational therapy interventions as this supports the commissioning of services.

In England, health services for older people are primarily provided through the general taxation and community charges. This differs significantly from the health insurance model where the individual purchases insurance to pay for their health or social care needs, or where insurance is linked to employment. Since the founding of the NHS and subsequent developments in social care, the majority of occupational therapists have worked within the state sector. This has been driven by legislation such as the Chronically Sick and Disabled Persons Act (UK Parliament 1970) which required local authorities to provide services to maintain disabled people within their communities. The employment of occupational therapists by local authorities enshrined the organisation split that existed between health and social care, which all subsequent reforms have tried to address through integrating services across agency boundaries. Recognising that there was a need to improve the services for older people, the government developed "The National Service Framework [NSF] for Older People" (Department of Health 2001) which established eight standards that the NHS was required to meet and these were:

- Routing out age discrimination
- Person-centred care
- Intermediate care
- General hospital care
- Stroke
- Falls
- Mental health in older people
- Promotion of active health in older age.

The first seven of these are discussed below. A policy document that needs to be considered alongside the NSF for Older People is the document 'The vision for a modern system of social care'. This is built on the principles of Personalisation, Partnership, Plurality, Protection, Productivity, and People (Department of Health 2010(a)).

Rooting out age discrimination and Protection

The NSF for older adults aims to ensure that older people are never unfairly discriminated against in accessing NHS or social care services as a result of their age. The next steps in implementing the National Service Framework for Older People (Department of Health 2006) launched Dignity in Care across all aspects of care, as one of the themes to improve standards of care for older people experienced across all aspects of care. A study by Harries et al. (2007) indicates that the issue of age discrimination has to be addressed, including the intrinsic attitudes of health care professionals, as this study demonstrates that patients aged over 65 years receive different management from younger patients, with less options for assessment and treatment. As occupational therapists, we need to consider if these societal attitudes and prejudices are reflected in our own practice and what this means in order to practise in a non-ageist way. Indeed, the document 'A vision for adult social care: Capable communities and active citizens' (Department of Health 2010(b)) has emphasised the need for healthcare professionals to ensure patents are protected. This refers not only to dignity of care and equality issues but also relates to safety, risk assessment and best practice.

Person-centred care and Personalisation

Person-centred care aims to ensure that older people are treated as individuals and that they receive appropriate and timely packages of care which meet their needs as individuals, regardless of health and social services boundaries. This aligns with a fundamental concept of client-centred practice. The key components of client-centred practice are the effective partnership between the occupational therapists and service users and where the users' own goals are central to the intervention (Sumsion 1999). The concept of Personalisation, whilst similar to person-centred care, emphasises the need for service users to be better informed and more empowered about decisions and that they need to be key decision makers in the treatment process. Thus, occupational therapists need to ensure that service users have access to information that is evidence-based and given choices (plurality) over care and/or interventions. Moreover, it is essential that the occupational therapy process is led by service users and that occupational therapy services are managed and delivered with 'skill, compassion and imagination' (people). Thus the need for occupational therapists to be actively involved within research and evaluation of service delivery.

Intermediate care and Partnerships

The NSF for older adults aims to provide integrated services to promote faster recovery from illness, prevent unnecessary acute hospital admissions, support timely discharge and maximise independent living. Services have been established throughout the UK that target the rapid discharge of patients from acute settings, and the role of the occupational therapist is very important in these services. Critically, these services provide the link between the hospital and the community services, with pooled budgets and integrated management. The pressures on the occupational therapist to provide a limited package of care can militate against the client-centred approach. However, older adults must be given a choice about the type of service they want to meet their needs. Indeed, the document 'A vision for adult social care' (Department of Health 2010(b)) has highlighted the need for occupational therapists to promote partnerships between the voluntary sector, academia and the local authority.

General hospital care and Productivity

The NSF for older adults aims to ensure that older people receive the specialist help they need in hospital and that they receive the maximum benefit from having been in hospital. Research by Hammond et al. (2009) concluded that there were unnecessary admissions to hospital, with prolonged stays, and recommended that the balance and structure of services in the sub-acute and community should be reviewed. This would appear to indicate the need for further restructuring of services. The planning and coordination of discharge from hospital remains a problem, with a continual stream of policy and practice guides from the Department of Health aiming to improve services (Department of Health 2010(d)). Historically, occupational therapists based within the acute hospital setting provided services through a medical model of practice. The shift to delivering integrated health and social care has required occupational therapists to work on an interagency basis incorporating a community-focused, social model of practice (COT 2002). However, the efficacy of pre-discharge home visits as part of the discharge planning process, with which occupational therapists are centrally involved, is in question

(Atwal et al. 2008). The information that occupational therapists provide is also not necessarily to an appropriate standard (Atwal et al. 2011). The importance of providing client-centred practice is also challenged by the complex interdisciplinary process of discharge planning (Crennan and MacRae 2010).

Productivity is one component of the document 'The vision for a modern system of social care'. Thus for occupational therapists it is about ensuring that occupational therapy services are both efficient and effective. This is particularly relevant since the NHS will need to make £20 billion of efficiency savings by 2014–2015, whilst still improving quality of care. This work scheme is known as QIPP (Quality, Innovation, Productivity and Prevention; Department of Health 2012).

Key conditions that were viewed as needing to be improved were outlined in the NSF for older adults (Department of Health 2001). Stroke, falls and mental health conditions are discussed further in Chapter 5.

Stroke: The aim is to reduce the incidence of stroke in the population and ensure that those who have had a stroke have prompt access to integrated stroke care services. Research by Rudd et al. (2007) indicated that access to stroke care for older patients was less likely to be given in line with the NSF standard, which could also highlight elements of covert discrimination. How healthcare outcomes are measured for older people is a vexed question; Mangin et al. (2007) questions the use of a single disease model for older people as used in the NSF, and suggests a more nuanced approach which recognises the complexity of the multiple pathologies that exist in the aging process. There is a significant amount of high-quality research that has established the value of occupational therapy intervention for people with stroke (Walker et al. 1999, 2004, Logan et al. 2004, Legg et al. 2006).

Falls: The aim is to reduce the number of falls which result in serious injury and ensure effective treatment and rehabilitation for those who have fallen. The falls standard has been of particular interest to occupational therapists as this links with the health promotion and preventative treatment approaches that are integral to practice. This legislation established fall prevention and intermediate care services which integrated health and social care, providing evidence of significant benefits in preventing falls for the participants in the research group (Spice et al. 2009). The importance of effective interprofessional teamwork also improved the care that the patients received (Waldron et al. 2011). There is emerging evidence of the value of occupational therapy in reducing the risk of falls, but further research is needed.

Mental health in older people: The aim is to promote good mental health in older people and to treat and support those older people with dementia and depression. Recent legislation connects with the human rights and client-centred societal conversation and has had a significant effect on how services are designed and delivered. This is evident through the expert patient programme and the service user inclusion in service design and delivery as required by the Health and Social Care Act (Department of Health 2001). The Mental Capacity Act (UK Parliament 2005) links the needs of clients with mental health problems and the context of human rights legislation. This Act attempts to clarify the complex concerns about capacity and mental health. The client should be included in decisions where possible and any decisions made on their behalf should be made in their best interests. All staff should have an awareness of their responsibilities under the Act. As occupational therapists, we need to consider how we balance best practice in relation to being client centred, enabling the empowerment of the client and what this means in relation to potential risks for the client and the practitioner. Practising as a member of a team should support the development of practice and enable the practitioner to make difficult judgements in a supported context. The effective use of reflective practice both as an individual and as a team is an opportunity for professional progression. We have added dementia since the dementia strategy (Department of Health 2009) describes the priorities for one of the most important issues for the aging population.

These priority objectives are:

- good-quality early diagnosis and intervention for all
- improved quality of care in general hospitals
- living well with dementia in care homes
- reduce use of antipsychotic medication.

In relation to the evidence base for this client the American Association of Occupational Therapists have published practice guidelines for adults with Alzheimer's disease and related disorders (Schaber 2010).

Collaborative practice

The process of continuing to learn together collaboratively in order to maintain health-care improvement for patients has been driven by government policy (Box 4.3). One of the central aspects of delivering effective care for older people is the multiplicity of agencies involved, which can be confusing for service users. This includes the statutory, voluntary and independent sectors working interprofessionally and across agencies. There are many subtle and some overt barriers to effective collaborative and interagency working, not the least being organisational and funding barriers.

This guidance places the service user and carers as participants at the centre of the process. The guidance highlights the learning that takes place within the team in order to achieve best practice and stresses the importance of skilled and effective leadership to allow collaborative working to occur. The focus on collaboration within teams is explored by Øveretveit (2002) through quality improvement approaches This study found that not

---

Box 4.3 A definition of collaborative practice

'Collaborative practice in health-care occurs when multiple health workers from different professional backgrounds provide comprehensive services by working with patients, their families, carers and communities to deliver the highest quality of care across settings.

Practice includes both clinical and non-clinical health-related work, such as diagnosis, treatment, surveillance, health communications, management and sanitation engineering' (WHO 2010(b)).

all teams were successful but that careful preparation and organisation by the leaders and supportive management are essential for success of collaborations. Atwal and Caldwell (2006) states that there are three barriers to effective teamwork, including: differing perceptions of teamwork; different levels of acquired skills to function as a team member; and the dominance of medical power that influences interactions in teams. A study by Baxter and Markle-Reid (2009) explored an interprofessional team's approach to fall prevention with home care providers. In this study, working interprofessionally was perceived to be positive by the care providers, with benefits for the professional, the patient and the family, but support from managers was considered essential for the success.

Attitudes within professions and towards others are very important in the process of understanding how teams work in health settings. Leipzig et al. (2002) compared attitudes of medical postgraduate residents, advanced nurses and social workers toward working in interdisciplinary healthcare teams with older people. This study identifies a crucial issue in team working, which is who should have the ultimate responsibilities for decisions taken. The doctors believed they had primary responsibility, which may reflect a practical reality but would appear to devalue the contribution of other members of the team. Research by Salhani and Coulter (2009) used a political analysis of interprofessional working and identified the struggle for professional autonomy by nurses in relation to medics. The various strategies used by the nurses and medics to assert power and authority are the antithesis of effective team working. A study of good practice in collaborative working highlights the collaborative commitment of the individuals in the team to work together (Nicholson et al. 2000).

Conclusion

This rich tapestry of global and national policy and research for older people could be viewed as a steady progression of provision. Acknowledging the historical context of UK provision within a culturally and ethnically diverse contemporary population, where significant inequalities exist, particularly in old age, presents challenges for policy makers and service providers. The themes in these policies include patient-centred care, health promotion, cultural competence, healthy life years, and personalisation of budgets. Services and interventions are expected to be based on evidence and delivered through quality-assured integrated provision.

How do these policies affect Isobel (Box 4.2)? She expects that, when she needs medical help, it is prompt, appropriate and respectful. However, her experience of the health service has often been confusing and negative. Effective collaborative and interagency working is a basic requirement of delivering care but there remain significant problems in achieving this, one of the most important being good leadership.

In these times of global economic insecurity the options and choices of democratic nations such as the UK for the management of health and social care for older people may be stark. We are at a point of transition in policy where the funding source for the NHS remains direct taxation, with the providers of services opened to consortia of GPs which offer the private sector the opportunity to undertake contracts. The Government is proving radical in their response to the financial crisis and is using this as an opportunity to realign and reduce the state sector. The private sector has recently been contracted to manage Hinchingbrook NHS Trust and this could be a harbinger of further independent sector developments. Social enterprise, which could include service users and the voluntary sector, will further increase the range of service providers. These initiatives will change the NHS and social care landscape.

Currently, there is no consensus about the funding for long-term social care and this is one of the most important debates the nation faces. What will be the vulnerability of older people in the global financial crisis as governments and families perhaps choose to reduce investment in services that promote inclusion and participation of older people in their communities? Indeed, the current economic climate presents particular challenges for social care with regard to maintaining services for older people. It is interesting to acknowledge the prescience of the World Health Organization, which promotes intergenerational interdependence as opposed to intergenerational conflict. Polemics that describe the post-war generation as having mortgaged the future through self indulgence are not helpful (Willetts 2010). The notion that older people are a burden on the younger generation will not assist in the development of policies that address the significant inequalities that persist in the UK, particularly as people age. The Kings Fund's (2010) recommendations for a new settlement for older people require radical reform and are urgent both in relation to the demographic changes but also to improve the quality of services provided. The contribution that occupational therapists make to the development of services, including the best practice guidance such as re-enablement, can have a profound influence on the shape of client-centred services for the future. As health professionals, we need to take responsibility as occupational activists, delivering the evidence for practice, shaping policy and practice developments and cherishing good practice for all the Isobels who we may encounter in practice.

References

Age UK (2010) Agenda for Later Life. Age UK London,. Available at: http://policy.helptheaged. org.uk/NR/rdonlyres/CA9B5B5F-3BD7-40EE-99AF-CE2531B6D413/0/AgendaforLater LifeMarch2010.pdf

Atwal, A. and Caldwell, K. (2006) Nurses' perceptions of multidisciplinary team work in acute health-care. *International Journal of Nursing Practice* **12(6)**, 359–365.

Atwal, A., McIntyre, A., Craik, C. and Hunt, J. (2008) Occupational therapists' perceptions of predischarge home assessments with older adults in acute care. *The British Journal of Occupational Therapy* **71(2)**, 52–58.

Atwal, A., Luke, A. and Plastow, N. (2011) Evaluation of occupational therapy pre-discharge home visit information leaflets for older adults *The British Journal of Occupational Therapy* **74(8)**, 383–386.

Baxter, P. and Markle-Reid, M. (2009) An interprofessional team approach to fall prevention for older home care clients 'at risk' of falling: Health care providers share their experiences. *International Journal of Integrated Care*, Apr–Jun, **9**, e15.

Clark, F., Azen, S., Zemke, R., Jackson, J., Carlson, M., Mandel, D., Hay, J., Josephson, K., Cherry, B., Hessel, C., Palmer, J. and Lipson, L. (1997) Occupational therapy for independent-living older people. *The Journal of the American Medical Association* **278(16)**, 1321–1326.

College of Occupational Therapists (2002) From Interface to Integration: a strategy for modernising occupational therapy services in local health and social care communities. College of Occupational Therapists. London.

College of Occupational Therapists (2009) Curriculum guidance for pre-registration education. College of Occupational Therapists. London.

College of Occupational Therapists (2010) A Manifesto. College of Occupational Therapists. London Available at: http://www.cot.co.uk/MainWebSite/Resources/Document/COT%20 Manifesto%202010.pdf

Crennan, M. and MacRae, A. (2010) Occupational therapy discharge assessment of elderly patients from acute care hospitals. *Physical and Occupational Therapy in Geriatrics* **28(1)**, 33–43.

Department of Health (2001) The National Service Framework for Older People. London: HMSO. Available at: http://www.dh.gov.uk/en/Publicationsandstatistics/Lettersandcirculars/ Healthservicecirculars/DH_4004832

Department of Health (2006) The next steps in implementing the National Service Framework for Older People. London: HMSO. Available at: http://www.dh.gov.uk/prod_consum_dh/groups/ dh_digitalassets/@dh/@en/documents/digitalasset/dh_4133947.pdf

Department of Health (2009) Living well with dementia: a National Dementia Strategy. London: HMSO Available at: http://www.dh.gov.uk/en/Publicationsandstatistics/Publications/Publications PolicyAndGuidance/DH_094058

Department of Health (2010a) *Equity and Excellence: Liberating the NHS*. London: HMSO.

Department of Health (2010b) *A Vision for Adult Social Care: Capable communities and active citizens*. London: HMSO.

Department of Health (2010c) Quality Improvement, Productivity, Prevention. London: HMSO. Available at: http://www.dh.gov.uk/en/Healthcare/Qualityandproductivity/QIPPworkstreams/ DH_115448

Department of Health (2010d) Ready to go? Planning the discharge and the transfer of patients from hospital and intermediate care. London: HMSO. Available at: http://www.dh.gov.uk/en/ Publicationsandstatistics/Publications/PublicationsPolicyAndGuidance/DH_113950

Department of Health (2011) Healthy lives, healthy people White Paper: Update and way forward. London: HMSO. Available at: http://www.dh.gov.uk/en/Publichealth/Healthyliveshealthypeople/ index.htm

Department of Health (2012) QIPP (Quality, Innovation, Productivity and Prevention). London: HMSO. Available at: http://www.dh.gov.uk/health/category/policy-areas/nhs/qipp/

European Union (2005) The Healthy Life Years. Available at: http://ec.europa.eu/health/ph_ information/reporting/docs/hly_en.pdf

European Union (2007) Together for Health: A Strategic Approach for the EU 2008–2013. Available at: http://ec.europa.eu/health/ph_overview/Documents/strategy_wp_en.pdf

European Commission (2009) Initiative on Alzheimer's disease and other dementias. Available at: http://ec.europa.eu/health/archive/ph_information/dissemination/documents/com2009_380_ en.pdf Accessed 15.12.10

Flannery, G. and Barry, M. (2003) An exploration of occupational therapists' perceptions of health promotion. *The Irish Journal of Occupational Therapy*, Winter, 33–41.

Hammond, C., Pinnington, L. and Phillips, M. (2009) A qualitative examination of inappropriate hospital admissions and lengths of stay. BMC. Health Service Research **9**:44.

Harries, C., Forrest, D., Harvey, N., McClelland, A. and Bowling, A. (2007) Which doctors are influenced by a patient's age? A multi-method study of angina treatment in general practice, cardiology and gerontology. *Quality and Safety in Health Care* **16(1)**, 23–27.

Health and Social Care Act (2012). Available at: http://www.legislation.gov.uk/ukpga/2012/7/ contents

Holmes, W.M. and Scaffa, M.E. (2009) An exploratory study of competencies for emerging practice in occupational therapy. *Journal of Allied Health* **38(2)**, 81–90.

Human Rights Act (1998) Available at: http://www.legislation.gov.uk/ukpga/1998/42/contents

Kings Fund (2010) Securing good care for more people. Available at: http://www.kingsfund.org.uk/publications/securing_good_care.html

Leipzig, R., Hyer, K., Ek, K., Wallenstein, S., Vezina, M., Fairchild, S., Cassel, C. and Howe, J. (2002) Attitudes toward working on interdisciplinary healthcare teams: A vomparison by fiscipline. *Journal of the American Geriatrics Society* **50(6)**, 1141–1148.

Legg, L., Drummond, A. and Langhorne, P. (2006) Occupational therapy for patients with problems in activities of daily living after stroke. Cochrane Database of Systematic Reviews 2006, Issue 4. Art. No.: CD003585, doi: 10.1002/14651858.CD003585.pub2

Lis, K., Reichert, M., Cosack, A., Billings, J. and Brown, P. (eds) (2008) *Evidence-based Guidelines on Health Promotion for Older People*. Vienna: Austrian Red Cross.

Logan, P.A., Gladman, J.R.F, Avery, A.J., Walker, M.F., Dyas, J. and Groom, L. (2004) Randomised controlled trial of an *occupational therapy intervention to increase outdoor mobility after stroke*. *BMJ* **329(7479)**, 1372–1375.

Mangin, D., Sweeney, K. and Heath, I. (2007) Preventive health care in elderly people needs rethinking. *BMJ* **335(7614)**, 285–287.

National Institute for Health and Clinical Excellence (NICE) (2008) NICE Public Health Guidance 16: Occupational therapy interventions and physical activity interventions to promote the mental wellbeing of older people in primary care and residential care. London: NICE.

Nicholson, D., Artz, S. and Armitage, A. (2000) Working relationships and outcomes in multidisciplinary collaborative practice settings. *Child and Youth Care Forum* **29(1)**, 39–73.

Øvretveit, J. (2002) *Action Evaluation of Health Programmes and Change*. Oxford: Radcliffe Medical Press.

Reagon, C., Bellin, W. and Boniface, G. (2010) Challenging the dominant voice: The multiple evidence sources of occupational therapy. *British Journal of Occupational Therapy* **73(6)**, 284–286.

Rudd, A,. Hoffman, A., Down, C., Pearson, M. and Lowe, D. (2007) Access to stroke care in England, Wales and Northern Ireland: The effect of age, gender and weekend admission. Available at: http://ageing.oxfordjournals.org/content/36/3/247.full.pdf+html

Salhani, D. and Coulter, I. (2009) The politics of interprofessional working and the struggle for professional autonomy in nursing. *Social Science and Medicine* **68(7)**, 1221–1228.

Schaber, P. (2010) *Occupational Therapy Practice Guidelines for Adults with Alzheimer's Disease and Related Disorders*. Bethesda, MD: AOTA Press.

Spice, C., Morotti, W., George, S., Dent, T., Rose, J., Harris, S., Christopher, J. and Gordon, C. (2009) The Winchester falls project: A randomized controlled trial of secondary prevention of falls in older people. *Age Ageing.* **38(1)**, 33–40.

Sumsion, T. (1999) *Client Centred Practice in Occupational Therapy: A guide to implementation*. London: Churchill Livingstone.

The Universal Declaration of Human Rights: 1948–2008 (2012) United Nations. Available at: http://www.un.org/events/humanrights/udhr60/

UK Parliament (1970) Chronically Sick and Disabled Persons Act 1970. Available at: http://www.legislation.gov.uk/ukpga/1970/44

UK Parliament (2005) The Mental Capacity Act (2005) Available at: http://www.legislation.gov.uk/ukpga/2005/9/contents

UK Parliament (2012) Health and Social Care Act 2001. The expert patient: A new approach to chronic disease management for the 21st century. Available at: http://www.dh.gov.uk/en/Publicationsandstatistics/Publications/PublicationsPolicyAndGuidance/DH_4006801

United Nations (UN) Universal Declaration of Human Rights (1948). Available at: http://www.
un.org/events/humanrights/2007/.../declaration%20_eng.pdf

United Nations (2002) Madrid International Plan of Action on Ageing. Available at: http://www.
un.org/ageing/documents/building_natl_capacity/guiding.pdf

Waldron, N., Dey, I., Nagree, Y., Xiao, J. and Flicker, L. (2011) A multi-faceted intervention
to implement guideline care and improve quality of care for older people who present to the
emergency department with falls. *BMC Geriatrics* **31(11)**, 6.

Walker, M.F., Leonardi-Bee, J., Bath, P., Langhorne, P., Dewey, M., Corr, S., Drummond, A.,
Gilbertson, L., Gladman, J.R.F., Jongbloed, L., Logan, P.A. and Parker, C. (2004) Individual
patient data meta-analysis of randomized controlled trials of community occupational therapy for
stroke patients. *Stroke* **35(9)**, 2226–223.

Walker, M.F., Gladman, J.R.F., Lincoln, N.B., Siemonsma, P. and Whiteley, P. (1999) Occupational
therapy for stroke patients not admitted to hospital: A randomised controlled trial. *Lancet*
354(9175), 278–280.

Wilcock, A.A. (1998) Occupations for health. *British Journal of Occupational Therapy* **61(8)**,
340–345.

Wilcock, A.A. (2002) *Occupation for Health, Volume 2: A Journey from Prescription to Self Health.*
London: College of Occupational Therapists.

Willetts, D. (2010) *The Pinch: How the Baby Boomers Took Their Children's Future – And Why
They Should Give it Back.* London: Atlantic Books.

World Health Organization (1996) WHOQOL-BREF Introduction, administration, scoring and
generic version of the assessment programme on mental health WHO. Geneva: WHO. Available
at: http://www.who.int/mental_health/media/en/76.pdf

World Health Organization (2002a) Active aging. A policy framework. Available at: *http://
whqlibdoc.who.int/hq/2002/WHO_NMH_NPH_02.8.pdf*

World Health Organization (2002b) Long term care tool kit for policy makers. Available at: http://
www.who.int/chp/knowledge/publications/ltctoolkit.pdf Accessed 15.12.10

World Health Organization (2007) Global age friendly cities. Available at: http://www.who.int/
mediacentre/news/releases/2010/age_friendly_cities_20100628/en/

World Health Organization (2010a) Perth framework for age-friendly community-based primary
health care. Available at: http://www.who.int/ageing/projects/perth/en/

World Health Organization (2010b). Framework for action on interprofessional education and
collaborative practice. Geneva: WHO. at:http://whqlibdoc.who.int/hq/2010/WHO_HRH_
HPN_10.3_eng.pdf

Yamada, T., Kawamata, H., Kobayashi, N., Kielhofner, G. and Taylor, R. (2010) A randomised
clinical trial of a wellness programme for healthy older people. *British Journal of Occupational
Therapy* **73(11)**, 540–548.

Chapter 5

Health conditions and active ageing

Melanie Manley, Rachel Bentley, Christina Richards, Kirsty Tattersall, Alison Warren, Alice Mackenzie, Anna L. Pratt, Alison Lillywhite, Mary Grant, Anne McIntyre, Jacqueline Lawson and Thérèse Jackson

In order to restore the functional health of older adults it is essential that therapists understand the medical conditions that can impact upon the rehabilitation process. Thus, occupational therapists need to understand how older adults respond to illness and disability. They need to be able to assess and evaluate how each health condition impacts upon an individual's health and wellbeing. This is particularly difficult as older adults often present with one or more chronic health conditions. Consequently, is it essential that older adults have access to appropriate skilled professionals who are both motivated and have expertise in working with older adults. The National Service Framework [NSF] for Older People (Department of Health (DH) 2001) realised that this did not always occur in practice, and had the ultimate aim of raising standards within health and social care in the United Kingdom. It also established performance measures against which progress was to be measured within a given time scale. The Framework was published in 2001 and, whilst it has influenced service delivery, there is still concern regarding the standards of care on general wards, lack of dignity and respect, and the amount of consideration given to the needs of older adults. The provision of end of life services was also found to be inconsistent (Healthcare Commission et al. 2006). Within the United Kingdom, real concerns exist regarding the management of older adults by healthcare professionals. In order to understand this better, it is useful to read patients' stories and/or experiences on the internet. Hence the importance of understanding the patients' experiences to enhance services for older adults.

In this chapter, we asked experienced occupational therapists to write evidence-based accounts using case studies to outline their practice with older adults. Some of the case studies highlight the importance of the risk of falls, and a specific section on falls management can be found at the end of the chapter. What should be noted is the importance of occupational therapists assessing not only for falls risks but for mood and cognitive changes. As an occupational therapist, the key area for assessment is function or occupational performance. Each therapist has used the International Classification of

Functioning (WHO 2001) as a framework. Since we are committed to the concept of evidence-based practice, we wanted to encourage therapists to utilise standardised assessments and outcome measures. Outcome measures enable therapists to demonstrate with confidence that a change in a client's wellbeing can be attributed to their intervention. The data generated by such assessments can be used not only by practitioners but also by managers to monitor quality assurance and to develop health and social care policy and research. However, occupational therapists need to try to find an outcome measure that is right for their client group and organisation. This is a difficult and challenging task (Stubbs et al. 2004). In this chapter, many of the outcome measures are not occupational therapy- or pathology-specific, such as the Canadian Occupational Therapy Performance Measure (COPM) (Law et al. 2005) and can be used by different team members. It is also important that occupational therapists consider using quality of life measures to ascertain the older person's perspectives on their health and wellbeing (Liddle and Mckenna 2000).

Bi-polar disorder

Melanie Manley

Joan is 68 years old and has a diagnosis of bi-polar disorder. She is a retired divorcee with one daughter who lives abroad.

Joan was diagnosed with bi-polar disorder in her late 20s following a number of episodes of both depression and mania. Joan made serious attempts on her life aged 39 and 45; in more recent years she has experienced severe episodes of mania.

During the manic phase of her illness Joan struggles to sleep, becomes sexually disinhibited, spends large amounts of money and has been known to become irritable and agitated with people. When manic, Joan tends to lack insight, stating she feels 'on top of the world' and is reluctant to accept the assistance of health and social care services.

Throughout her illness Joan has been admitted on numerous occasions, both informally and under sections of the Mental Health Act.

Due to physical health concerns, Joan has recently been taken off her long-standing mood stabiliser drug, Lithium. A change in medication regime has precipitated a voluntary admission to trial alternative medications. Since her admission, Joan has begun to display some symptoms of mania; her sleep has deteriorated and she has been noted to be 'overly' talkative.

Occupational therapy input has been indicated to monitor and sustain occupational performance skills during the admission. Although research into bi-polar disorder is widespread, there is relatively little information available in relation to the older population (Bartels et al. 2008), particularly when considering occupational performance and functioning.

When core diagnostic criteria are applied, prevalence of bi-polar disorder of adults in the community living population is approximately 1%. This figure drops to 0.1% of the elderly population (Depp and Jeste 2004). However, this may not be an accurate representation of prevalence in this age group. When care home and hospital communities are considered, it has been suggested the figures change and that 10% of the older population in such settings are diagnosed (Vasudev and Thomas 2010). This raises the question of whether the ageing individual with this diagnosis is more likely to be admitted to long-term care or whether symptoms decrease over time The literature indicates that an older individual with bi-polar disorder is at a more significant risk of developing a dementia over time. This could in part account for the disparity in community living for adult and older populations.

Currently, late life bi-polar disorder accounts for 8–10% of hospital admissions (Depp and Jeste 2004). With an increasingly ageing population arising from improved healthcare and life expectancy, this figure is expected to increase significantly. In turn, this will only serve to place an ever-increasing burden on healthcare services (Depp et al. 2006).

Bi-polar disorder is a chronic, progressive disease with several contributing factors including physical, environmental and social. It is also known to be caused by chemical imbalances in the brain. In particular, neurotransmitters such as serotonin and dopamine are affected.

Bi-polar disorder as a diagnosis falls into two clear categories:

Bi-polar I: This requires episodes of both depression and mania to have been experienced before a diagnosis is made.

Bi-polar II: This diagnosis may be made when the individual has experienced episodes of depression and hypomania (a milder form of mania) with no evidence of mania itself required (National Institute for Health and Clinical Excellence 2006(b)).

Due to her age, Joan could now be considered to be at increased risk of relapsing into depressive symptoms when recovering from a manic episode, although Coryell et al. (2009) suggest that this may not be the case and that there is simply a poor recall of historical episodes. This is particularly relevant to Joan as she has made a number of serious attempts on her life in the past. Additionally, Joan is now likely to experience protracted episodes of mood disturbance with shorter periods of respite that are 'symptom free', although this may be disputed (Box 5.1). It has also been suggested that ageing individuals are less likely to respond to psychopharmacological intervention (Depp and Jeste 2004) and that poor management will lead to longer admissions to hospital.

Box 5.1   Joan's difficulties with functioning due to bi-polar disorder.

Mental functions: irritable and agitated with people, symptoms of mania.

Activity limitations: limited sleep so loss of routine, ability to form relationships with persons, manage and pay bills.

Participation restrictions: unable to keep appointments with health and social care professionals, difficulty maintaining and forming relationships, difficulty managing routines and everyday tasks.

Contextual factors: Joan tends to lack insight and has been admitted on numerous occasions both informally and under sections of the Mental Health Act.

Bi-polar disorder is recognised as likely to cause a degree of occupational and psycho-social dysfunction whether the individual is in relapse (manic or depressive) or considered to be euthymic. The most significantly impacted areas are executive functioning, verbal and visual memory, information processing and attention (Brissos et al. 2008). Indeed, 30–60% of diagnosed individuals experience such challenges (Mur et al. 2009). Occupational therapy is in a strong position to assist individuals like Joan to adapt occupational behaviour and choices during an admission (and following discharge) in order to sustain occupational performance.

Research indicates that working with the individual to recognise their relapse indicators, prompting a request for treatment will increase the period of time relapse phases, thus decreasing the number of episodes experienced. In turn, it would be reasonable to expect an improvement in psycho-social functioning and occupational performance (Perry et al. 1999). This is considered to be particularly effective when working with the individual to recognise indicators of a manic relapse.

Occupational therapy has a significant role to play in facilitating the individual to recognise their relapse indicators and put appropriate coping strategies or action plans into place. It will also have an important role in assisting the individual to identify obstacles to occupational participation and adapt occupational performance through working in partnership to identify their ability, areas of skill deficits, prioritising and goal setting (Woodside et al. 2006).

When considering Joan's narrative, the occupational therapist should recognise that she is currently exhibiting prodromal symptoms for a relapse into an episode of mania. At this stage,it might be able to conduct an AMPS (Assessment of Motor and Process Skills) assessment with Joan's chosen tasks, to obtain a baseline indication of the quality of her occupational performance and identify specific areas of skills deficit. This could then be repeated at stages throughout her admission to indicate progress and assist with evaluation and adaptation of intervention. It could also be conducted as she prepares for discharge, as an outcome measure. The occupational therapist may also choose with Joan to use the recovery star as a means of measuring global improvement.

Once a baseline measurement is achieved, the occupational therapist will be able to work with Joan to identify her priorities and potential discharge location before negotiating an intervention plan with her and agreeing timely and realistic short-, medium- and long-term goals. As part of the occupational therapy process, the therapist may wish to use a number of standardised assessments such as OCAIRS, OSA, AOF-CV (Assessment of Occupational Functioning – Collaborative Version) and the VQ (Volitional Questionnaire) as a means of gathering relevant information to inform their treatment planning and assist Joan in achieving her goals (Table 5.1). Initially, as Joan is showing early signs of a manic relapse the occupational therapist is likely to work toward establishing a good therapeutic relationship with Joan and focus on short-term achievable goals to prevent Joan disengaging from services.

When revisiting the figures relating to the percentage of hospital admissions attributed to the older persons with bi-polar disorder there is a strong case, not only for occupational therapy to support an inpatient admission, but for the role of the occupational therapist to continue in the community. Here, they may work closely with the individual to maintain occupational performance and prevent readmission to hospital. Evidence also

Table 5.1   Assessment and outcome measures for persons with bi-polar disorder.

Assessment of Motor and Process Skills (AMPS): An observational, functional assessment tool that examines both the motor and process elements of the activity. Training is required from a specific AMPs course (Fisher 1995). Further information about the AMPS can be found at http://www.medicine.mcgill.ca/strokengine-assess/module_amps_intro-en.html

Assessment of Occupational Functioning Collaborative Version: The AOF-CV is a screening tool designed to collect a broad range of information believed to influence and be indicative of a person's occupational performance and to identify areas which require further investigation or analysis. Further information about the tool and how it should be administered can be found at http://www.sahp.vcu.edu/occu/ot/aofinstrument2.pdf

Volitional Questionnaire (De las Heras et al. 2007): This is an observational tool that aims to enable therapists to gain further understanding of a person's inner motives and how the environment impacts upon participation in his or her occupations. Further information about the tool can be found at http://www.uic.edu/depts/moho/assess/vq.html

suggests that active engagement with occupational therapy services could have influence on delaying or avoiding placement in long-term care.

Cancer

Rachel Bentley

> Mr Archer is an 80-year-old man who is the main carer for his 78-year-old wife. He lives in an owner-occupied bungalow and his son and daughter live locally.
>
> He has undergone palliative chemotherapy for non-small-cell lung cancer diagnosed six months ago and is receiving supportive and palliative care.
>
> Mr Archer has been referred to the community occupational therapist by his daughter, who is concerned about how he is coping at home. He has become weaker and is finding toilet transfers and bathing difficult. He suffers from shortness of breath on exertion and fatigue. Subsequently, he is finding caring for his wife difficult and is not managing his daily activities. His family assist with shopping and cleaning but don't feel able to provide any further assistance at present. Mr Archer also feels withdrawn as he can no longer go to the pub to meet his friends once a week. He is a lifelong Arsenal fan.

Cancer predominantly occurs in people aged 60 and over, with 75% of cases diagnosed in those aged 60 and over and a third in individuals over the age of 75. Prostate cancer is the most common cancer in men (24%), followed by lung cancer (15%) and colorectal (14%). In women, breast cancer is by far the most common cancer (31%), followed by colorectal (12%) and lung (12%); other cancers in both sexes have smaller incidences (Cancer Research 2010).

Tumours can be benign or malignant. Cancer is the name given to a malignant tumour; this consists of cells that have the ability to spread beyond the original area. If left untreated, the cells will not only spread and destroy surrounding tissue but have the potential to break off and spread to other parts of the body via the lymphatic system or blood stream to form new tumours known as metastasis (Macmillan Cancer Support 2007).

The cancer reform strategy suggests that over half of all cancers could be prevented by lifestyle changes (Department of Health 2007). Risk factors for developing cancer include: smoking; excessive alcohol consumption; obesity; ultraviolet radiation; and exposure to chemicals. Health promotion in these areas will help improve cancer outcomes. Other measures to improve outcomes include vaccination schemes and screening as it is thought the earlier a cancer can be detected the greater the chance of a cure (Department of Health 2007). Ngune et al. (2009) found that, despite evidence suggesting that modifying risk factors at any age can reduce the risk of cancer, many older people fail to take preventative actions, not perceiving them as being beneficial after the age of 60. Occupational therapists have a role here when working with older people in health promotion and promoting the benefits of cancer prevention. The College of Occupational Therapists (2008) suggests that health promotion activities should be included in therapists' everyday practice.

Older people who are diagnosed with cancer often present with a number of other conditions and increased frailty associated with older age, making it difficult to define the effects the cancer and its treatment have on the individual. The multidisciplinary team needs to work together to identify and support patients' needs, taking into account other factors of aging (Gosney 2009). High-quality communication skills are essential to assessing the older person and delivering client-centred practice. Improving supportive and palliative care for adults with cancer guidelines also highlights the importance of this, suggesting that good communication and well-coordinated services are required to meet the needs of patients (National Institute of Clinical Excellence 2004(a)).

Occupational therapists make a valuable contribution in symptom management (Cooper 2007). Interventions that can be used by therapists include:

* Lifestyle management
* Fatigue management
* Breathlessness management
* Relaxation and anxiety management
* Problem solving

The role of occupational therapy is to enhance wellbeing and quality of life through engagement in meaningful occupation. For Mr Archer (Box 5.2), the occupational therapy interventions would include provision of assistive technology and advice to enable him to carry out toilet and bath transfers independently. Other interventions could be

---

Box 5.2   Mr Archer's difficulties with functioning due to cancer.

Body functions: increased shortness of breath. Increased fatigue. Reduced mobility.

Activity limitations: self care, transfers, cooking and laundry.

Participation restriction: unable to care for his wife and visit his friends in the pub due to limiting body functions.

Contextual factors: family are unable to provide any further support.

Table 5.2 Assessment and outcome measures for persons with cancer.

The Canadian Occupational Performance Measure (COPM) is a client-centred outcome measure used to detect change in a client's self-perception of occupational performance over time. It is carried out by a semi-structured interview which takes about 30–40 minutes. The COPM has been tested for validity and reliability (Law et al. 2005).

Westcotes Individualised Outcome Measure (WIOM) was designed to measure the outcome of occupational therapy in achieving patients' goals. After initial assessment, problems are identified and placed into categories using an agreed goal list. Goals are negotiated with the patient and, following intervention, the goals are measured against an outcome code (Eames et al. 1999).

Goal setting, e.g. Goal Attainment Scale (GAS), is a method of scoring the extent to which patients' goals are achieved in the course of intervention and can be used by the multidisciplinary team. The outcomes can be statistically analysed (Turner-Stokes 2009).

fatigue and breathlessness management, and addressing the issue of social isolation by liaison/ team working with other agencies to provide care and support for him and his wife to enable them to remain at home. Again, the importance of good communication with Mr Archer and his family is paramount to ensure his needs and wishes are being addressed.

There is a big drive for patients like Mr Archer, who are palliative, to be cared for in their own homes. The College of Occupational Therapists' guidance on intervention in cancer highlights that there is a move towards community-based care and supporting individuals to live as independently as possible, even if life expectancy is short (College of Occupational Therapists 2004). Therefore, it is important that patients at the palliative stage of cancer care are able to access occupational therapy services in the community (Kealey and Mcintyre 2005).

It is important as occupational therapists that the services and interventions provided are evaluated to ensure practice is evidence based. Eva (2007) suggests a number of ways to achieve this, including conducting service audits, carrying out patient satisfaction surveys and measuring outcomes of an intervention using a data collection tool.

Some possible outcome measures that can be used to evaluate occupational therapy interventions with cancer patients are outlined in Table 5.2.

Chronic obstructive pulmonary disease

Christina Richards

Mrs Watson is 85 years old and was admitted to hospital with increased shortness of breath. She has previously been diagnosed with chronic obstructive pulmonary disease (COPD) and has both oxygen and a nebuliser at home. She was referred to the in-patient occupational therapy team for further assessment of her ability to manage at home on discharge from hospital. Mrs Watson enjoys activities such as completing crosswords and knitting.

She has two sons and lives with the oldest son. She has a good relationship with both of them but is concerned she is becoming a burden to them both. Mrs Watson reports feeling low in mood which she feels is due to her inability to participate in activities outside the home.

She lives in a two-storey house with her son, who provides assistance for all domestic tasks. Due to her shortness of breath, she is no longer able to access the upstairs of her property. Mrs Watson states she often feels anxious, especially when attempting to mobilise and this has further restricted her participation in activities. She is finding carrying out personal care activities difficult, especially washing and dressing her lower half due to her breathlessness. Mrs Watson has stated she would like to be able to manage basic kitchen activities whilst her son is at work.

Box 5.3   Mrs Watson's Problems with functioning due to COPD

Bodily function/structures: low mood, poor exercise tolerance, anxiety, poor sleep pattern causing difficulties with cognitive functioning, poor respiratory function.

Activity limitations: restricted mobility indoors, personal care activities – unable to wash and dress lower half, unable to manage domestic tasks, unable to mobilise outdoors.

Participation restrictions: unable to socialise with friends, unable to attend family gatherings.

Occupational therapists in both primary and secondary care will see patients with respiratory disease such as chronic obstructive pulmonary disease (COPD). In the case of COPD, the obstruction within the airways is caused by damage to both the airways and parenchyma and is generally progressive (National Institute of Clinical Excellence (2010(a)). The main cause of this disease is long-term smoking. In 2004, approximately 27,000 people died as a result of COPD; respiratory disease is responsible for the death of 1 in 5 people and currently costs around £6 billion per year in NHS, mortality, and morbidity costs (British Thoracic Society 2006). The symptoms experienced by people with obstructive respiratory disease include breathlessness on exertion, cough, wheeze and regular sputum production. There are other consequences of this disease which include:

- Anxiety and depression
- Poor nutrition
- Social isolation

All of these were seen in the case of Mrs Watson (Box 5.3) and can be a factor in determining readmissions to hospital for an exacerbation of the condition. Occupational therapy assessment should form a holistic approach which considers the physical, psychological and social effects of the disease on the ability of the person to perform meaningful occupations. There are a number of different assessments that can be used by occupational therapists, some of which are disease-specific, some more occupation-focused.

Energy conservation techniques are an important part of the occupational therapy intervention with this client group. Evidence suggests that energy conservation, especially in

Table 5.3 Assessment and outcome measures for persons with COPD.

Hospital Anxiety and Depression Scale [HAD] (Zigmund and Snaith 1994): a bi-dimensional self-report instrument. It is divided into two subsections. Section HADS-A is divided into anxiety subscales and a depression subscale (HADS-D). It was originally designed for an hospital in-patient setting but there is evidence that it can be used with older adults (Helvik et al. 2011).

St Georges Respiratory Questionnaire (SGRQ): the SGRQ is a self-administered questionnaire in two parts designed to measure health impairment in patients with asthma and COPD. Part 1 (Questions 1–8) addresses the frequency of respiratory symptoms. Part 2 (Sections 9–16) addresses the patient's current state The Manual is available at: http://www.healthstatus.sgul.ac.uk/SGRQ_download/SGRQ%20Manual%20June%20 2009.pdf

Borg Scale of Perceived Exertion (Borg 1982): the Borg Rating of Perceived Exertion (RPE) is a subjective measure for measuring physical activity intensity level.

Canadian Occupational Performance Measure [COPM] (Law et al. 2005).

Assessment of Motor and Process Skills [AMPS] (Fisher 1995)

terms of teaching good use of body position, can reduce both energy use and perceptions of breathlessness when completing activities of daily living (Velloso and Jardim 2006). The role of the occupational therapist is mainly educative in terms of providing information on energy conservation. This has been shown to be effective in terms of improving outcomes for patients admitted following an exacerbation of COPD (Lorenzi et al. 2004), reducing fear and increasing reported ability to perform activities of daily living (Rubí et al. 2010). Energy conservation techniques can be based around the principles of positioning, planning daily routines and prioritisation of meaningful occupation.

This could take the form of discussing with a person how they currently manage their daily routine as well as talking about activities that need to be prioritised and those that could be delegated to others. MrsWatson chose being able to prepare drinks and snacks as an activity of importance to her but was willing to accept assistance for other personal care tasks to conserve her energy. An important aspect of energy conservation is activity analysis – being able to analyse an activity as performed by a person and working with them to find more efficient ways of completing this activity.

Currently, much of the role within the hospital setting focuses on compensating for deficits caused by the illness as well as considering the impact of the environment as this can also have either a enabling or disabling effect on a person's ability to carry out their normal activities. It may also be necessary to consider the role of the use of equipment to increase or maintain participation. In the case of Mrs Watson, a kitchen trolley was provided to increase her confidence when mobilising and enable her to prepare drinks and snacks.

Community teams also have an important role with this population in terms of promoting and maintaining independence and self-management. One way in which this can be achieved is through a pulmonary rehabilitation programme (National Institute of Clinical Excellence 2010b). Pulmonary rehabilitation is a multidisciplinary programme providing both exercise and education Table 5.3.

Coronary heart disease

Kirsty Tattersall

> *Mrs Rose Smith is a 79-year-old lady who has been referred to the occupational therapist whilst she is in hospital. Mrs Smith has a history of coronary artery disease and frequent hospital admissions, having recently been diagnosed with heart failure. She lives with her husband, a retired accountant, in their own house, and has one daughter who is a full-time mum and lives nearby. Her husband and daughter are concerned about her shortness of breath on activity, and her extreme tiredness. They now assist with most of the housework and cooking. Mrs Smith finds it difficult to walk around the supermarket and has stopped going to her bridge club because of the flight of stairs to get there. She is spending much of her time at home and reports feeling quite low.*

Heart failure is a common chronic condition, the prevalence of which increases markedly with age. It is the only major cardiovascular disease with increasing prevalence, incidence and mortality. This is due in particular to better overall treatment of coronary heart disease amongst younger people and an ageing population. Heart failure accounts for about 5% of all medical admissions and readmission rates are the highest for any common condition in the UK (Department of Health 2000).

Heart failure occurs when the heart muscle is unable to maintain an effective pumping action to meet the body's needs and the heart does not function with maximum efficiency. By looking at Mrs Smith's narrative, she is displaying some of the main symptoms of heart failure, i.e. fatigue and breathlessness. Loss of energy is a common problem, making it difficult to carry out normal everyday activities. Failure on the left side of the heart to pump blood into the arteries results in 'back pressure' in the circulation. This can cause fluid to accumulate in the air spaces of the lungs, resulting in breathlessness (British Heart Foundation (BHF) 2009).

The impact of heart failure on a person's life may be related as much to psychological adaptation to the disease as to impairment in physical functioning. The effects of heart failure, particularly on women's ability to perform activities such as shopping and housework, have been found to have a profound effect on their self esteem and quality of life (Riedinger et al. 2001). Symptoms such as breathlessness can severely limit activity and cause avoidance of situations that might precipitate it. This can lead to further problems such as disuse atrophy and social isolation, both of which are evident for Mrs Smith (Box 5.4). Psycho-social function is also commonly affected; with depression being more common in heart failure patients than in the general population (National Institute of Clinical Excellence 2003). For Mrs Smith, the negative impact of heart failure on her ability to carry out her roles of homemaker and caregiver could be having a profound effect on her feelings of self-worth and quality of life (Box 5.4).

Occupational therapists have an important role to play in the assessment and treatment of people with heart failure due to their holistic approach and ability to analyse activity, with a major occupational therapy aim being to assist clients in making a positive

---

Box 5.4 Mrs Smith's difficulties with functioning due to her heart failure.

Body function/structures: low mood, breathlessness, poor exercise tolerance, disuse atrophy, fatigue, swollen ankles and feet.

Activity limitations: Difficulty completing heavier domestic tasks, difficulty climbing stairs, difficulty walking outdoors.

Participation restriction: Social isolation, loss of role within household.

Table 5.4 New York Heart Association classifications.

Class I: No symptoms

Class II: Symptoms of fatigue, palpitation, dyspnoea or angina pain on ordinary physical activity

Class III: Symptoms in less than ordinary activity. Comfortable at rest

Class IV: Symptoms at rest and unable to carry out physical activity without discomfort.

Table 5.5 Assessment and outcome measures for Mrs Smith.

Assessment of Motor and Process Skills [AMPS] (Fisher 1995)

Canadian Occupational Performance Measure [COPM] (Law et al. 1998)

MOS 36-Item Short-Form Health Survey [SF-36] (Ware and Sherbourne 1992): SF-36 measures 8 aspects of functional health status: physical function, social function, pain, general health, mental health, vitality, and role functional limitations due to physical or emotional problems Concerns have been expressed about the suitability of SF-36 for all patient groups (Jenkinson et al. 1993). Brazier et al. (1992) and Parker et al. (1998) reported a lower response rate for the SF-36 amongst older adults, although Singleton and Turner (1993) suggest that the SF-36 can be used with older adults if care and attention is paid to the layout of the questionnaire and that help could be available if necessary.

Hospital Anxiety and Depression Scale [HAD] (Zigmund and Snaith 1994).

---

adjustment to their condition. An older person has to adjust to living with new limitations and the knowledge that life expectancy may be shortened.

It is recommended that persons with heart failure care should receive care from a multidisciplinary team (NICE 2003). The occupational therapist is an integral member of the multidisciplinary team, working closely with the specialist heart failure nurses to advocate the person's self-care, which can improve outcomes from heart failure (American Heart Association 2009).

Assessments will be undertaken by the multidisciplinary team, assessing both the symptoms of the disease and the effects they are having on the person. People with heart failure (Table 5.4) are routinely categorised by the cardiologist on discussion of symptoms according to the New York Heart Association (NYHA) classifications (American Heart Association 2009).

Occupational therapists can add to the quality of information about the person's functional ability in the areas of self-care, productivity and leisure through the use of observations and standardised assessment and outcome measures (Table 5.5). It is important to also assess the person's view of their quality of life and mood as these are known to be poor in people with heart failure.

Occupational therapy interventions target the symptoms of fatigue and breathlessness that affect occupational performance. Dyspnoea on exertion and fatigue are expected symptoms of heart failure, and for Mrs Smith and her family, knowing this can alleviate some of the anxiety when performing activities. Teaching energy conservation techniques through the use of pacing, time management and cycles of rest and activity can lead to a marked reduction in breathlessness and fatigue. This will help Mrs Smith regain some of her roles within the house and feel a valued member of her family.

Assistive products and technology might achieve energy conservation, but also increase independence and safety. Anxiety can trigger dyspnoea and tax cardiopulmonary function. The teaching of breathing control techniques such as diaphragmatic breathing and promotion of a relaxed and gentle breathing pattern should be considered along with other types of relaxation techniques. These are effective for the relief of anxiety and help in slowing breathing patterns (Keable 1997).

Exercise can improve symptoms, exercise performance and quality of life in people with heart failure and referral to a cardiac rehabilitation programme may be appropriate. Programmes that combine exercise, psychological support and education are of greater benefit than those providing only one of the components (National Institute of Clinical Excellence 2003). As well as becoming more physically active, Mrs Smith can undertake other health promotion strategies such as eating a healthy balanced diet, particularly concentrating on reduced salt, fluid management and a reduced alcohol intake, also working towards a sensible body weight and, if she did smoke, to stop. Reassessment of psychological status should be undertaken once treatment for the symptoms has been carried out to determine if any depression was precipitated by the symptoms. This will assist the multidisciplinary team to plan future treatment if needed.

Current treatment for heart failure does not arrest progression of the disease. A palliative care approach may need to be considered for end-stage heart failure. The team's approach should be one of aiming to maintain quality of life and good symptom control (British Heart Foundation 2009).

Dementia and older adults

Alison Warren

> *Mr Darragh Kelly is a 78-year-old widower, who was referred to the specialist community mental health team for older adults. His daughter, Breda, had become concerned as Darragh was tearful, forgetting appointments and was having difficulty problem-solving tasks, e.g. organising shopping lists. Darragh is losing confidence in his abilities and now relies on Breda to go shopping with him. Breda finds herself visiting or phoning Darragh every day. This is having an impact on Breda who has given up an evening class and is considering working part time. Until recently, Darragh had enjoyed going to support the local rugby team, visiting his sister in Ireland and helping neighbours.*

It is estimated that 1 in 88 of the entire population of the United Kingdom has dementia (Alzheimer's Society 2007). Dementia is described as a syndrome caused by a variety of diseases of the brain which is progressive (WHO 2012). Alzheimer's disease is the most common form of dementia, followed by vascular dementia (Alzheimer's Society 2007). Dementia leads to disturbance of cognition, emotion and behaviour, all of which are evident in Mr Kelly.

In the United Kingdom, 55.4% of people with dementia have mild dementia, with 36.5% living in institutional care settings (Alzheimer's Society 2007). Building on the dementia care strategy for England, the government has prioritised quality early diagnosis and intervention for all (Department of Health 2010). This indicates a need to focus occupational therapy intervention at the earlier stages of the disease process as well as in the moderate-to-severe stages of dementia.

It has been an exciting time with research into community occupational therapy for people with dementia (Graff et al. 2006, 2007, Bennett and Liddle 2008). Occupational therapists have a valuable contribution to make when working with people who have dementia at all stages. We should be viewed as core contributors in the dementia care pathway in order to provide occupation-focused interventions that support the achievement of clients' goals and enhance an individual's wellbeing. However, occupational therapists have struggled to apply traditional models of adaptation and rehabilitation in dementia care (Perrin et al. 2008).

Mr Kelly is experiencing difficulties which may indicate the early stage of a dementia (Box 5.5). Mr Kelly would benefit from a multidisciplinary assessment and, because his symptoms are recent, this assessment could take place in a memory clinic. A role for occupational therapists in memory clinics has been highlighted for several decades (Robinson 1992). In recent years, occupational therapists have become part of the multidisciplinary team in some memory clinics. Key interventions include assessment, programmes on coping strategies and new techniques for completing activities of daily living. This can also include the provision of equipment including telecare.

The ICF enables the therapist to gain an understanding of the impact of these impairments (difficulty in problem-solving, being tearful) on his ability to complete activities of daily living (shopping) and any restriction caused in participation in daily life (visiting friends, supporting rugby, travelling to Ireland). There are many assessments available to occupational therapists in dementia care (Table 5.6). Occupational therapists in dementia care

---

Box 5.5   Darragh's difficulties with functioning due to dementia.

Mental functions: short-term memory loss, difficulty problem solving and emotional functions, e.g. tearful and losing confidence in abilities.

Activity limitations: shopping, keeping appointments.

Participation restrictions: unable to visit friends, support the local rugby team or, travel to Ireland to visit sister due to loss of confidence in his own abilities.

Contextual factors: lives alone with a daughter who visits or telephones every day.

Table 5.6 Outcome measures for persons with dementia.

Large Allen's Cognitive Level Screen (LACLs): One of several assessment tools designed to be used in conjunction with the Cognitive Disabilities Model (Allen et al. 1992). The client is given a rectangular piece of leather with holes around the edge and instructed to complete three different types of stitch and to correct certain errors. This screening tool identifies a client's cognitive ability, which should always be backed up by a practical assessment and by talking to carers. The client's intervention is planned in order to maintain or maximise the client's functional performance. Further information can be found on the website where there is a specific video for occupational therapists: www.allencognitivelevelscreen.org

Assessment of Motor and Process Skills [AMP] (Fisher 1995): Further information about the AMPS can be found on this website: https://www.ampsintl.com/AMPS/

Canadian Occupational Performance Measure [COPM] (Law et al. 2005)

Model of Human Occupational Screening Tool (MOHOST): This screening uses several methods to collate information which the occupational therapist then rates, addressing the client's motivation for occupation, pattern of occupation, communication, environment, process and motor skills (Parkinson et al. 2006). Further information about the tool can be found on the MOHO Clearinghouse: http://www.uic.edu/depts/moho/assess/mohost.html

Pool Activity Level Instrument (PAL): Developed to engage people with dementia in meaningful occupation. Comprises of a checklist completed by both formal and informal carers to recognise the activity level of an individual and promote appropriate activities to increase wellbeing (Pool 2008).

need to focus on the achievement of client-centred goals and the wellbeing of individuals and caregivers. Traditionally, the Mini Mental State examination (Folstein et al. 1975) is used to assess cognitive function and a standardised assessment to rate activities of daily living can also be useful to gain information from Mr Kelly and his daughter, for example, the Bristol Activities of Daily Living (Bucks et al. 1996).

Occupational therapy intervention is valuable for individuals at any stage of dementia. The holistic, client-centred approach with problem solving leads to a variety of interventions. With Mr Kelly, the occupational therapists would adapt his environment with visual cues to assist with his memory loss and problem-solving difficulties. They would also work with Mr Kelly to encourage him to explore his loss of confidence and introduce or reintroduce him to organisations in the community as a social outlet. Occupational therapy interventions range from completing occupation-focused individual or group work to providing equipment.

Driving is a controversial topic and occupational therapists could be involved in assessing a person's ability with this complex activity of daily living. Liddle et al. (2008) in a study with older people, identified interventions that occupational therapists can offer at the pre-decision, decision and post-driving cessation time. These are relevant when working with older people with dementia and links to the assessment of risk with this older client group. When completing risk assessments and risk-reducing interventions it is essential that a multidisciplinary approach is taken involving the views of the individual and caregivers.

Depression

Alice Mackenzie

> Mr James is 86 years old. His wife died six years ago. Approximately a year ago, Mr James moved into a sheltered housing complex. Mr James has two adult children: a married son living in Australia and a married daughter living nearby. Mr James has Type II diabetes and suffered a stroke approximately six months ago as a result of high blood pressure. He made a reasonable recovery from the stroke; he is able to walk independently using a stick, and after six weeks of rehabilitation was independent in personal activities of daily living such as washing, dressing, grooming and being able to move around his flat and sheltered housing independently. He has home care two times a week to help with shopping, laundry and household cleaning.
>
> Mr James worked as bus driver for a local bus company working for most of his working life. After retirement he and his wife enjoyed a variety of activities such as going to an over 60's club, working on their allotment and taking the occasional holiday. He continued going to his club and working on his allotment after his wife's death.
>
> Over the last 2–3 months, Mr James's daughter has noticed changes in her father's appearance; appearing dishevelled, wearing grubby clothes and on occasions being unshaven, and he appears to have lost weight. He has needed more persuasion to go out with her when she visits at the weekend and complains of feeling tired and is not watching his usual television programmes. His home carer has also noticed that he does not initiate as much conversation as he used to.

Clinical depression is medically diagnosed when a number of symptoms have occurred regularly over a period of time, usually two weeks or more (National Institute for Health and Clinical Excellence [NICE] 2009). One in seven people over the age of 65 will have major depression and one in four older people will experience some level of depression in which symptoms impair the person's quality of life (Rodda et al. 2011). However, depression among older people is often under-recognised and under-treated compared to other age groups. In addition, proportionally more people over the age of 65 who have major depression will commit suicide (Moussavi et al. 2007, Rodda et al. 2011). The risk factors associated with depression in old age are:

- Living in institutional care
- Moving accommodation
- Migrated from country of origin
- Loss of social contacts
- Increased social isolation
- Being a carer
- Changes in role or social status
- Bereavement or loss
- Major physical illness such as Parkinson's disease, diabetes, stroke or cardio-vascular disease
- Chronic pain

- Functional impairment
- Previous history of depression
- Cognitive impairment
- Receiving high levels of home care
- Poor defences against death anxiety.

Depression is often a multifactorial illness with biological, social and psychological factors (refer to Box 5.6 for the DSM-IV Criteria).

A diagnostic assessment of Mr James would need to consider any risk factors contributing to his depression, such as moving accommodation. An occupational therapist would need to ascertain whether Mr James is less able to perform everyday tasks as a result of his stroke, and whether he is experiencing feelings of loss, social isolation, etc. as a result of moving and/or as a result of his stroke. It would also be necessary to establish to what extent Mr James is able to contribute to the decision about receiving home-care. Because of Mr James's co-morbidity it would be important to ascertain if any of the symptoms listed above were related to his diabetes or his stroke or depression, for example experiencing tiredness could be due to the diabetes and/or because of his stroke (Box 5.7).

Prior to commencing the assessment, it is important to take into account the individual client factors as outlined in Table 5.7. Carrying out the Canadian Occupational Performance Measure (COPM) would enable Mr James and the occupational therapist to agree what activities were most important for them both to focus on. In addition, the

---

Box 5.6   DSM-IV Criteria

- Depressed mood for most of the day
- Decreased interest or pleasure in nearly all activities for most of the day over a period of time, i.e. two weeks.
- Marked loss or gain of weight or markedly increased or decreased appetite
- Excessive sleep or not enough sleep
- Observable psychomotor agitation or retardation
- Tiredness or loss of energy
- Feelings of guilt or worthlessness
- Poor concentration or indecisiveness
- Thoughts of dying or suicide and/or suicide attempt.

Box 5.7   Classification of Mr James's problems.

Activity limitations: shopping and cooking, gardening – attending his allottment, socialising at the pub

Participation restriction: going to the pub – Mr James feels unable to talk about how he is feeling with his friends; this type of conversation may not be part of his social norm

Contextual factors: social – recently widowed after a 46-year relationship, daughter visits at weekends, son lives abroad.

Table 5.7 Assessment and outcome measures for Mr James.

Canadian Occupational Performance Measure [COPM] (Law et al. 1998)

The Geriatric Depression scale: The GDS was developed to assess depression in older people. The original 30-item scale (cut-off of 10 points) was developed by Yesavage et al. (1983) and more recently a 15-item (cut-off 5 points) version has been validated. It is also sensitive to depression among elderly persons suffering from mild-to-moderate dementia and physical illness. It has also been found to be useful as a screening tool for minor depression in the post-stroke population (Sivrioglu et al 2009). A copy of the scale can be found at http://www.chcr.brown.edu/GDS_SHORT_FORM.PDF

Patient Health Questionnaire-9 (PHQ-9): The patient health questionnaire developed out of the more detailed PRIME-MD (Spitzer et al. 1994). A copy of the questionnaire can be found at http://steppingup.washington.edu/keys/documents/phq-9.pdf

occupational therapist would need to ensure that there is no suicidal intent and, with members of the multidisciplinary team, determine whether any of his additional medical problems are related to his low mood. In relation to the non-pharmaceutical management of depression for older adults the evidence suggests that the most effective treatments for depression are cognitive behavior therapy (CBT), behavioural activation, interpersonal therapy, or guided self-help based on CBT or behavioural principles (Scottish Intercollegiate Guidelines Network Guidelines (SIGN) 2010). Whilst there is no high evidence to support lifestyle advice, it is recommended that advice should address alcohol and drug use, diet and eating behaviours, maintenance of social networks and personally-meaningful activities and sleep problems (Department of Health 2007, Scottish Intercollegiate Network 2010(a)).

Fractures and osteoporosis

Anna L. Pratt

Val is a 68-year-old widow who volunteers at her local charity shop and looks after her grandchildren, who live a short car journey from her home, two days a week.

Val has been independent until seven weeks ago, when she fell whilst getting up from her kitchen chair and sustained a colles fracture (fracture of the distal radius) of her dominant side. Following diagnosis and initial treatment of the fracture she was referred for bone density scanning and a positive diagnosis of osteoporosis was confirmed.

On the removal of her plaster-of-paris (POP) Val had limited range of motion at her wrist, digits and overall grip strength combined with increased oedema and pain. This lack of motion and strength resulted in difficulty completing most activities she would normally carry out bilaterally or with her dominant hand. This has ultimately meant that she has been unable to resume her charity work or driving which gives her the independence she enjoys. She is having to live with her daughter some of the time to continue her childcare commitments to her grandchildren.

Table 5.8   Assessments and outcome measures commonly used for older people following upper limb fractures.

Disabilities of Arm, Shoulder, Hand Questionnaire (DASH). A self-administered questionnaire of 30 items concerned with upper limb functional activities over previous week to measure disability regardless of which arm, shoulder or hand used. Questions are also concerned with work, sleep, social life, pain and symptoms (Hudak et al. 1996). Further information about the tool can be found at http://www.dash.iwh.on.ca/

Jamar Grip Dynamometry: A calibrated tool administered using a standardised protocol to measure grip strength (Fess 1992). This is commonly used as an indication of possible hand function (Goa et al. 2007).

Goniometry: A method of assessing joint range of motion in degrees with reliability depends on placement position and protocol use (Pratt et al. 2004).

Tape measure: Joint girth measurements to establish size or volumeter water displacement for overall hand size due to oedema (Pellecchia 2003).

Pain: Visual analogue scale to establish the pain level and allow simple reassessment to plot changes (Scudds 2001). Further information can be found at www.cebp.nl/vault_public/filesystem/?ID=1478

Osteoporosis is a chronic, progressive skeletal disease which weakens bone strength. It is characterised by low bone density and deterioration of bone tissue, and affects one in three women and one in 12 men over the age of 50 (World Health Organization 2003) and helps to explain why Val sustained such an injury from a small height. It has been reported that fractures of the distal forearm are strong predictors of subsequent fractures (Thompson et al. 2010) and therefore occupational therapists are well placed to advise patients of preventative measures.

Fractures of the distal radius are usually treated conservatively, involving a reduction of the fracture and immobilisation in a plaster of paris (POP) for usually six weeks (Handoll et al. 2006). An occupational therapist would usually only see a patient with this type of injury in Accident and Emergency (A&E) if their function was greatly compromised due to the fall or treatment. Following assessment of activities of daily living, assistive technology may be issued to enable safe and independent discharge.

Following a period of 6–8 weeks immobilisation, when the POP is removed it is not uncommon that the joints, grip and range of motion are usually compromised. In the older adult, such complications are generally more persistent and often require rehabilitation to regain function. Referral to an occupational therapist is usually received following an outpatient appointment when the POP is removed.

Following the removal of Val's POP, occupational therapists and physiotherapists would work as part of the multidisciplinary team to reach the treatment goals using a variety of assessments and outcome measures to guide their treatments as illustrated in Table 5.8. Additionally, it is good clinical practice to take a history of the injury to determine the force to the fracture site and identify other areas that might also have been compromised (Table 5.8).

In order to improve function and independence following such an injury, it is important to address the problems as illustrated using Val's situation (Box 5.8) and the International

---

Box 5.8 Val's difficulties with functioning due to upper limb fracture.

Body functions: reduced hand mobility and stiffness, increased oedema, pain and fatigue, reduced bone structure.

Activity limitations: driving, self care, shopping, cooking and cleaning.

Participation restriction: unable to volunteer in charity shop due to limiting body functions.

Contextual factors: lives with daughter a few days a week to continue collecting grandchildren from school, etc.

Classification of Functioning Disability and Health (ICF) framework (World Health Organization 2001).

Following the Val's assessment of her specific upper limb limitations treatment should include:

- Wrist, finger and thumb flexion, extension, span and opposition retraining
- Grip improvement/retraining
- Oedema management
- Encouragement to use hand functionally with minor assistive equipment to assist initially if required
- Osteoporosis preventive education including introduction of physical activity exercise programmes.

Thompson et al. (2010) highlighted the importance for therapists to not assume that patients with an upper limb injury from a fall have been screened for osteoporosis by other health care professionals. With this in mind, if osteoporosis screening hadn't been initiated for Val the occupational therapist should complete a Fracture Risk Assessment tool (FRAX) which was devised by the World Health Organisation in 2008. Further information about the tool is available on the FRAX website at http://www.shef.ac.uk/FRAX/tool.jsp.

Learning disability

Alison Lillywhite

Maureen is a 58-year-old lady with Down's Syndrome who lived with her sister and brother-in-law in a three-bedroom house. Maureen attended day services five days a week where she enjoyed observing people both within the services and out in the community. She also liked completing jigsaws, looking in magazines and making marks in a book. Maureen was able to undertake some personal care independently, but once dementia progressed she became increasingly passive and less motivated to complete tasks. Maureen was recently found on the floor and admitted to hospital with a fractured neck of femur and is currently in supported living accommodation.

Box 5.9   Maureen's difficulties with functioning.

Body functions: moderate learning disabilities, uses both hand gestures and vocalisation to communicate, limited vision, perceptual deficits, disorientated, reduced motivation, dysphagia, limited coordination.

Activity limitations: difficulty in communicating needs, needs assistance with mobility including transfers and steps, difficulties with eating and drinking, Self care – difficulties with washing and dressing, unable to perform domestic tasks.

Participation restriction: as dementia progressed unable to attend day services and increased assistance required with all personal and domestic activities of daily living.

Contextual factors: moved from living with family to a residential accommodation.

As life expectancy has increased, people with learning disabilities are living longer and these impact on the role of the occupational therapist. Consideration needs to be given to the person's age as well as their learning disability when occupational therapy assessments are undertaken. The National Service Framework for Older People (Department of Health 2001) emphasises that services need to be responding to the needs of older people with a learning disability. This is particularly important as persons with a learning disability often start the ageing process at an earlier age than the general population. Indeed, persons diagnosed with Down's Syndrome are at a greater risk of developing dementia and one in three people with Down's Syndrome may develop dementia in their 50s. Consequently, it is recommended that from the age of 30, persons with Down's Syndrome should have regular assessments to help identify any signs or symptoms of dementia (Alzheimer's Society 2011).

In this case study, Maureen has fractured her right neck of femur and is currently in supported living accommodation. This triggered a referral to the learning disability occupational therapists for advice around transfers. Maureen had difficulties accessing mainstream services due to her dementia and Down's Syndrome. The learning disability occupational therapist was based in an integrated community learning disability team which consisted of a variety of health professionals and those employed by social care. In many of these teams, the occupational therapist is a sole practitioner (Lillywhite and Haines 2010).

The importance of interagency work to ensure closer cooperation is important (Department of Health 2006, Alzheimer's Society 2011). Close collaboration will occur with the physiotherapist, the occupational therapists employed from social care and the support workers to ensure Maureen's physical needs are met. When the physiotherapist feels Maureen's mobility has reached a plateau, the occupational therapist could complete the Assessment of Motor and Process Skills (Fisher 1995) which has been discussed in Table 5.1. The Assessment of Motor and Process Skills assessment was used to gain a baseline assessment of Maureen's skills alongside broad functional assessment to ensure that her future accommodation needs were met (Lillywhite and Haines 2010).

Throughout the assessment process, it was noted that Maureen (Box 5.9) had significant difficulties with depth distance perception so it was important that access was level both internally and externally. Level access accommodation additionally catered for a potential deterioration in her mobility as the dementia progressed. Suitable accommodation for older people with a learning disability was identified for Maureen by the social worker.

During the transition process of moving home the occupational therapist worked with the support workers to identify suitable activities. Goodman and Locke (2009) emphasise the importance of enabling individuals to try new occupations that are meaningful and valued by them. These include maintaining family contact as well as using lights and sound to provide visual and auditory stimuli. Contact was made with learning disability employment services to establish if there was a volunteer who could visit Maureen and talk to her as she appeared to enjoy social contact.

As her physical skills were reduced, closer working relationships were established with the wheelchair services and social care occupational therapists. A joint assessment was completed with speech and language therapy, physiotherapy and occupational therapy to assess her eating and drinking skills following concerns regarding her aspirating on food.

Musculoskeletal problems/arthritis

Mary Grant

> *Betty Johnson is an 81-year-old woman who lives alone, with a long history of osteoarthritis. Her back, knees, ankles and hands are most affected. She is in a lot of pain and gets very stiff but is reluctant to take analgesic medication because of the side effects. However, she does take glucosamine tablets and other natural remedies. She has always been active and used to run her own corner shop. She is very fond of knitting, reading, watching films, doing jigsaws and is involved in her local church. Gardening is a great passion but she is no longer able to do it herself. She has quite a large family who she sees regularly. She used to go into town on the bus but has not done this since she had a fall in her kitchen a year ago. One of her daughters takes her shopping every week and she finds it hard to get in and out of the car. She is finding it increasingly difficult to get up and down the stairs in her house and also struggles to get up from her chair and toilet. Betty has just been referred to the community therapy team.*

Betty Johnson's narrative describes the impact of osteoarthritis on her life. Osteoarthritis is the most common form of arthritis and is a major cause of functional limitation, reduced participation in activities and decreased health-related quality of life in older people. Symptoms include pain, aching, stiffness and discomfort and management comprises pharmacological and non-pharmacological interventions such as surgery (Hochberg 2010). Osteoarthritis is characterised by a gradual degenerative process and low-grade inflammation but the abnormal changes that occur in the articular cartilage of people with the disease differ from the typical changes associated with joint ageing. Risk factors include lifestyle issues (obesity, engagement in manual labour) and risk is higher in women (Moskowitz 2009). Rheumatoid arthritis can present as a new onset disease in old age, but often is seen as a sequel to earlier onset disease and its impact is very similar to osteoarthritis and they can occur together (Jakobsson and Hallberg 2002).

Table 5.9   Key assessment and outcome measures used by occupational therapists with older people in musculoskeletal care.

Canadian Occupational Performance Measure [COPM] (Law et al. 1998)
Health Assessment Questionnaire (HAQ): A well-researched and evaluated self-report functional status measure (Bruce and Fries 2003)
Arthritis Impact Measurement Scales (AIMS2): A self-administered health status questionnaire tested on a mixed arthritis population. It measures functional ability, activity levels and psychosocial status (Meenan et al. 1992)

Occupational therapists work with people with arthritis in a number of different settings including secondary care (rheumatology, orthopaedics, hand therapy), primary care and social services. The scope of the intervention offered is very broad and includes activities of daily living (teaching new techniques and advice on assistive devices), pain management, splinting, psychosocial support, work and leisure adaptations and education on joint protection, energy conservation and self management techniques (Grant 2005). Occupational therapists work as part of a multidisciplinary team to provide services for people with arthritis which has shown to be effective in maintaining functional ability in community settings (Helewa et al. 1991, Hakala et al. 1994).

Betty Johnson is being seen by a community therapy team and her difficulties are described using the ICF (WHO 2001; also see Box 5.10). Table 5.9 outlines some assessments and outcome measures commonly used by occupational therapists in the musculoskeletal care of older people.

Occupational therapy aims for Betty are:

• To restore, maintain and enhance meaningful occupations
• To prevent loss or further loss of use of the joints affected by arthritis
• To teach pain management strategies
• To maintain health and wellbeing through health promotion and lifestyle strategies.

The provision of assistive devices such as chair raisers, raised toilet seat, stair rail, and grab rail at the back door into the garden will make daily occupations more manageable for Betty and less stressful for the joints and muscles. There is evidence that a focused home visit can prevent falling by reducing hazards in the home environment (Steultjens 2009). In addition, a Cochrane review concluded that occupational therapy has a positive effect on functional ability of patients with rheumatoid arthritis and that there is strong evidence for the effectiveness of instruction on joint protection (Steultjens et al 2004). Joint protection education is often provided by occupational therapists with the aim of reducing stress on the joints whilst participating in daily occupations. The principles of joint protection include:

• Awareness and respect for pain
• Distributing the load over several joints
• Using stronger and larger joints
• Using joints in their most stable and functional positions
• Avoiding positions of deformity.

Box 5.10   Betty's difficulties with functioning due to arthritis.

Body function/structures: pain and stiffness of back, knees, ankles and hands, fear of falling.

Activity limitations: difficulty getting off chair and toilet, difficulty managing stairs, difficulty getting into back garden.

Participation restriction: unable to do gardening, unable to use public transport to do her own shopping.

It is important to use an educational behavioural approach when teaching joint protection to increase its effectiveness (Hammond and Freeman 2004).

Occupational therapists teach energy conservation, work simplification techniques and pain management, including relaxation, to reduce pain and improve psycho-social functioning (Kessler 2001). The assessment and provision of splints is also a common occupational therapy role, with evidence of reduction in pain and also improved grip strength (Weiss et al. 2000, Steultjens et al. 2004).

Self management is continuing to be a popular concept and occupational therapists may refer people to the Expert Patient Programme which has shown to be a cost-effective way of helping people to maintain their independence and maximise their wellbeing (Plews 2005).

Occupational therapists have an important health promotion role, with other team members, incorporating education about musculoskeletal conditions and ways of preventing further deterioration of the joints whilst at the same time participating in balanced and meaningful occupations.

Parkinson's disease

Anne McIntyre

Mrs Wright's parkinsonian symptoms began 10 years ago. However, it was five years later, as a result of a fall in her garden and subsequent shoulder injury which required a visit to her local hospital A&E department, that she was diagnosed as having Parkinson's disease. Until this time, Mrs Wright was living alone in her own house, and was busy with her voluntary driving for the WRVS meals on wheels service, helping in the classroom at her local primary school and going out to various social activities with her friends.

After her fall, Mrs Wright moved out of her local area and went to live with her daughter and family. Although Mrs Wright enjoys her role as mother and grandmother, she feels a loss of autonomy and social isolation. Her bradykinesia, rigidity and tremor have got worse and she is now increasingly experiencing 'on-off' phenomena. A recent deterioration in her motor function has meant that she can no longer climb the stairs in her daughter's three-bedroomed house, and requires help with bed, chair and toilet transfers as well as getting dressed. Her loss of independence has led to her feeling low in mood and being slightly confused and anxious. However, Mrs Wright's daughter feels that this is because she is no longer interested in reading the newspaper or watching the television. She no longer wants to leave the house to visit friends or go shopping.

Parkinson's disease (PD) is the most common neuro-degenerative disease after Alzheimer's Disease, affecting 4 million people worldwide and 1% of over-60s and 2% of over-80-year-olds in the UK. The disease commonly starts between the ages of 40 and 70 and the cause is unknown. Parkinson's disease leads to extensive disability and is a frequent cause of falls, subsequent fractures and death. Diagnosis still depends on identification by signs and symptoms and, unfortunately, Parkinson's disease is often wrongly diagnosed (National Institute for Clinical Excellence [NICE] 2006, Scottish Intercollegiate Guidelines Network (SIGN) 2010). The cost of health and social care for people with Parkinson's disease in the UK is £3.3 billion annually (Porter et al. 2010).

The pathological changes that occur in PD are depletion of dopamine in the basal ganglia and the reticular formation, and it is said that Parkinson's disease symptoms manifest when there is approximately 50% loss of dopamine producing cells in these areas. It has been observed that the pathology of Parkinson's disease starts in the brain stem and progressively ascends to the cerebral cortex (Brooks 2000, Gibb 1997, Herrero et al. 2002, Parkinson's Disease Society 2007).

Like many other people, Mrs Wright's diagnosis was based upon what are considered the cardinal signs of Parkinson's disease – bradykinesia, tremor, rigidity and postural instability (Parkinson's Disease Society 2007, Jankovic 2008). There are other motor and non-motor signs and symptoms of Parkinson's disease that can be seen in Box 5.11.

Interestingly, some of the non-motor signs can predate the motor signs and diagnosis. Perhaps this is not too surprising as the basal ganglia are also involved in emotional, motivational, associative and cognitive functions.

Whilst there is no cure for PD, the management of the disease needs a multidisciplinary approach, involving both pharmacological and rehabilitative approaches. In the early stages of her PD, Mrs Wright was given Levodopa to manage her symptoms. Unfortunately, six years later, Mrs Wright is experiencing fluctuating motor control (on–off phenomenon) and some involuntary movements, which she finds upsetting and painful at times (Macphee and Stewart 2007).

The College of Occupational Therapists has recently published practice guidelines for people with PD (Aragon and Kings 2010). Although these are based upon best practice, feedback from clients and carers and the available evidence base, there is no high-level evidence to support (or refute) the efficacy of many of the therapies in Parkinson's disease (Dixon et al. 2009). Disappointingly, the content of occupational therapy interventions is not fully explained within the literature and the incidence and timing of client referrals to occupational therapy need to be investigated (Deane et al. 2001a, 2001b, Kale and Menken 2004, NICE 2006, Dixon et al. 2009). Despite the lack of evidence for occupational therapy, it is recommended that people with PD should receive occupational therapy and that the following should be considered (NICE 2006, p. 7):

- Maintenance of work and family roles, employment, home care and leisure activities
- Improvement and maintenance of transfers and mobility
- Improvement of personal self-care activities, such as eating, drinking, washing and dressing
- Environmental issues to improve safety and motor function
- Cognitive assessment and appropriate intervention.

Box 5.11   Example of motor and non-motor signs and symptoms of Parkinson's disease.

Early motor symptoms

Tremor*   )

Rigidity*   )   cardinal signs

Akinesia/bradykinesia*   )

Postural Instability   )

Hypokinesia

Asymmetric onset

Upper limb involvement

(*For diagnosis, bradykinesia MUST be present plus either rigidity or tremor)

Early non-motor symptoms

Mental health problems

Depression[§] (20–50% of PD population)

Anxiety[§] (25–40% of PD population)

Psychosis (visual hallucinations) (20–40% of PD population)

Cognitive impairment (30% of PD population) – switching attention, divided attention, selective attention, task management, motor planning

Fatigue[§] (30–60% of PD population)

Apathy[§]

Sleep disturbance[§] (incl. daytime somnolence)

Constipation[§]

Olfactory dysfunction[§]

(§ Can pre-date motor symptoms and diagnosis)

Later symptoms

Motor

Motor fluctuations (end-of-dose/on-off)

Dyskinesias, freezing, gait festination, postural instability, postural deformity, Dysphagia

Non-motor

Psychosis (paranoia), Impulsive control disorders (compulsive gambling or eating, hypersexuality), tip of the tongue phenomena

Dementia (50–80% of PD population)

Falls (66% of PD population)

Autonomic dysfunction – weight loss, constipation, bladder dysfunction, urinary incontinence, sexual dysfunction, orthostatic hypotension, excessive sweating, drooling and pain (40% of PD population)

(Horstinck et al. 2006a, 2006b, National Institute of Clinical Excellence 2006, Taylor et al. 2006, Friedman et al. 2007, Lieberman 2006, Macphee and Stewart 2007, Parkinson's Disease Society 2007, Jankovic 2008).

It is apparent that Mrs Wright would benefit from occupational therapy as she is experiencing many problems that are impacting upon her occupational performance (Box 5.12). For example, occupational therapists are particularly involved with managing mobility problems, especially in relation to preventing falls. An awareness of Mrs Wright's propensity to 'freeze in doorways or at steps' and her 'on-off' experiences mean that the occupational therapist needs to reinforce the falls prevention techniques given to Mrs Wright as well as providing acceptable environmental adaptations. Mobility difficulties in relation to dressing and other self-care activities also need to be addressed and a good

---

Box 5.12   Mrs Wright's problems in functioning with Parkinson's disease.

Body functions: bradykinesia and rigidity in both upper and lower limbs, with tremor in her upper limbs.

Activity limitations: Mobility and transfers – particularly climbing stairs, moving in bed, transferring on and off bed, chair or toilet. No longer able to drive her car or walk outdoors unassisted. Has help with dressing and cutting up food. Has limited leisure occupations

Participation restrictions: Not wanting to socialise with friends, not carrying out chosen occupations, such as reading and watching television.

Contextual factors: lives with her daughter and grandchildren in a 3-bedroomed house with stairs. Does not know the local environment that well and has no links with local community. Has a loss of autonomy and feelings of independence.

Table 5.10   Assessment and outcome measures for persons with Parkinson's disease.

Movement Disorder Society (MDS)-sponsored revision of the Unified Parkinson's Disease Rating Scale (MDS-UPDRS). The MDS-UDPRS has four parts: (Part 1) Non-motor Experiences of Daily Living; (Part 2) Motor Experiences of Daily Living; (Part 3) Motor Examination; (Part 4) Motor Complications. Twenty questions are completed by the patient/caregiver (Goetz et al. 2008).
The Parkinson's Disease Questionnaire [PDQ 39 and PDQ 8] (Jenkinson et al. 2008). Patients are asked to think about their health and general wellbeing and to consider how often in the last month they have experienced certain events. The PDQ 8 is the shorter version of the PDQ 39. It is frequently used in research studies. Further information is available at http://www.publichealth.ox.ac.uk/research/hsru/PDQ/Intropdq

resource to guide intervention is the COT guide by Aragon and Kings (2010). It is also important that the occupational therapist considers Mrs Wright's leisure and social activities to facilitate her health and wellbeing and also be cognisant of the needs of Mrs Wright's daughter in her role as carer. Fatigue has been noted people with PD and excessive daytime sleepiness (EDS) is also common in patients with Parkinson's disease (Tandberg et al. 1999, Miwa and Miwa 2011). In this event, it is essential that a multidisciplinary approach is taken and that the team examines factors which could result in excessive daytime sleepiness including depression, poor sleep hygiene, and drugs associated with altered sleep pattern (Scottish Intercollegiate Network 2010b).

As with all older adults, occupational therapists need to assess and be aware of signs of dementia with this client group. One study found that over a period of three to five years, 10% developed dementia (Williams-Gray et al. 2007). In the case of Mrs Wright, it is essential that the occupational therapist, along with other members of the team, obtains a detailed history and assesses both memory and mood. In addition, occupational therapists need to beware of psychosis and, in PD, visual hallucinations are the most prevalent manifestation occurring between 30–40% of hospital-based patients (Williams-Gray et al. 2006). Depression is common in persons with Parkinson's and various assessment tools can be used, including the Geriatric Depression Scale (GDS) and Hospital Anxiety and Depression Scale (HADS). See Table 5.10 for assessment and outcome measures for persons with Parkinson's disease.

Schizophrenia

Jacqueline Lawson

> *Frank is a 77-year-old gentleman with a diagnosis of paranoid schizophrenia. Frank is retired, has never been married and does not have any children, his next of kin is a brother with whom he has no contact. Frank was diagnosed with schizophrenia at the age of 30 following a serious incident of deliberate self-harm whereby he stabbed himself in the belief he was possessed by evil spirits. Frank has been admitted to hospital on numerous occasions throughout his life due to repeated paranoid delusions that his home is bugged and that his thoughts have been projected so that others can hear them. Frank also suffers from auditory hallucinations that inform him it is not safe to eat and drink.*

Studies and research into schizophrenia in older people are limited; indeed, only 6% of the literature relates to the study of schizophrenia in later life (Jeste 1996). Prevalence of schizophrenia in older adults is unclear. Using the core diagnostic criteria amongst the general adult population, schizophrenia is said to have a mean incidence of approximately 0.11 per 1000 (National Institute for Clinical Excellence 2010(b)). In older people, schizophrenia has been stated to affect a similar proportion of people, approximately 1% of the population (Gurland and Cross 1982); however, it has been suggested that true prevalence figures have been underestimated (Palmer et al. 1999) and the number of older people with a diagnosis of schizophrenia is anticipated to substantially increase (Cohen et al. 2000).

It is important to recognise Frank was diagnosed with schizophrenia in his 30s and does not have the condition frequently termed 'late onset paraphrenia' or late onset psychosis. This term is used to describe older people who develop a psychotic condition for the first time in their older years; over the age of 55 (Clare and Giblin 2008).

Symptoms of schizophrenia are usually classified as either positive or negative (Turner 1997, Comer 1998, Gelder et al. 1998). Positive symptoms refer to the presence of hallucinations and delusions (Gelder et al. 1999) – in Frank's case his beliefs about being possessed, his house being bugged, his thoughts being projected and his auditory hallucinations. The term 'negative symptoms' generally refers to loss of functioning (Gelder et al. 1999); Frank is displaying these symptoms through his self-neglect, social isolation and possible inability to continue living independently (Box 5.13).

A diagnosis of schizophrenia has been defined in the 4th edition of the *Diagnostic and Statistical Manual of Mental Disorders* (DSM-IV) as:

> "…a disorder that lasts for at least 6 months and includes at least 1 month of active-phase symptoms (i.e., two [or more] of the following: delusions: hallucinations, disorganised speech, grossly disorganised or catatonic behaviour, negative symptoms." (American Psychiatric Association 2000)

Frank has a diagnosis of paranoid schizophrenia. A diagnosis for paranoid-type schizophrenia may be made if preoccupation with one or more delusions or frequent auditory

---

Box 5.13   Frank's difficulties with functioning due to schizophrenia.

Temperament and personality functions: mild impairment of psychic stability, moderate impairment in confidence, moderate impairment in motivation, moderate impairment in content of thought.

Activities and participation: mild difficulty in thinking, specifically decision making.

Self care: mild difficulty in washing whole body, moderate difficulty in preparing simple meals, severe difficulty in forming relationships.

Environmental factors: no immediate family available to provide support and also no friends to provide ongoing and mutual support.

---

hallucinations is present, but disorganised speech, disorganised or catatonic behaviour, or flat or inappropriate affect is not prominent (American Psychiatric Association 2000).

It is suggested that the severity of negative symptoms worsen as people with schizophrenia age (Gur et al. 1996). Alongside this worsening of negative symptoms is the concern of medication side effects. Anti-psychotic medication (such as the Clozapine prescribed to Frank) may have multiple side effects; however, of specific concern in older people is the adverse effect these medications may have upon motor functioning. The most commonly-reported side effects are related to motor functioning including abnormal, involuntary movements such as tardive dyskinesia (Palmer et al. 1999). In older people this can greatly influence occupational performance and the ability to engage with activities of daily living. Anti-psychotic medications also increase the risk and incidence of falls amongst older people (National Institute of Clinical Excellence 2004b).

Frank evidently has a treatment-resistant schizophrenia in order for Clozapine to have been prescribed. This anti-psychotic is prescribed to those who demonstrate treatment resistance (Bazire 2003); it is not the initial drug of choice due its potential to severely affect white blood cell count. For this reason, people who are prescribed Clozapine require regular blood tests and physical health checks. Side effects of anti-psychotics also need to be closely monitored, and this is achieved through the use of rating scales such as the Liverpool University Neuroleptic Side Effect Rating Scale (LUNSERS) (Day et al. 1995).

Schizophrenia can cause occupational dysfunction (Bejerholm 2010). This decrease in functional ability, whether it is caused by mere presence or worsening of symptoms or medication side effects, may often necessitate the need for occupational therapy intervention. Occupational therapists can have a substantial role to play in aiding the individual recognise their abilities and also to problem solve, adapt and recommend assistance with certain activities the individual feels he or she are no longer able to manage.

With current drives in mental health to focus upon recovery (Department of Health 2009b, Future Vision Coalition 2009), it is important to maintain a strengths focus with individuals. Recovery might happen even after many years and it should also be recognised that, despite continued symptoms, many people with schizophrenia can achieve meaningful lifestyles (National Institute for Health and Clinical Excellence 2010b). Maintaining this strengths focus and acknowledgement of abilities could also serve as a preventative measure against additional, more common mental illnesses such as depression in old age, and promote concepts such as active ageing as recommended by the World Health Organization (WHO 2002). Ongoing symptoms of psychosis can be monitored by the multidisciplinary team, through the use of tools such as the Brief Psychiatric Rating Scale (BPRS) (Overall and Gorham 1962, 1988).

In the case of Frank, the occupational therapist would initially need to establish his preferences regarding the future, including his individual long- and short-term goals. This could be done through a variety of means, including the use of the Occupational Self Assessment (OSA) (Baron et al. 2006) or through the Recovery Star (Mackeith and Burns 2010); both of these measures can also be utilised to outcome interventions.

If Frank identified a preference for returning to his home environment, his occupational performance would need to be ascertained. This could be achieved informally through conversation with Frank, provided he has good insight, or through more standardised means such as use of the Model of Human Occupation Screening Tool (MOHOST) (Parkinson et al. 2006) or Assessment of Motor and Process Skills (AMPS) (Fisher 2006). Once a baseline level of performance is established, Frank and the occupational therapist can devise a treatment/intervention plan which support his goals and promotes his recovery. Both the MOHOST and the AMPS can be repeated and utilised as an outcome measure of occupational therapy intervention. Following intervention, the repeat MOHOST or AMPS may establish whether there has been any improvement in occupational performance, whereas use of the Recovery Star could demonstrate more global improvements in life domains such as relationships and responsibilities.

Frank has been working with the psychologist, learning to ignore the impulses he has to act upon his auditory hallucinations. In addition, Frank has expressed that he would like to return to his home environment but, in order to do so, feels he needs to take control and improve his nutritional intake, ensuring his daily dietary needs are met. Whilst he remains an in-patient, Frank attends the supper cooking group run jointly by the occupational therapist and the dietician. This group intervention has multiple aims for Frank, improving his occupational performance in cooking tasks but also teaching him how to manage healthy eating on a budget, encouraging him to form and maintain social relationships and reduce his social isolation. A single observation MOHOST (see Table 5.1: Bi-polar) is completed post each group intervention and Frank's progress is monitored. The occupational performance scores produced by the MOHOST also serve to advise the multidisciplinary team on how much assistance Frank requires with other activities of daily living (such as washing and dressing).

After he had attended a number of supper cooking groups, Frank reported feeling more confident in the kitchen but that he also enjoyed the social aspect of the group, forming a friendship with another gentleman from the same ward. The occupational therapist liaised with the social worker and community mental health team and recommended attendance at a luncheon club twice per week post discharge. As Frank's discharge date approached he was encouraged to go on leave from the ward and attend the identified luncheon group to ease transition from hospital to the community. Initially, Frank was escorted to the luncheon club by the occupational therapist to ease his anxiety, build his self-confidence and ensure practicalities of attendance were addressed, for example which bus to catch and that he had the correct finances available.

The role of the occupational therapist may extend beyond Frank being an in-patient. Although not related specifically to older people, the literature suggests there is a role for OTs working with people with schizophrenia to establish levels of occupational engagement (Bejerholm and Ecklund 2006, 2007), ensure an optimal level of occupational balance is achieved (Bejerholm 2010), and to advise upon occupational choice and the implications of this choice upon wellbeing, including stress and life satisfaction (Minato and Zemke 2004).

Stroke

Thérèse Jackson

James Clark is a 68-year-old man who had a left hemisphere Total Anterior Circulation Stroke (TACS) 18 months ago, resulting in a right-sided hemiplegia with motor and sensory deficits. He has increased tome in his right arm and leg. He also has a homonymous hemianopia, expressive dysphasia, and apraxia which affects his ability to plan and execute movements effectively.

Mr Clark is retired and lives at home with his wife in a privately-owned bungalow. They have a daughter who lives nearby. Mr Clark's wife is fit and healthy. She is able to help him with personal care and can attend to domestic activities at home, such as cooking and housework.

Mr Clark is able to stand for limited periods and is mobile over short distances indoors. He requires the use of a wheelchair for longer distances and when outdoors. He is able to transfer on and off his toilet and chair, but requires assistance for bath transfers and with washing and dressing. He has recently been finding it difficult to get out of the house and enjoy some of their free time together. He has become less independent than he was on discharge from hospital 15 months ago.

Stroke is a clinical syndrome characterised by an acute loss of focal cerebral function with symptoms lasting for more than 24 hours or leading to death. It is thought to be due to either spontaneous haemorrhage into the brain substance (haemorrhagic stroke) or inadequate cerebral blood supply to part of the brain (ischaemic stroke) (Warlow et al. 2007). Stroke can be sub-classified according to the area of damage, i.e. Total Anterior Circulation Stroke (TAC); Lacunar Stroke (LAC); Partial Anterior Circulation Stroke (PAC); and Posterior Circulation Stroke (POC). To determine stroke type, a last letter is added, e.g. S – Syndrome,. TACS; I – Infarct, TACI, H – Haemorrhage, TACH (Bamford et al. 1991). Globally, stroke is the second most common cause of death, after heart disease. Annually, almost 10% of worldwide deaths (over 5 million) are caused by stroke. A significant and lasting impact of stroke is long-term disability and it is the most common cause of severe physical disability amongst adults in the UK (Wolfe 2000, Adamson et al. 2004).

The strongest risk factor for ischaemic stroke is increasing age, with an 80-year-old having 30 times the risk of ischaemic stroke as a 30-year-old. (Rothwell et al. 2005). The symptoms of stroke can include: unilateral weakness or sensory disturbance; visual

---

Box 5.14   Mr Clark's difficulties with functioning due to stroke.

Body function/structures: mental functions, apraxia – cognitive motor planning disorder which affects his ability to sequence complex movements, aphasia – language problem, fatigue.

Sensory functions: homonymous hemianopia (visual field loss to his right), sensory loss on the right side of the body.

Muscle functions: weakness/loss of power on the right side of the body, altered muscle tone on the right side of the body

Activity limitations:
communicating: difficulty with both verbal and written communication
mobility: lifting and carrying objects, walking and moving around
self care: problems with eating, washing and dressing
Domestic life: unable to perform most household tasks, e.g. cooking and cleaning

Participation restrictions:
interpersonal interactions and relationships, loss of role within family structure, i.e. father and husband
community, social and civic life: unable to participate in previous social and leisure atcivities

---

disturbance; problems with speech and language; swallowing difficulty (dysphagia); cognitive and perceptual disorders; and emotional and psychological problems.

Stroke can be a long-term condition and the occupational therapist may intervene at any stage of the person's pathway, from acute to community care. The issues that might need to be addressed are demonstrated in terms of the ICF. Following stroke, people may experience difficulties performing everyday activities and participating in meaningful activities. The varied and often complex nature of occupational dysfunction experienced as a result of stroke requires specialised assessment and treatment, provided by an occupational therapist with expertise in stroke care (Box 5.14).

Occupational therapy assessment of stroke at any stage of recovery mighty include a detailed analysis of motor, sensory, cognitive, psychological and social performance skills, and the impact of any deficits on a person's ability to perform self care, domestic, work and leisure activities within a defined environment, i.e. physical, social and cultural.

The occupational therapist could use a combination of observation and standardised assessments to identify performance deficits (Table 5.11). National Clinical Guidelines for Stroke produced for England (Intercollegiate Stroke Working Party 2008) and for Scotland (Scottish Intercollegiate Network [SIGN] 2010(c)) make several evidence-based, best practice recommendations for stroke care. These include the need for early access to coordinated and specialised multidisciplinary stroke care, provided on a stroke unit. Specialised therapy-based community rehabilitation services, including early supported discharge, if a specialised stroke team is available, are also advised. Rehabilitation should be goal-focused and patient-centred. Both of these national stroke guidelines highlight the need for all patients who have problems with activities of daily living following stroke to have access to an occupational therapist with specific knowledge and expertise in neurological care. More specifically, personal activity of daily living (ADL)

Table 5.11 Key assessment tools used by occupational therapists in stroke care.

AMPS – Assessment of Motor and Process Skills (Fisher 1995)

BADS – Behavioural Assessment of Dysexecutive Syndrome (Wilson et al. 1996);
http://www.dwp.gov.uk/docs/no2-sum-03-test-review-2.pdf

CAM – Cognitive Assessment of Minnesota (Rustard et al. 1993); http://www.worldcat.org/
title/cognitive-assessment-of-minnesota-examiners-guide/oclc/28947896?tab=details

COTNAB – Chessington Occupational Therapy Neurological Assessment Battery (Tyerman
et al. 1986); http://www.saetrahealth.co.za/cognitive_assessment/cotnab.html

MEAMS – Middlesex Elderly Assessment of Mental State (Golding 1989)
http://www.pearsonclinical.co.uk/Psychology/AdultCognitionNeuropsychologyandLanguage/
AdultGeneralAbilities/MiddlesexElderlyAssessmentofMentalState(MEAMS)/Middlesex
ElderlyAssessmentofMentalState(MEAMS).aspx

Rivermead Behavioural Inattention Test (Wilson et al. 1987)

Rivermead Perceptual Assessment Battery (Whiting et al. 1985)

Rivermead Behavioural Memory Test-111 (Wilson et al. 2008)
https://www.pearsonclinical.co.uk/Psychology/AdultCognitionNeuropsychologyandLanguage/
AdultAttentionExecutiveFunction/BehaviouralInattentionTest(BIT)/BehaviouralInattention
Test(BIT).aspx

TEA – Test of Everyday Attention (Robertson et al. 1994) http://www.pearsonassessments.
com/HAIWEB/Cultures/en-us/Productdetail.htm?Pid=015-8054-458

training by an occupational therapist is recommended as part of in-patient and community rehabilitation. Patient-centred goals and a programme of purposeful activity are usual in stroke rehabilitation settings. Occupation is used as a therapeutic medium in the treatment of stroke by occupational therapists and a combination of restorative and functional approaches are used.

A systematic review produced by Legg et al. (2007) included nine trials with 1258 participants to assess the effectiveness of occupational therapy interventions for patients with problems in ADL after a stroke. The review found that people were more independent in personal activities such as feeding, dressing, bathing, toileting and moving about, and were more likely to maintain these abilities if they received treatment from an occupational therapist. The detail of the interventions is still, however, not fully defined. Walker et al. (2004) carried out a meta-analysis of randomised controlled trials of community occupational therapy for stroke patients and found that it significantly improved personal and extended activities of daily living and leisure activity in patients with stroke. They also concluded that targeted interventions produced better outcomes, e.g. leisure therapy improved leisure scores.

Whilst there is good evidence to support occupational therapy for people with stroke, there remain many other treatment approaches and methods which have insufficient evidence to either support or refute their effectiveness. The most common physical treatment approaches used by occupational therapists in the UK, often in combination with a functional approach, include facilitation of motor performance in activities using Bobath or Motor relearning (Carr and Shepherd 1989). The evidence does not support one treatment over the other, so a combination is often used within the multidisciplinary team.

A systematic review of the evidence found insufficient evidence to either support or refute the effectiveness of hand splinting for adults after stroke (Lanin and Herbert 2003). A randomised controlled trial found that hand splints did not demonstrate short-term ability to manage contracture. They advised that other methods of stretch, which provided a greater degree of intensity of stretch through the muscles, might be more beneficial (Lanin et al. 2007). Use of specific cognitive strategies could be incorporated in to a treatment plan. These may be remedial or compensatory, to adapt for lost performance components and to aid more independent functioning. Interventions are generally more effective if they are task-orientated and performed in an appropriate and relevant environment.

A functional approach using meaningful and purposeful activity would be appropriate for James. To address his physical problems, facilitation of normal movement in activities of daily living and fatigue management is recommended. James's positioning and seating could be addressed by the occupational therapist to ensure comfort, safety and maximal function. A goal-orientated approach is advocated and practice of daily living activities with an occupational therapist experienced in stroke care is likely to enable him to better perform and maintain self-care tasks and to reduce the risk of deterioration.

Constraint Induced Movement Therapy (CIMT) is emerging as an evidence-based intervention for people who have developed a learned non-use of their upper limb (Sitori et al. 2009) but have some motor return (10 degrees of finger extension, intact balance) and intact cognition. CIMT would not be advised in James's case as he does not meet the criteria for these interventions. For James's cognitive problems (apraxia) the evidence suggests using principles of cognitive rehabilitation, including: using activities in context; task-specific training (nongeneralisation of skills); practice and repetition; goal-directed activity and structured tasks (Edmans 2010). Multidisciplinary team-working and involvement of family and carers is usually appropriate if the patient agrees.

Falls in older people

Anne McIntyre

Many of the case studies within this chapter have discussed falling as part of their story. For older people like Darragh with dementia, Maureen with learning disability, Mrs Wright with PD and James with stroke, their health conditions are predisposing factors for falls. However, in Val's situation, her colles fracture occurred as a result of a fall. For all of these individuals, interventions should be offered to prevent further falls and any subsequent injury or psychological consequences.

Falls are considered one of the giants of health and social care because of the consequentially high rates of physical trauma, disability, admission to hospital or long-term care, or death. With the increase in the average age of the global population, falls and their consequences are predicted as an increasing burden on health and social care (Rubenstein 2006, Gilbert et al. 2009). Falls management is therefore perceived to be an important part of healthcare provision for older people.

Box 5.15   Definition of a fall.

A fall is:

"an unexpected event in which the participant comes to rest on the ground, floor or lower level."
(Lamb et al. 2005, p. 1619)

Falls are the fifth leading cause of death in older people (Rubenstein 2006). It is estimated that approximately 25% of people aged 70+ and 50% of those aged 80+ fall at least once a year. However, this is considered a conservative estimate as not all falls are reported (Martin 2009) and there is no consensus definition of a fall within the research literature and policy documents (Hauer et al. 2006). However, Lamb et al. (2005) have attempted to provide a definition of falls that has international consensus (see Box 5.15).

Another issue is that it is difficult to identify the cause of most falls, and falls management is therefore often problematic (Close 2005). It is recognised that multiple risk factors increase the likelihood of falls (National Institute of Clinical Excellence 2004(b)), with the greater the number of risk factors, the higher the risk (Close et al. 2003, United States of America Centres for Disease Control and Prevention 2008, American Geriatric Society and British Geriatric Society 2010). The National Institute of Clinical Excellence (2004b) state the following as the most common multiple-risk factors:

- Poly-pharmacy
- Mobility problems, especially as a result of balance problems and/or muscle weakness
- Chronic health conditions (e.g. stroke, Parkinson's disease)
- Sensory impairments (e.g. visual or proprioceptive)
- Reduced ability in carrying out everyday activities
- Environmental hazards and/or incorrect use of assistive technology.

However, it is acknowledged that single-risk factors such as cognitive impairment also significantly increase the risk of falling (Tinetti and Williams 1998). Therefore, it can be seen that many of the people described in the case studies within this chapter would be at high risk of falling.

There are also psychological consequences of falls, such as fear of falling, depression, loss of self-efficacy, and autonomy (Lord et al. 2007). There are also consequences for carers when their older care-recipient falls, such as increases in carer burden and carer strain (Saltz et al. 1999, Kuzuya et al. 2006), and for carers of people with dementia that fall, changes in relationship and also loss of identity of the carer (McIntyre and Reynolds 2012).

Occupational therapy plays an integral part in falls management and prevention, as part of a multidisciplinary team. For older people who fall, multifactorial interventions are perceived as being the most effective by Cochrane reviews (Gillespie et al. 2009). A recent randomised control trial of community-living older people who had fallen (Logan et al. 2010) was seen to significantly reduce further falls by 55% in the following 12 months, whilst also reducing fear of falling, the number of calls to the ambulance service asking for help with getting up off the floor, and improving everyday activity.

This study specifically identified occupational therapy elements to the multifactorial intervention, which had individualised intervention goals for each participant. The key areas for intervention in the study that are pertinent to occupational therapy are (Logan et al. 2010):

- Strength and balance training
- Health and safety checks
- Provision of equipment and home adaptation
- Teaching getting up off the floor and group training.

Although these multifactorial interventions work with cognitively normal older people, there is little evidence for their use with older people with cognitive impairment, such as Darragh with dementia or Maureen with learning disability (Jensen et al. 2003, Shaw et al. 2003, Hauer et al. 2006). However, many international policies advocate a client-centred and individualised approach to falls management with older people with cognitive impairment (Australian Commission on Safety and Quality in Health Care [ACSQHC] 2009) and that research evidence must be built for this group of older people who fall (Shaw 2007, Gillespie et al. 2009, American Geriatric Society and British Geriatric Society 2010).

There are many policies and guidance written about falls management (American Geriatric Society and British Geriatric Society (2010), National Institute of Clinical Excellence (2004b – reviewed in 2011). The College of Occupational Therapists also produces professional guidance to therapists on falls management (College of Occupational Therapists 2006) which advocates the use of evidence-based practice in assessment intervention and evaluation. What is advocated is a client-centred approach to identify the individual needs of the older person who has fallen, to identify those at risk and those with occupational performance difficulties. Therefore, many of the assessments suggested in the guidelines have already been described in this chapter in relation to the differing health conditions discussed. However, more specific outcome measures can also be used, with these relating to psycho-social aspects of falling. See Table 5.12 for assessment and outcome measures for falls.

Sadly, none of these measures are validated for older people with dementia or cognitive impairment and therefore, although they might be appropriate to be used with Val, Mrs Wright and James, they would not be valid or reliable measures to be used with Darragh or Maureen.

It is also interesting to note that, although the evidence for falls intervention is increasing, the uptake of falls management programmes by older people can be low, with approximately 30–70% of older people refusing to participate or not adhering to the intervention. It would seem that participating in falls programmes or taking up of environmental adaptations threaten older people's perceptions of identity and autonomy (Simpson et al. 2003). Yardley et al. (2006a,b) identified that falls carry the stigma of associated ageing and frailty, with falls advice and intervention being seen as irrelevant, patronising and interfering. It therefore seems even more important for occupational therapists to carry out falls management and prevention that are 'user-friendly', client-centred and individualised to each older person's needs and fit within the principles of occupational justice, active and successful ageing.

Table 5.12   Assessment and outcome measures for falls.

Balance confidence
Activities-specific Balance Confidence (ABC) Scale (Powell and Myers 1995)
http://www.pacificbalancecenter.com/forms/abc_scale.pdf

CONFBal (Simpson et al. 1998) http://www.feedslibrary.scot.nhs.uk/media/CLT/
ResourceUploads/4002429/CONFbal.pdf

Fear of falling
Falls Efficacy Scale (Tinetti et al. 1990) http://consultgerirn.org/uploads/File/trythis/try_
this_29.pdf

Falls Efficacy Scale International [FES-1] (Yardley et al. 2005) http://eprints.soton.ac.
uk/40199/1/6.pdf

Survey of Activities of Fear of Falling – SAFFE (Lachman et al. 1998) http://www.ecu.edu/
cs-dhs/encfpc/upload/17-SAFFE.pdf

Environmental assessments
HOME FAST (Mackenzie et al. 2000, 2002, 2003) http://www.bhps.org.uk/falls/documents/
HomeFast.pdf

Safety Assessment of Function and the Environment for Rehabilitation – SAFER
(Oliver et al. 1993) http://www.caot.ca/cjot_pdfs/cjot60/60.2oliver.pdf

Westmead Home Safety Assessment (Clemson 1997)

Summary

The challenge for occupational therapists is to ensure that all interventions are based on best evidence. Moreover, outcome measures need to be utilised in practice to demonstrate that outcomes and/or goals have been achieved. Older adults and their carers must be given choices about the types of interventions that are available, and must play an active part in decision making and empowered to do so.

References

Adamson, J., Beswick, A. and Ebrahim, S. (2004) Is stroke the most common cause of disability? *Journal of Stroke and Cerebrovascular Diseases* **13**, 171–177.

Allen, C.K., Earhart, C.A. and Blue, T. (1992) *Occupational Therapy Treatment Goals for the Physically and Cognitively Disabled*. USA: The American Occupational Therapy Association.

Alzheimer's Society (2007) *Dementia UK: The full report*. London: Alzheimer's Society.

Alzheimer's Society (2011) *Learning Disabilities and Dementia*. London: Alzheimer's Society. Available at: http://alzheimers.org.uk/site/scripts/documents_info.php?documentID=103

American Geriatric Society and British Geriatric Society (2010) Prevention of falls in older persons: AGS/BGS clinical practice guideline. Available at: http://www.americangeriatrics.org/health_care_professionals/clinical_practice/clinical_guidelines_recommendations/2010/

American Heart Association (2009) Classification of functional capacity and objective assessment. American Heart Association. Available at: http://circ.ahajournals.org/content/116/3/329.full.pdf

American Psychiatric Association (2000) *Diagnostic and Statistical Manual of Mental Disorders*, 4th edition, text revision). Washington, DC: American Psychiatric Association.

Aragon A. and Kings, J. (2010) Occupational therapy for people with Parkinson's disease: Best practice guidelines. London: College of Occupational Therapists. Available at: http://www. parkinsons.org.uk/pdf/OTParkinsons_guidelines.pdf

Australian Commission on Safety and Quality in Health Care (2009) Preventing falls and harm from falls in older people: Best practice guidelines for Australian community care. Commonwealth of Australia: Department of Health and Ageing.

Bamford., J., Sandercock, P., Dennis, M. et al. (1991) Classification and natural history of clinically identifiable subtypes of cerebral infarction. *Lancet* **337(8756)**, 1521–1526.

Baron, K., Kielhofner, G., Iyenger, A., Goldhammer, V. and Wolenski, J. (2006) Occupational Self Assessment (OSA) Version 2.2, 2006. Available at: http://www.uic.edu/depts/moho/assess/ osa.html

Bartels, S.J., Forester, B., Miles, K. and Joyce, T. (2008) Mental health service use by elderly patients with bipolar disorder and unipolar major depression. *American Journal of Geriatric Psychiatry* **8(2)**, 160–166.

Bazire, S. (2003) *Psychotropic Drug Directory 2003/04: The professionals' pocket handbook and aide memoire.* Wiltshire: Fivepin Publishing.

Bejerholm, U. (2010) Occupational balance with schizophrenia. *Occupational Therapy in Mental Health* **26**, 1–17.

Bejerholm, U. and Ecklund, M. (2006) Profiles of occupational engagement in people with schizophrenia, POES: Development of a new instrument based on time-use diaries. *British Journal of Occupational Therapy* **69(2)**, 58–68.

Bejerholm, U. and Ecklund, M. (2007) Occupational engagement in persons with schizophrenia: Relationships to self-related variables, psychopathology and quality of life. *American Journal of Occupational Therapy* **61(1)**, 21–32.

Bennett, S. and Liddle, J. (2008) Community-based occupational therapy improved daily functioning in people with dementia. *Australian Occupational Therapy Journal* **55(1)**, 73–74.

Borg, G.A. (1982) Psychophysical bases of perceived exertion. *Medicine and Science in Sports and Exercise* **14(5)**, 377–381.

Brazier, J.E., Harper, R., Jones, N.M.B., O'Cathain, A., Thomas, K.J., Usherwood, T. et al. (1992) Validating the SF-36 health survey questionnaire: New outcome measure for primary care. *British Medical Journal* **305**, 160–164.

Brissos, S., Videira, Dias V. and Kapczinski, F. (2008) Cognitive performance and quality of life in bipolar disorder. *Canadian Journal of Psychiatry* **53(8)**, 517–524.

British Heart Foundation (BHF) (2009) Living with heart failure. Available at: http://www.bhf.org. uk/publications/view-publication.aspx?ps=1000873

British Thoracic Society (2006) The burden of lung disease: A statistic report from the British Thoracic Society. Available at: http://www.brit-thoracic.org.uk/Portals/0/Library/BTS%20 Publications/burden_of_lung_disease.pdf

Brooks, D.J. (2000) Imaging basal ganglia function. *Journal of Anatomy* **196(4)**, 543–554.

Bruce, B. and Fries, J.F. (2003) The Stanford Health Assessment Questionnaire: Dimensions and practical applications. *Health and Quality of Life Outcomes* **1**, 1–20.

Bucks, R.S., Ashworth, D.L., Wilcock, G.K. and Siegfried, K. (1996) Assessment of Activities of Daily Living in Dementia: Development of the Bristol Activities of Daily Living Scale. *Age and Ageing* **25(2)**, 113–120.

Cancer Research (2010) Summary of Cancer Incidence and Mortality in the UK Cancer Research UK. Available from: http://www.cancerresearchuk.org

Carr, J.H. and Shepherd, R.B. (1989) A motor learning model for stroke rehabilitation. *Physiotherapy* **75(7)**, 372–380.

Clare, L. and Giblin, S. (2008) Late onset psychosis. In: Woods, R. and Clare, L. (eds) *Handbook of the Clinical Psychology of Aging*, 2nd edition. Chichester: John Wiley and Sons.

Clemson, L. (1997) *Home Fall Hazards and the Westmead Home Safety Assessment*. West Brunswick: Coordinates Publications.

Close, J.C.L. (2005) Prevention of falls in older people. *Disability and Rehabilitation* **27(18–19)**, 1061–1071.

Close, J., Hooper, R., Glucksman, E., Jackson, S.H.D. and Swift, C.G. (2003) Predictors of falls in a high risk population: Results from the prevention of falls in the elderly trial. *Emergency Medicine Journal* **20(5)**, 421–425.

Cohen, C.L., Cohne, G.D., Blank, K., Gaitz, C., Katz, I.R., Leuchter, A., Maletta, G., Meyers, B., Sakauye, K. and Shamoian, C. 2000. Schizophrenia and older adults. *American Journal of Geriatric Psychiatry* **8(1)**, 19–28.

Comer, R.J. (1998) *Abnormal Psychology*, 3rd edition. New York: Freeman and Company.

College of Occupational Therapists (2004) *Occupational Therapy Intervention in Cancer: Guidance for professionals, managers and decision-makers*. London: College of Occupational Therapists.

College of Occupational Therapists (2006) *Guidance: Falls management*. London: College of Occupational Therapists.

College of Occupational Therapists (2008) *Health Promotion in Occupational Therapy*. London: College of Occupational Therapists.

Cooper, J. (2007) *Occupational Therapy in Oncology and Palliative Care*, 2nd edition. Chichester: John Wiley & Sons.

Coryell, W., Fiedorowicz, J., Solomon, D. and Endicott, J. (2009) Age transitions in the course of bipolar I disorder. *Psychological Medicine* **39(8)**, 1247–1252.

Day, J.C., Wood, G., Dewey, M. and Bentall, R.P. (1995) A self-rating scale for measuring neuro-leptic side effects. Validation in a group of schizophrenic patients. *British Journal of Psychiatry* **166(5)**, 650–653.

Deane, K.H.O., Ellis-Hill, C., Playford, E.D., Ben-Shlomo, Y. and Clarke, C.E. (2001a) Occupational therapy for Parkinson's disease (review). Cochrane Database of Systematic Reviews.

Deane, K.H.O., Jones, D., Ellis-Hill, C., Clarke, C.E., Playford, E.D. and Ben-Shlomo, Y. (2001b) Physiotherapy for Parkinson's disease: A comparison of techniques (review). Cochrane Database of Systematic Reviews.

De las Heras, Carmen Gloria, Geist, R. Kielhofner, G. and Li, Y. (2007) The Volitional Questionnaire (VQ) Version 4.1. MOHO Clearinghouse. Available at: http://www.uic.edu/depts/moho/assess/vq.html

Department of Health (2000) National Service Framework for Coronary Heart Disease. London: Department of Health.

Department of Health (2001) National Service Framework for Older People. London: Department of Health.

Department of Health (2006) Our Health, Our Care, Our Say: A new direction for community services. London: Department of Health.

Department of Health (2007) Cancer Reform Strategy. London: Department of Health.

Department of Health (2009) New Horizons: A shared vision for mental health. London: Department of Health.

Department of Health (2010) Quality Outcomes for People with Dementia: Building on the work of the National Dementia Strategy. London: Department of Health. Available at: www.dh.gov.uk/publications

Depp, C.A., Jeste, D.V. (2004) Bipolar disorder in older adults: A critical review. *Bipolar Disorders* **6(5)**, 343–367.

Depp, C.A., Lindamer, L.A., Folsom, D.P., Gilmer, T., Hough, R.L., Garcia, P. and Jeste, D.V. (2006) Differences in clinical features and mental health service use in bipolar disorder across the lifespan. *American Journal of Geriatric Psychiatry* **13(4)**, 290–298.

Dixon, L., Duncan, D.C., Johnson, P., Kirkby, L,. O'Connell, H., Taylor, H.J. and Deane, K. (2009) Occupational therapy for patients with Parkinson's disease. *Cochrane Review* 3:CD002813.

Eames, J., Ward, G. and Siddans, L. (1999) Clinical audit of the outcome of individualised occupational therapy goals. *British Journal of Occupational Therapy* **62(6)**, 257–260.

Edmans, J. (2010) *Occupational Therapy and Stroke*. Oxford: Wiley Blackwells.

Eva, G. (2007) Measuring occupational therapy outcomes in cancer and palliative care. In: Cooper, J. (ed.) *Occupational Therapy in Oncology and Palliative Care*, 2nd edition. Chichester: John Wiley & Sons.

Fess E.E. (1992) Grip strength. In: Casanova, J.S. (ed.) Clinical Assessment Recommendations, 2nd ed. Chicago, pp. 41–45.

Fisher, A.G. (1995) Assessment of Motor Process Skills. Fort Collins, CO: Three Star Press.

Fisher, A.G. (2006) Assessment of Motor and Process Skill, 6th edition. Fort Collins, CO: Three Star Press.

Folstein, M.G., Folstein, S.E. and McHugh, P.R. (1975) Mini-mental state: A practical method for grading the cognitive state of patients for the clinician. *Journal of Psychiatric Research* **12(3)**, 189–198.

Freidman, J.H., Brown, R.G., Cornella, C., Garber, C.E., Krupp, L.B., Lou, J.-S., Marsh, L., Nail, L., Shulman, L. and Taylor, C.B. (2007) Fatigue in Parkinson's disease: A review. *Movement Disorders* **22(3)**, 297–308.

Future Vision Coalition (2009) A Future Vision for Mental Health. London: NHS Confederation.

Gelder, M., Gath, D., Mayou, R. and Cowen, P. (1998) *Oxford Textbook of Psychiatry*, 3rd edition. Oxford: Oxford University Press.

Gelder, M., Mayou, R. and Geddes, J. (1999) Psychiatry, 2nd edition. Oxford: Oxford University Press.

Gibb, W.R. (1997) Functional neuropathology in Parkinson's Disease. *European Neurology* **38(suppl2)**, 21–25.

Gilbert, R., Todd, C., May, M., Yardley, L. aaand Ben-Shlomo, Y. (2009) Socio-demographic factors predict the likelihood of not returning home after hospital admission following a fall. *Journal of Public Health* **32(1)**, 117–124.

Gillespie, L., Robertson, M., Gillespie, W., Lamb, S., Gate, S., Cumming, R. and Rowe, B. (2009) Interventions for preventing falls in older people. The Cochrane Collaboration. The Cochrane Library Issue 2.

Goa, F., Latash, M.L. and Zatsiorsky, V.M. (2007) Similar motion of hand held objects may trigger non-similar grip force adjustments. *Journal of Hand Therapy* **20(4)**, 300–308.

Goetz, C.G., Tilley, B.C., Shaftman, S.R., Stebbins, G.T., Fahn, S., Martinez-Martin, P., Poewe, W., Sampaio, C., Stern, M.B., Dodel, R., Dubois, B., Holloway, R., Jankovic, J., Kulisevsky, J., Lang, A.E., Lees, A., Leurgans, S., LeWitt, P.A., Nyenhuis, D., Olanow, C.W., Rascol, O., Schrag, A., Teresi, J.A., van Hilten, J.J., LaPelle, N. Movement Disorder Society UPDRS Revision Task Force (2008) Movement Disorder Society-sponsored revision of the Unified Parkinson's Disease Rating Scale (MDS-UPDRS): Scale presentation and clinimetric testing results. *Journal of Movement Disorders* **23(15)**, 2129–2170.

Goodman, J. and Locke, C. (2009) Occupations and the occupational therapy process. In: Goodman, J., Hirst, J. and Locke, C. (eds) *Occupational Therapy for People with Learning Disabilities*. London: Churchill Livingstone.

Golding, E. (1989) *The Middlesex Elderly Assessment of Mental State*. London: Pearson Assessment.

Graff, M.J.L., Vernooij-Dassen, M.J.M., Thijssen, M., Dekker, J., Hoefnagels, W.H.L. and Olde Rikkert, G.M. (2006) Community based occupational therapy for patients with dementia and their care givers: Randomised controlled trial. *BMJ* **333(7580)**, 1196–1199.

Graff, M.J., Vernooij-Dassen, M.J., Thijssen, M., Dekker, J., Hoefnagels, W.H. and Olderikkert, M.G. (2007) Effects of community occupational therapy on quality of life, mood, and health status in dementia patients and their caregivers: A randomized controlled trial. *Journals of Gerontology Series A: Biological Sciences and Medical Sciences* **62(9)**, 1002–1009.

Grant, M. (2005) Occupational therapy for people with osteoarthritis: Scope of practice and evidence base. *International Journal of Therapy and Rehabilitation* **12(1)**, 7–13.

Gosney, M. (2009) General care of the older cancer patient. *Clinical Oncology* **21(2)**, 86–91.

Gurland, B.J. and Cross, P.S. (1982) Epidemiology of psychopathology in old age: Some implications for clinical services. *Psychiatric Clinics of North Americ*, **5**, 11–15.

Gur, R.E., Petty, R.G., Bruce, I., Turetsky, B.I. and Gur, R.C. (1996) Schizophrenia throughout life: Sex differences in severity and profile of symptoms. *Schizophrenia Research* **21(1)**, 1–12.

Hakala, M., Nieminen P. and Kolvist, O. (1994) More evidence from a community based series of better outcome in rheumatoid arthritis. Data on effect of multidisciplinary care on the retention of functional ability. *Journal of Rheumatology* **21(8)**, 1432–1437.

Hammond, A. and Freeman, K. (2004) The long-term outcomes from a randomised controlled trial of an educational-behavioural joint protection programme for people with rheumatoid arthritis. *Clinical Rehabilitation* **18(5)**, 520–528.

Handoll, H.H.G., Madhokr, R. and Rowe, T.E. (2006) Rehabilitation for distal radial fractures in adults. *Cochrane Database of Systematic Reviews* **19(3)**, CD003324.

Hauer, K., Lamb, S.E., Jorstad, E.C., Todd, C. and Becker, C. (on behalf of the ProFaNE group) (2006) Systematic review of definitions and methods of measuring falls in randomised controlled fall prevention trials. *Age and Ageing* **35(1)**, 5–10.

Healthcare Commission, CSCI, Audit Commission (2006) Living well in later life: A review of progress against the National Service Framework for Older People. London: The Healthcare Commission.

Helvik, A.S., Engedal, K., Skancke, R.H. and Selbæk, G. (2011) A psychometric evaluation of the Hospital Anxiety and Depression Scale for the medically hospitalized elderly. *Nordic Journal of Psychiatry* **65(5)**, 338–344. Epub Feb 22, 2011.

Helewa, A., Goldsmith, C., Lee, P., Bombardier, C., Hanes, B., Smythe, H.A. and Tugwell, P. (1991) Effects of occupational therapy home service on patients with rheumatoid arthritis. *The Lancet* **337(8755)**, 1453–1456.

Herrero, M.-T., Barcia, C. and Navarro, J. (2002) Functional anatomy of the thalamus and basal ganglia. *Child's Nervous System* **18(8)**, 386–404.

Hochberg, M.C. (2010) Opportunities for the prevention of osteoarthritis. *Seminars in Arthritis and Rheumatism* **39(5)**, 321–322.

Horstink, M., Tolosa, E., Bonuccelli, U. et al. (2006a) Review of the therapeutic management of Parkinson's disease. Report of a joint task force of the European Federation of Neurological Societies and the Movement Disorder Society – European Section. Part 1: Early (uncomplicated) Parkinson's disease. *European Journal of Neurology* **13(11)**, 1170–1185.

Horstink, M., Tolosa, E., Bonuccelli, U. et al. (2006b) Review of the therapeutic management of Parkinson's disease. Report of a joint task force of the European Federation of Neurological Societies and the Movement Disorder Society – European Section. Part 2: Late (complicated) Parkinson's disease. *European Journal of Neurology* **13(1)**, 1186–1202.

Hudak, P., Amadio, P., Bombardier, C. and the Upper Extremity Collaborative Group (1996) Development of an upper extremity measure: The DASH (Disability of the Arm, Shoulder and Hand). *American Journal of Industrial Medicine* **29(6)**, 602–608.

Intercollegiate Stroke Working Party (2008) *National Clinical Guideline for Stroke*, 3rd edition. London: Royal College of Physicians.

Jakobsson, U. and Hallberg, I.R. (2002) Pain and quality of life among older people with rheumatoid arthritis and/or osteoarthritis: A literature review. *Journal of Clinical Nursing* **11(4)**, 430–443.

Jankovic, J. (2008) Parkinson's disease: Clinical features and diagnosis. *Journal of Neurology, Neurosurgery and Psychiatry* **79(4)**, 368–376.

Jenkinson, C.; Coulter, A. and Wright, L. (1993) Short form 36 (SF36) health survey questionnaire: Normative adults of working age. *BMJ* **306(6890)**, 1437–1440.

Jenkinson, C., Fitzpatrick, R., Peto, V., Harris, R. and Saunders, P. (2008) *New User Manual for the PDQ-9, PDQ-8 and PDQ Index*, 2nd edition. Oxford: Health Services Research Unit, University of Oxford.

Jensen, J., Nyberg, L., Gustafson, Y. and Lundin-Olsson, L. (2003) Fall and injury prevention in residential care – effects in residents with higher and lower levels of cognition. *Journal of the American Geriatric Society* **51(5)**, 627–635.

Jeste, D.V. (1996) Growing disparity between need and reality: Research in geriatric psychiatry. *Current Opinion in Psychiatry* **9(4)**, 279–280.

Kale, R. and Menken, M. (2004) Who should look after people with Parkinson's disease? *BMJ* **328(7431)**, 62–63.

Keable, D. (1997) The Management of Anxiety. A guide for Therapists, 2nd edition. London: Churchill Livingstone.

Kealey, P. and Mcintyre, I. (2005) An evaluation of the domiciliary occupational therapy service in palliative cancer care in a Community Trust: A patient and carers perspective. *European Journal of Cancer Care* **14(3)**, 232–243.

Kessler, R. (2001) CBT added to medical management improved clinical outcomes in rheumatoid arthritis. *Evidence-Based Mental Health* **4(3)**, 89.

Kuzuya, M., Masuda, Y., Hiarkawa, Y., Iwata, M., Enoki, H., Hasegawa, J., Izawa, S. and Iguchi, A. (2006) Falls of the elderly are associated with burden of caregivers in the community. *International Journal of Geriatric Psychiatry* **21(8)**, 740–745.

Lachman, M., Howland, J., Tennstedt, S., Jette, A., Assman, S. and Peterson, E. (1998) Fear of falling and activity restriction: The Survey of Activities and Fear of Falling in the Elderly (SAFFE). *Journal of Gerontology* **53(1)**, 43–50.

Lamb, S.E., Jørstad-Stein, E.C., Hauer, K. and Becker, C. (2005) Development of a common outcome data set for fall injury prevention trials: The Prevention of Falls Network Europe Consensus. *Journal of the American Geriatrics Society* **53(9)**, 1618–1622.

Lanin, N.A. and Herbert, R.D. (2003) Is hand splinting effective for adults following stroke? A systematic review and methodological critique of published research. *Clinical Rehabilitation* **17(8)**, 807–816.

Lanin, N.A., Cusick, A., McCluskey, A. and Herbert, R.D. (2007) Effects of splinting on wrist contracture after stroke: A randomised controlled trial. *Stroke* **38(1)**, 111–116.

Law, M., Baptiste, S., Carswell, A., McColl, M., Polatajko, H. and Pollock, N. (2005) *Canadian Occupational Performance Measure*. Toronto, ON: Canadian Association of Occupational Therapists Publications, ACE.

Legg, L.A., Drummond, A.E. and Langhorne, P. (2007) Occupational therapy for patients with problems in activities of daily living after stroke. *Cochrane Database of Systematic Reviews* **18(4)**, CD003585.

Liddle, J. and McKenna, K. (2000) Quality of Life: An overview of issues for use in occupational therapy outcome measurement. *Australian Occupational Therapy Journal* **47(2)**, 77–85.

Liddle, J, Turpin, M., Carlson, G. and McKenna, K. (2008) The needs and experiences related to driving cessation for older people. *British Journal of Occupational Therapy* **71(9)**, 379–388.

Lieberman, A. (2006) Depression in Parkinson's disease: A review. *Acta Neurologica Scandinavia* **113(1)**, 1–8.

Lillywhite, A. and Haines, D. (2010) *Occupational Therapy and People with Learning Disabilities.* London: College of Occupational Therapists.

Logan, P.A., Coupland, C.A.C., Gladman, J.R.F., Sahota, O, Stoner-Hobbs, V., Robertson, K., Tomlinson, V., Ward, M., Sach, T. and Avery, J. (2010) Community falls prevention for people who call an emergency ambulance after a fall: Randomised controlled trial. *BMJ* **340**, c2102.

Lord, S., Sherrington, C., Menz, H. and Close, J. (2007) *Falls in Older People*, 2nd edition Cambridge: Cambridge University Press.

Lorenzi, C., Cilione, C., Rizzardi, R., Furino, V., Bellantone, T., Lugli, D. and Clini, E. (2004) Occupational therapy and pulmonary rehabilitation of disabled. *COPD Patients Respiration* **71(3)**, 246–251.

Mackeith, J. and Burns, S. (2010) *Mental Health Recovery Star.* London: Mental Health Providers Forum.

Mackenzie, L., Byles, J. and Higginbotham, N. (2000) Designing the Home Falls Assessment and Screening Tool (HOME FAST). *British Journal of Occupational Therapy* **62**, 260–269.

Mackenzie, L., Byles, J. and Higginbotham, N. (2002) Reliability of the Home Falls Assessment and Screening Tool (HOME FAST) for identifying older people at increased risk of falls. *Disability and Rehabilitation* **24(5)**, 266–274.

Mackenzie, L., Byles, J. and Higginbotham, N. (2003) Professional perceptions about home safety: Cross-validation of the Home Falls and Accidents Screening Tool (HOME FAST). *Journal of Allied Health* **31(1)**, 22–28.

Macmillan Cancer Support (2007) What is Cancer? Available from: www.macmillan.org.uk/cancerinformation.

Macphee, G.J.A. and Stewart, D. (2007) Parkinson's disease. *Reviews in Clinical Gerontology.* Online. Cambridge University Press.

McIntyre, A. and Reynolds, F. (2012) There's no apprenticeship for Alzheimer's: The caring relationship when an older person with dementia falls. *Ageing and Society* **32(5)**, 873–896.

Martin, F.C. (2009) Next steps for falls and fracture reduction. *Age and Ageing* **38(6)**, 640–643.

Meenan, R.F., Mason, J.H., Anderson, J.J., Guccione, A.A. and Kazis, L.E. (1992) AIMS2: The content and properties of a revised and expanded Arthritis Impact Measurement Scales Health Status Questionnaire. *Arthritis and Rheumatism* **35(1)**, 1–10.

Minato, M. and Zemke, R. (2004) Occupational choices of persons with schizophrenia Living in the community. *Journal of Occupational Science* **11(1)**, 31–39.

Miwa, H. and Miwa, T. (2011) Internal medicine. Fatigue in patients with Parkinson's disease: Impact on quality of life. *Internal Medicine* **50(15)**, 1553–1558.

Moskowitz, R.W. (2009) The burden of osteoarthritis: Clinical and quality of life issues. *American Journal of Managed Care* **15(8 Suppl)**, 5223–5229.

Moussavi, S., Chatterji, S., Verdes, E., Tandon, A., Patel, V. and Ustun, B. (2007) Depression, chronic diseases, and decrements in health: Results from the World Health Surveys. *The Lancet* **370(9590)**, 851–858.

Mur, M., Portella, M., Martinez-Aran, A., Pifarre, J. and Vieta, E. (2009) Influence of clinical and neuropsychological variables on the psychosocial and occupational outcome of remitted bipolar patients. *Psychopathology* **42(3)**, 148–156.

National Institute of Clinical Excellence (2003) *Chronic Heart Failure: National Clinical Guideline for diagnosis and management in primary and secondary care.* London: National Institute of Clinical Excellence. Available at: http://guidance.nice.org.uk/CG108

National Institute of Clinical Excellence (2004a) *Improving Supportive and Palliative Care for Adults with Cancer.* London: National Institute for Clinical Excellence.

National Institute of Clinical Excellence (2004b) *Clinical Practice Guideline for the Assessment and Prevention of Falls in Older People*. London: National Institute for Clinical Excellence.

National Institute for Health and Clinical Excellence (2006a) *Parkinson's Disease: Diagnosis and management in primary and secondary care*. London: National Institute for Health and Clinical Excellence. Available at: http://www.nice.org.uk/nicemedia/pdf/cg035fullguide line.pdf

National Institute for Health and Clinical Excellence (2006b) *Bipolar Disorder. The management of bipolar disorder in adults, children and adolescents, in primary and secondary care*. London: National Institute for Health and Clinical Excellence. Available at: http://www.nice.org.uk/ nicemedia/pdf/CG38niceguideline.pdf

National Institute for Health and Clinical Excellence (2009) *Depression. The treatment and management of depression in adults*. NICE clinical guideline 90. London: NICE. Available at: www. nice.org.uk

National Institute of Clinical Excellence (2010a) *Chronic Obstructive Pulmonary Disease: Management of chronic obstructive pulmonary disease in adults in primary and secondary care (partial update)*. Clinical Guideline 101. London: National Institute of Clinical Excellence. Available at: http:// publications.nice.org.uk/chronic-obstructive-pulmonary-disease-cg101/introduction

National Institute of Clinical Excellence (2010b) *Schizophrenia: The NICE guideline on core interventions in the treatment and management of schizophrenia in adults in primary and secondary care*. Updated edition. National Clinical Guideline. London: The British Psychological Society and The Royal College of Psychiatrists.

National Institute for Health and Clinical (2011) Review of Clinical Guideline (CG21) – Clinical practice guideline for the assessment and prevention of falls in older people. NICE: National Institute of Clinical Excellence. Available at: http://www.nice.org.uk/CG021

Ngune, I. Howat, P. Maycock, B. and Slevin, T. (2009) Do older people perceive cancer prevention and early detection to be worthwhile? Implications for prevention. *Australian Journal of Primary Health* 15(2),139–145.

Oliver, R., Blathwayt, J., Brackley, C. and Tamaki, T. (1993) Development of the Safety Assessment of Function and the Environment for Rehabilitation (SAFER) tool. *Canadian Journal of Occupational Therapy* 60(2), 78–82.

Overall, J.E. and Gorham, D.R. (1962) The Brief Psychiatric Rating Scale. *Psychological Reports* 10, 799–812.

Overall, J.E. and Gorham, D.R. (1988) The Brief Psychiatric Rating Scale: Recent developments in ascertainment and scaling. *Psychopharmacological Bulletin* 24, 97–99.

Palmer, B.W., Heaton, S.C. and Jeste, D.V. (1999) Older patients with schizophrenia: Challenges in the coming decades. *Psychiatric Services* 50(9),1178–1183.

Parker, S.G., Peet, S.M., Jagger, C., Farhan, M. and Castleden, C.M. (1998) Measuring health status in older patients. The SF-36 in practice. *Age and Ageing* 27(1), 13–18.

Parkinson, S., Forsyth, K. and Kielhofner, G. (2006) *The Model of Human Occupation Screening Tool (MOHOST): Version 2*. Chicago: Model of Human Occupational Clearing House.

Parkinson's Disease Society (2007) *The Professional's Guide to Parkinson's Disease*. London: Parkinson's Disease Society.

Pellecchia, G.L. (2003) Figure of eight method of measuring hand size: Reliability and concurrent validity. *Journal of Hand Therapy* 16(4), 300–304.

Perrin, T., May, H. and Anderson, E. (2008) *Wellbeing in Dementia*, 2nd edition. London: Churchill Livingstone Elsevier.

Perry, A., Tarrier, N., Morriss, R., McCarthy, E. and Limb, K. (1999) Randomised controlled trial of efficacy of teaching patients with bipolar disorder to identify early symptoms of relapse and obtain treatment. *BMJ* 318(7177), 149–153.

Plews, C. (2005) Expert Patient Programme: Managing patients with long-term conditions. *British Journal of Nursing* **14(20)**, 1086–1089.

Pool, J. (2008) *Pool Activity Level (PAL) Instrument for Occupational Profiling: A practical resource for carers of people with cognitive impairment*, 3rd edition. London: Jessica Kinglsey Publishers.

Porter, B., Henry, S.R., Gray, W.K. and Walker, R.W. (2010) Care requirements of a prevalent population with idiopathic Parkinson's disease. *Age and Ageing* **39(1)**, 57–61.

Powell, L.E. and Myers, A.M. (1995) The Activities-specific Balance Confidence (ABC) Scale. *Journal of Gerontology* **50A(1)**, 28–34.

Pratt, A.L., Burr, N. and Stott, D. (2004) An investigation into the degree of precision achieved by a team of hand therapists and surgeons using hand goniometry with a standardised protocol. *British Journal of Hand Therapy* **10(4)**, 116–112.

Riedinger, M.S., Dracup, K.A., Brecht, M.L., Padilla, G. and Sarna, L. (2001) Quality of life in patients with heart failure: Do gender differences exist? *Heart and Lung* **30(2)**,105–116.

Robertson, I.H., Ward, T., Ridgeway, V. et al. (1994) *Test of Everyday Attention*. London: Pearson Assessment.

Robinson, S. (1992) Occupational therapy in a memory clinic. *British Journal of Occupational Therapy* **55(10)**, 394–396.

Rodda, J., Walker, Z. and Carter, J. (2011) Depression in older adults. *BMJ* **343**, d5219.

Rothwell, P.M., Coull, A.J., Silver, L.E. et al. (2005) Population-based study of event-rate, incidence, case fatality, and mortality for all acute vascular events in all arterial territories (Oxford Vascular Study). *Lancet* **366(9499)**, 1773–1783.

Rubenstein, L.Z. (2006) Falls in older people: Epidemiology, risk factors and strategies for prevention. *Age and Ageing* **35(2)**, 37–41.

Rubí, M., Renom, F., Ramis, F., Medinas, M., Centeno, M.J., Górriz, M., Crespí, E., Martín, B. and Soriano, J.B. (2010) Effectiveness of pulmonary rehabilitation in reducing health resources use in chronic obstructive pulmonary disease. *Archives of Physical Medicine and Rehabilitation* **91(3)**, 364–368.

Rustard, A., DeGroot, T.L., Jungkunz, M.L. et al. (1993) *The Cognitive Assessment of Minnesota*. London: Psychological Corporation.

Saltz, C.C., Zimmerman, S., Tompkins, C., Harrington, D. and Magaziner, J. (1999) Stress among caregivers of hip fracture patients. *Journal of Gerontological Social Work* **30(3)**, 167–181.

Scottish Intercollegiate Network (2010a) Non-pharmaceutical management of depression in adults. Edinburgh: SIGN.. Available at: http://www.sign.ac.uk/pdf/sign114.pdf

Scottish Intercollegiate Network (2010b) Diagnosis and pharmacological management of Parkinson's disease. A national clinical guideline. Edinburgh: SIGN. Available at http://www. sign.ac.uk/pdf/sign113.pdf

Scottish Intercollegiate Guidelines Network (SIGN) (2010) Management of patients with stroke: Rehabilitation, prevention and management of complications, and discharge planning. A national clinical guideline. Edinburgh: SIGN. Available at: http://www.sign.ac.uk/pdf/sign118.pdf

Scudds, R. (2001) Pain outcome measures. *Journal of Hand Therapy* **14(2)**, 86–90.

Shaw, F.E. (2007) Prevention of falls in older people with dementia. *Journal of Neural Transmission* **114(10)**, 1259–64.

Shaw, F.E., Bond, J., Richardson, D.A., Dawson, P., Steen, I.N., McKeith, I.G. and Kenny, R.A. (2003) Multifactorial intervention after a fall in older people with cognitive impairment and dementia presenting to the accident and emergency department: Randomised controlled trial. *BMJ* **326(7380)**, 73–79.

Simpson, J.M., Worsfield, C., Hawke, J. (1998) Balance confidence in elderly people: The CONFbal Scale. *Age and Ageing* **27**(suppl **2**), 57-b-57.

Simpson, J.M., Darwin, C. and Marsh, N. (2003) What are older people prepared to do to avoid falling? A qualitative study in London. *British Journal of Community Nursing* **8(4)** 152–159.

Singleton, N. and Turner, A. (1993) SF36 is suitable for elderly patients. *BMJ* **307(6896)**, 12612–126127.

Sivrioglu, E.Y., Sivrioglu, K., Ertan, T., Ertan, F.S., Cankurtaran, E., Aki, O., Uluduz, D., Inc,e B. and Kirli, S. (2009) Reliability and validity of the Geriatric Depression Scale in detection of poststroke minor depression. *Journal of Experimental and Neuropsychology* **31(8)**, 999–1006.

Sitori, V., Corbetta, D., Moja, I. and Gatti, R. (2009) Constraint-induced movement therapy for upper extremities in stroke patients. *Cochrane Database of Systematic Reviews*, Issue **4**.

Spitzer, R.L., Williams, J.B.W., Kroenke, K., Linzer, M., deGruy, F.V., Hahn, S.R., Brody, D. and Johnson, J.G. (1994) Utility of a new procedure for diagnosing mental disorders in primary care: The PRIME-MD 1000 study. *The Journal of the American Medical Association* **272(22)**, 1749–1756.

Steultjens, E.M.J. (2009) Focussed, comprehensive home visits, prevent falling when targeted to specific groups of older people at high risk of falls. *Australian Journal of Occupational Therapy* **56(2)**, 144–146.

Steultjens, E.M.J., Dekker, J., Bouter, L.M., van Schaardenburg, D., van Kuyk, M.A.H. and van den Ende, C.H.M. (2004) Occupational therapy for rheumatoid arthritis. *Cochrane Review* **1**, CD003114.

Stubbs, R., Atwal, A. and Mckay, K. (2004) Searching for the Holy Grail. *International Journal of Therapy and Rehabilitation* **11(6)**, 281–286.

Tandberg, E., Larsen, J.P. and Karlsen, K. (1999) Excessive daytime sleepiness and sleep benefit in Parkinson's disease: A community-based study. *Movement Disorders* **14(6)**, 922–927.

Taylor, B.P., Bruder, G.E., Stewart, J.W., McGrath, P.J., Halperin, J., Ehrlichman, H. and Quitkin, F.M. (2006) Psychomotor slowing as a predictor of fluoxetine non-response in depressed outpatients. *American Journal of Psychiatry* **163(1)**, 73–78.

Thompson, M., Evitt, C.P. and Whaley, M. (2010) Screening for falls and osteoporosis: Prevention practice for the hand therapist. *Journal of Hand Therapy* **23**(2), 212–229.

Tinnetti, M.E. and Williams, C.S. (1998) The effect of falls and fall injuries on functioning in community dwelling older persons. *Journal of Gerontology: Medical Sciences* **53A(2)**, M112–9.

Tinetti, M.E., Richman, D. and Powell, L. (1990) Falls efficacy as a measure of fear of falling. *Journal of Gerontology: Psychological Sciences* **45(6)**, 239–243.

Turner, T. (1997) ABC of mental health: Schizophrenia. *BMJ* **315**, 108–111.

Turner-Stokes, L. (2009) *Goal Attainment Scaling (GAS) in Rehabilitation: A practical guide.* London: Kings College London and The North West London Hospitals. Available from: http://www.csi.kcl.ac.uk/files/Goal%20Attainment%20Scaling%20in%20Rehabilitation%20%20a%20practical%20guide.pdf

Tyerman, R., Tyerman, A., Howard, P.L. and Hadfield, C. (1986) *Chessington Occupational Therapy Neurological Assessment Battery.* Leicestershire: Nottingham Rehabilitation Supplies.

United Kingdom Department of Health (2009) *Fracture Prevention Services: An economic evaluation.* London: HMSO.

United States of America Centers for Disease Control and Prevention [CDC] (2008) A CDC Compendium of Effective Fall Interventions: What works for community-wwelling older adults. Atlanta, Georgia: CDC National Center for Injury Prevention and Control.

Vasudev, A. and Thomas, A. (2010) Bipolar disorder in the elderly: What's in a name? *Maturitas* **66(3)**, 231–235.

Velloso, M. and Jardim, J.R. (2006) Study of energy expenditure during activities of daily living using and not using body position recommended by energy conservation techniques in patients with COPD. *Chest*; **130(1)**, 126–132.

Walker, M.F., Leonardi-Bee, J., Bath, P. et al. (2004) Individual patient data meta-analysis of randomized controlled trials of community occupational therapy for stroke patients. *Stroke* **35(9)**, 2226–2232.

Ware, J.E. and Sherbourne, C.D. (1992) The MOS 36-Item Short-Form Health Survey (SF-36). *Medical Care* **30(6)**, 473–481.

Warlow, C., van Gijn, J., Dennis, M. et al. (2007) *Stroke: Practical management*, 3rd edition. Oxford: Blackwell Publishing.

Weiss, S., LaStayo, P., Mills, A. and Bramlet, D. (2000) Prospective analysis of splinting the first carpometacarpal joint: An objective, subjective and radiographic assessment. *Journal of Hand Therapy* **13(93)**, 218–226.

Whiting, S., Lincoln, N.B., Bhavnani, G. and Cockburn, J. (1985) Rivermead Perceptual Assessment Battery. Windsor: NFER-Nelson.

Williams-Gray, C.H., Foltynie, T., Lewis, S.J.G. and Barker, R.A. (2006) Cognitive deficits and psychosis in Parkinson's disease: A review of pathophysiology and therapeutic options. *CNS Drugs* **20(6)**, 477–505.

Williams-Gray, C.H., Foltynie, T., Brayne, C.E., Robbins, T.W. and Barker, R.A. (2007) Evolution of cognitive dysfunction in an incident Parkinson's disease cohort. *Brain* **30(Pt 7)**,1787–1798.

Wilson, B.A. Cockburn, J. and Halligan, P.W. (1987) *Behavioural Inattention Test*. Oxford: Pearson Assessment.

Wilson, B.A., Alderman, N., Burgess, P.W. et al. (1996) *Behavioural Assessment of Dysexecutive Syndrome*. London: Pearson Assessment.

Wilson, B.A., Greenfield, E., Clare, L. et al. (2008) *Rivermead Behavioural Memory Test*, 3rd edition. London: Pearson Assessment.

Wolfe, C.D.A. (2000) The impact of stroke. *British Medical Bulletin* **56(2)**, 275–286.

Woodside, H., Schell, L. and Allison-Hedges, J. (2006) Listening for recovery: The vocational success of people living with mental illness. *The Canadian Journal of Occupational Therapy* **73(1)**, 36–43.

World Health Organization (2001) *The International Classification of Functioning Disability and Health*. Geneva: WHO.

World Health Organization (2002) Active Ageing: A Policy Framework. Geneva: World Health Organization.

World Health Organization (2003) Prevention and management of osteoporosis. World Health Organization Scientific Group. Available at: http://whqlibdoc.who.int/trs/who_trs_921.pdf

World Health Organization (2007) *WHO Global Report on Falls Prevention in Older Age*. Geneva: World Health Organization.

World Health Organization (2012) Fact Sheet 362. What is dementia? Available at: http://www.who.int/mediacentre/factsheets/fs362/en/index.html

Yardley, L., Beyer, N., Hauer, K., Kempen, G., Piot-Ziegler, C. and Tood, C. (2005) Development and initial validation of the Falls Efficacy Scale-International (FES-I). *Age and Ageing* **34(6)**, 614–619.

Yardley, L., Donovan-Hall, M. , Francism K, and Todd, C. (2006a) Older people's views of advice about falls prevention: A qualitative study. *Health Education Research* **21(4)**, 508–517.

Yardley, L., Bishop, F.L., Beyer, N., Hauer, K., Kempen, G.I.J.M., Piot-Ziegler, C., Todd, C.J., Cuttelod, T., Horne, M., Lauta, K. and Rosell Holt, A. (2006b) Older people's views of falls preventions in six European countries. *The Gerontologist* **46(5)**, 650–60.

Yesavage, J.A., Brink, T.L., Rose, T.L., Lum, O., Huang, V., Adey, M.B. and Leirer, V.O. (1983) Development and validation of a geriatric depression screening scale: A preliminary report. *Journal of Psychiatric Research* **17(1)**, 37–49.

Zigmond, A.S. and Snaith, R.P. (1994) The Hospital Anxiety and Depression Scale. Windsor: Nfer-Nelson.

Chapter 6

The ageing body – body functions and structures: Part 1

Stephen Ashford and Anne McIntyre

Previous chapters have introduced how an older person's opportunity to age successfully in an occupationally just way relates to their person–environment interaction. This chapter and the following (Chapter 7) discuss the ageing of body functions and structures that impact on an individual's ability to perform activities and participate in meaningful occupations. The World Health Organization (WHO) (2001) classifies these as body functions and structures within the International Classification of Functioning (ICF) and these are defined as follows:

> "Body functions are the physiological functions of body systems, including psychological functions.
>
> Body structures are anatomical parts of the body such as organs, limbs and their components." (WHO 2001, p. 10)

Current practice within occupational therapy advocates that assessment and intervention should have a 'top-down' approach, so that an individual's occupational needs and performance are ascertained (American Occupational Therapy Association [AOTA] 2002). Therefore, occupation, activity and participation are our core business rather than impairment of body function or structure. However, in many instances it is necessary for us to have a 'bottom-up' approach and consider the impact an impairment of body function or structure has on activity or participation (and therefore occupational performance).

Deconstruction of an activity (activity analysis) should identify not only the demands of the activity (what, where, how often, how quickly and with what), and the context of the activity, but also the body functions and structure required to successfully carry out the activity. These are also referred to as 'client factors' (AOTA 2008) and 'performance components' (Law and Baum 2001) within the occupational therapy literature.

It is important to be able to ascertain whether an older person's impairments of body structure and function have arisen from pathological processes such as those discussed in Chapter 5, or are a result of the normal ageing process. Indeed, these pathological changes may often be superimposed upon normal age-related changes to body structure and function. Health professionals working with older people therefore have a responsibility to possess knowledge of these normal changes and their relationship to functional performance,

Occupational Therapy and Older People, Second Edition. Edited by Anita Atwal and Anne McIntyre.
© 2013 Blackwell Publishing Ltd. Published 2013 by Blackwell Publishing Ltd.

whilst also understanding the additional impact of pathologies (often multiple) in this age group. It is important to remember that many individual factors impact upon the rate and extent of age-related changes – such as those personal and social factors already discussed in previous chapters, as well as heredity and lifestyle.

Physiological ageing has its basis in cellular and sub-cellular change. The physiological theories of ageing discussed in Chapter 2 help us understand what might happen to body structures. Some cells, notably skeletal muscle fibres, cardiac fibres and neurons, do not replicate at all, so these cell populations decline with age and cells are not replaced if tissue damage occurs. Also with ageing, the spontaneous binding of glucose to proteins both inside and outside cells occurs, forming irreversible links between molecules, and contributing to stiffening and loss of elasticity of tissues. An accumulation over time of oxidative damage – the action of free radicals in 'stealing' electrons from other, stable atoms to render them unstable – can lead to toxicity and chemical imbalances, cell membrane disruption and eventual cell death.

From the cellular level of organisation, cells become organised and grow to form tissues, which then become organised into organs (identifiable structures composed of two or more tissues). Organs are organised into systems culminating in a complex multisystem organism capable of coordinated functions that sustain life and all its features. Ultimately, changes at the cellular level culminate in the variety of age-related changes manifest in the organism, observable by others and experienced by the individual.

Box 6.1   Body functions and structures.

- Structures of the nervous system
  - Central nervous system
  - Peripheral nervous system
- Structures and functions of voice and speech
- Mental functions
  - Global mental functions
    - consciousness and sleep
    - orientation
    - intellect
    - energy and motivation
    - personality and temperament
  - Specific mental functions
    - attention
    - memory
    - executive functions
    - psychomotor performance
    - emotion
    - perception
    - language
- Structures and functions of the sensory system
    - touch
    - pain
    - eye
    - ear
    - balance

In Chapter 7, the integrative and mutual functioning of body systems and the importance of homeostasis are highlighted.

The ICF has been used as a classification to discuss the body functions and structures considered in this chapter (listed in Box 6.1) and other body functions and structures will be discussed in Chapter 7.

The nervous system

The function of the nervous system is to control the body by acquiring and processing information from extrinsic and intrinsic sources and activating an appropriate response. These responses involve movement, cognitive functioning and communication. The control of human movement is a complex task and requires the interaction of a number of systems. Key to the production and control of movement is the structure and function of the nervous system. Likewise, sensory perception is required to perceive the environment and allow for appropriate responses and meaningfully-controlled movement that produce useful behaviours to the individual.

Neurological damage to the brain, for example as a result of stroke or trauma, typically leads to paralysis or weakness of the opposite side of the body (hemiparesis), which may be partial or complete. Therefore, movement of this side of the body is affected, so that at best fine movement is impaired or, at worst, gross movement is compromised. In the early stages after injury, the affected limbs are often flaccid (low-toned paresis), but after a few weeks muscle tone might start to return and can lead to the development of muscle over-activity or 'spasticity'. Spasticity will often have unwanted effects, such as pain, and result in secondary problems such as muscle stiffness and contracture. However, significant weakness will often persist and is commonly the most significant impairment contributing to activity limitation. Even if return of active movement occurs, spasticity in addition to weakness could still interfere with the fine motor coordination required for highly-skilled tasks.

The nervous system comprises of the central nervous system (CNS) and the peripheral nervous system (PNS). The CNS has two main component parts: the brain and the spinal cord. The PNS consists of peripheral nerves which connect the CNS to the muscles or

---

Before reading further, it would be useful for you to review the general structure and function of the nervous system. In particular, it would be useful to be aware of the general anatomy and principal functions of the following:
   The brain's four principal regions:

(1) Cerebral hemispheres
(2) Diencephalon (thalamus, hypothalamus and eipithalamus)
(3) Brain stem (mid-brain, pons and medulla)
(4) Cerebellum

   The spinal cord:

(1) Principle regions
(2) Motor and sensory connections to peripheral nervous system

sensory receptors. Nerves linking the CNS to muscles are termed 'motor nerves' and those linking sensory receptors to the CNS are termed 'sensory nerves'. Many of the nerves in both the CNS and PNS are surrounded by myelin, an insulating material that improves the speed of nerve conduction.

Apoptosis is a normal process by which cells are allowed to die. It is not a patholo- gical process, but necessary to ensure appropriate development of connections between neurones (Joaquin and Gollapudi 2001). Apoptosis is important to consider related to normal ageing because evidence suggests that changes occur in this process, causing increased numbers of cells to die as people get older (Volloch et al. 1998, Savory et al. 1999, Fillenbaum et al. 2001, O'Sullivan 2009).

Other factors are also thought to contribute to normal ageing at a neural cell level. Some processes might also contribute to certain pathological states such as Alzheimer's disease and vascular dementia (van Paasschen et al. 2009). These processes are thought to include oxidation of free radicals, calcium homeostasis, and variations in gene expres- sion, mitochondrial dysfunction and alterations in hormone levels (Troller and Valenzuela 2001, O'Sullivan 2009).

All of these processes have a similar result in that they produce increased levels of cell death as people become older; and in some cases this might produce a pathological state. For example, hypoestrogenism has been linked to a higher incidence of Alzheimer's disease in postmenopausal women (Richards et al. 1999). This was given further support by a study which demonstrated that administration of hormone replacement therapy reduced the incidence of alterations in the brain associated with Alzheimer's disease and maintained cognitive performance (Maki and Resnick 2000). Levels of homocysteine (a plasma-based amino acid) in the CNS have been demonstrated to increase with age and are indicated as a risk factor for increased incidence of cardiovascular disease, stroke and peripheral vascular disease (Perry 1995, Selhub et al. 1995).

In terms of brain structure, a number of changes have been documented to occur with normal ageing. It has been demonstrated through imageing studies that the lateral ventricles of the brain increase in size as people get older (Raz 1996, O'Sullivan 2009), indicating that atrophy is occurring in the cerebral hemispheres. Magnetic Resonance Imaging (MRI) studies demonstrate that cerebral volume decreases with age, indicating again that atrophy occurs throughout large regions of the brain, and in particular in the cerebral hemispheres (Raz 2000). It has been demonstrated in a number of studies that the frontal region of the cortex (frontal lobe) shows increased atrophy as people get older (Cowell et al. 1994, Raz et al. 1997). In particular, it has been identified that, while neural cells as a whole are lost, white matter representing the axon (neural) connections between cells are lost at a greater rate. This has again been identified in the frontal and prefrontal regions of the cortex (Ylikoski et al. 1995).

The other area of significant cell loss is the hippocampus in the medial temporal lobe where, like the frontal lobe, cell loss is significant for many aspects of cognitive function (O'Sullivan 2009). The hippocampus is an area of early cell loss in the development of Alzheimer's disease and has therefore been used as a focus in imageing studies to enable earlier diagnosis (Pruessner et al. 2000). Diagnosis based on imageing of this type has been shown to have high correlation with the density of neurofibrillary tangles used to confirm diagnosis at post-mortem (O'Sullivan 2009).

Changes in myelinated (white matter) areas of the frontal and prefrontal lobe have been inversely correlated with reduced performance in tasks involving executive function, for example higher planning and organisation of task performance (Valenzuela et al. 2000, van Paasschen et al. 2009). Speed of information processing seems to be particularly affected in individuals with white matter loss in this area (Ylikoski et al. 1993).

The presence of senile plaques in intracellular spaces and neurofibrillary tangles within cells occur in the ageing brain from the age of 60 onwards; however, larger numbers of these are seen in the brains of adults with Alzheimer's disease (like Millie in Chapter 5) and also those people with learning disability from the age of 50 onwards – like Jean who we met in chapter 5 (Selkoe 1992, Jones and Ferris 1999, Holland 2000, Pruessner et al. 2000, O'Sullivan 2009).

Neurotransmitters have also been implicated in being involved in the normal ageing process and in some instances have been linked to pathological states. Neurotransmitters allow the transmission of an action potential across a synapse (from one neurone to the next) and are chemicals released by the terminal part of the neurone. Different neurotransmitters are involved with conduction in different areas of the CNS and PNS.

The neurotransmitter acetylcholine, found in some of the cortical regions, is said to impact on learning and memory in people with Alzheimer's disease (Op den Velde 1976, Sims et al. 1980). It has been suggested that even in normal human ageing, reduction in cholinergic transmission may account for some of the identified decline in learning and memory (Trollor and Valenzuela 2001). Such research has also led to the use of cholinergic medication to enhance cognitive function in those people with mild Alzheimer's disease (Forette and Rockwood 1999).

Dopamine is another neurotransmitter found predominantly in the basal ganglia. Dopamine transmission is required to allow the initiation of movement, whereas the basal ganglia (lateral to the thalamus) are involved in controlling movement. Reduction in dopamine in the basal ganglia and loss of the striatal cells responsible for its production are associated with Parkinson's disease. However, studies using positron emission tomography have indicated significant alterations in dopamine neurotransmission with age (Volkow 1996). Further studies have also correlated loss of dopamine-producing cells with normal ageing and reduction in ability to perform motor tasks such as finger tapping tests (Volkow et al. 1998). Thus significant evidence is provided that reduction in the ability to manufacture dopamine is associated with decreases in motor performance, and particularly reaction times. Other neurotransmitters such as serotonin and glutamate also undergo age-related changes and a reduction in the number of available receptors sensitive to them (Mattson et al. 2004). Changes in the availability of a number of neurotransmitters therefore seem to occur with normal ageing and may be one of the factors producing alterations in brain function as individuals get older.

The evidence presented suggests that changes in the CNS are a normal product of ageing and are linked to decline in the functional ability of the brain in particular. Gross measures such as reduction in brain volume with age support the hypothesis that normal ageing produces changes in structure, which has implications for CNS function. However, it is important to note that recent evidence suggests that the 'normal' ageing brain can still show signs of plasticity (Selkoe 1992, Sofroniew 1997). It is important to consider whether this potential plasticity can be harnessed in intervention with a client.

The Peripheral Nervous System (PNS)

The PNS consists of both motor and sensory nerves. The motor nerves synapse with muscles via connections called motor end plates. Motor nerves are then able to stimulate the muscle to contract. Sensory nerves, on the other hand, have more varied connections to different types of sensory receptors. However, the principle of these different types of receptors is similar in that they convert mechanical (touch or pressure), thermal (temperature changes), light (as in the eye), chemical (taste or smell) or potentially damaging stimuli (producing pain) into electrical impulses or action potentials for transmission via peripheral sensory nerves to the CNS.

Peripheral nerves are also responsible for connections allowing autonomic responses within the body. Peripheral nerves connect to sweat glands, smooth muscles surrounding veins (allowing venous constriction and dilation) and body hair. This allows these effector organs to be linked to the autonomic nervous system (ANS) and assist in the regulation of body temperature.

An important factor in the function of nerves is the speed at which the nerve can conduct the impulse (or action potential) along its length. A number of body functions depend on this conduction occurring at a fast velocity or speed (see Box 6.2).

A number of electrophysiological studies have demonstrated that the speed at which nerve impulses travel decreases with age, using animal models of human nerve ageing (Dorfman and Bosley 1979, Buchthal et al. 1984, Mattson et al. 2004). Verdu et al. (2000) also found that the number of myelinated and unmyelinated nerve fibres (in animal models) tend to reduce in the PNS with age, with myelinated nerve fibres being affected more slowly than unmyelinated fibres.

A peripheral nerve injury might cause the loss of motor, sensory and autonomic control of target organs. These deficits may be regained if adequate regrowth of the nerve takes place, allowing the nerve to reconnect to the target organ. Parhad et al. (1995) indicate that the ability of peripheral nerves to regenerate following injury is reduced with advancing age. In particular, they indicate that the production of chemicals that encourage damaged nerves to grow (nerve growth factors) are reduced as an individual gets older. This work was done in animals, but has also been replicated in humans (Mattson et al. 2004).

Box 6.2   Mechanisms to correct balance when tripping over an object.

- In this situation, your muscles need to react quickly and in sequence so that you can prevent yourself from falling.
- This requires the CNS to react very quickly to the situation; therefore a number of 'spinal' reflexes are involved and much of the correction may have taken place before the brain is consciously aware of it.
- If this is to take place fast enough, then the speed of conduction in the peripheral nerves must be very fast indeed.
- In Mrs Wright's situation (see Chapter 5), the speed of nerve conduction could be slightly reduced because of her age, and in the majority of people of this age group this would not be too significant. However, Mrs Wright has Parkinson's disease, and the associated pathological impairments combined with slowing of nerve conduction as part of normal ageing might contribute to an increasing tendency to fall.

Therefore, in older people, if injuries occur then it is likely that the rate and degree of recovery will decrease (Vaughan 1992, Verdu et al. 1995).

Voice and speech production

Ageing of body functions and structures also impacts upon speech and voice production. A complex coordination of sensory and motor processes involving the respiratory, laryngeal, resonatory and articulatory systems are all involved in speech and voice production, and are referred to as the subsystems for speech.

> The reader is recommended to refer to anatomy and physiology textbooks to consider the anatomical structures and physiological processes involved in speech production.

Alongside other body structures, the larynx experiences changes due to the normal ageing process. Ossification and calcification of laryngeal cartilages and cartilage joints lead to less flexibility of the vocal cords which can lead to the perceptual voice quality being affected. Muscle wasting of the intrinsic muscles of the larynx and degeneration of the laryngeal mucosa also lead to reduced functioning of the vocal cords as part of normal ageing, contributing to the loss of quality of voice production and also a drop in pitch of the voice (Linville 2004, Baken 2005). It is important to note, however, that if there are any changes in the quality of the voice, a referral to a general practitioner is advised, especially when there is a history of heavy smoking or drinking. The presence of a carcinoma can have a similar presentation and therefore every permanent change in the quality of the voice should always be fully investigated.

As already stated, other body functions and structures impact upon voice production. These include loss of elasticity within lung tissue, resulting in loss of lung capacity and efficiency which in turn impact upon the volume and rate of speech production, causing speech to be breathy, hoarse or rough in quality (Robertson and Thompson 1987). Other involved body structures include the pharynx, the face and the structures of the mouth (including tongue, gums and teeth). These structures all atrophy as part of the normal ageing process and therefore contribute to changes in articulation and vocal resonance (Robertson and Thompson 1987, Murdoch 1998, Linville 2004).

Mental functions

Deterioration in mental function is seen by many old people as the true marker of the onset of old age and the most feared, with the belief that dementia is the only outcome. The phrase 'you can't teach an old dog new tricks' is commonly heard from both young and old alike to describe mental functioning in older age. However, current policy and guidance acknowledges the need for lifelong cognitive and emotional good health

(Foresight Mental Capacity and Wellbeing Project 2008). Indeed, Deary et al. (2009, p. 136) state '...the state of the brain in old age is the summary of effects across the life-course, from conception'.

Cognitive impairment is perceived as a global major health and social issue, with 40% of admissions to long-term care in the UK occurring as a result of cognitive impairment (Deary et al. 2009). However, a decline in mental functioning into dementia is not an inevitable part of old age – but part of disease processes (Hayden et al. 2011). Decline in cognitive function varies, and evidence is often conflicting, with Hayden et al. (2011) suggesting that methodological issues within research are a contributory factor. It must be remembered that older people are a heterogeneous group and therefore evidence (and recruitment to studies) has to be considered within this context. However, there is strengthening evidence for the positive relationship of physical activity with cognitive functioning, even in the oldest-old (Sumic et al. 2007). This is related to cardio-respiratory functioning (Angevaren et al. 2008, Middleton et al. 2008). Mentally and intellectually stimulating activities also positively contribute to cognitive functioning, with a 'use it or lose it' ethos. It is hypothesised that such activities add to an individual's cognitive reserve across their lifespan, thus protecting or delaying cognitive impairment (Verghese et al. 2003, Deary et al. 2009). Other predictors are poor general health (including midlife high blood pressure, cholesterol, blood glucose, and body mass) associated with generalised cognitive decline (Christensen 2001, Gilhoolly et al. 2003) and feelings of psychological wellbeing (Llewellyn et al. 2008).

Global mental functions

Consciousness and sleep

Arousal and sleep are seen as opposite ends of a continuum of consciousness, because they have common neurophysiological and neurochemical mechanisms. Therefore, these two states will be considered together. Consciousness is not often formally assessed by occupational therapists, unless intervening with those with traumatic brain injury (TBI) or observing drowsiness when working with an older person.

Arousal is necessary for most cognitive functions to take place, especially memory, learning and attention. Social and behavioural phenomena also impact on arousal and sleep, with the onset of retirement causing abrupt changes to routine, altered cognitive and physical demands and therefore sleep. The frontal lobe has an inhibitory role on the ascending reticular arousal system in the brain stem and therefore any reduction in frontal lobe function will cause changes in arousal and sleep patterns (Woodruff-Pak 1997). Interestingly, evidence to support changes in daytime arousal, as part of normal ageing, is limited (Kim et al. 2000).

Levels of consciousness are affected by stimulants such as alcohol, nicotine and caffeine, as well as barbiturates, narcotics and hallucinogens. The use of illicit substances is increasing in the older age group as the baby boomers enter old age. The misuse of prescription and over-the-counter medication is also high within the older population and a significantly high number of older people consume dangerously high levels of alcohol. Indeed, it is calculated that substance abuse in older people will double in the next 10–20 years. Unfortunately, substance abuse in older people is commonly overlooked and there are high levels of unmet needs (Christensen et al. 2006, Crome et al. 2011, Royal College of Psychiatrists 2011, Wu and Blazer 2011).

Other factors that influence consciousness in older people are:

* Syncope – caused by cardiac disease, hypotension, reflex activity, CNS disease, hypoglycaemia (Lipsitz and Jonsson 1992)
* Epilepsy – where symptoms are commonly mistaken for other diseases in older people (Kilpatrick and Lowe 2002)
* Delirium (Acute Confusional State) – often undiagnosed, causing impairment in attention, orientation, memory and executive functions (Schuurmans et al. 2001).
* General anaesthesia – can cause post-operative cognitive dysfunction and pain (Selwood and Orrell 2004).

An increase in sleep-related disorders is observed to occur as part of the ageing process (Wolkove et al. 2007). Typical sleep changes with older age are a decline in total hours of night-time sleep (although this is disputed by Ancoli-Israel 2009), a delayed onset and greater disturbance in sleep, an increase in daytime napping and somnolence (Münch et al. 2005, Wolkove et al. 2007). Sleep and wakefulness are determined by the biphasic circadian rhythm (our internal body clock), which is regulated by the suprachiasmatic nuclei of the hypothalamus – another area of the brain sensitive to age-related cell death (Hastings 1998, Münch et al. 2005). Alterations to sleep are not always inevitable but sleep disturbances are commonly associated with depression (early morning wakening and difficulty falling asleep), Alzheimer's disease (fragmented patterns of sleep and wakefulness at night and sleep during the day), cardiac and respiratory conditions, and musculo-skeletal conditions (e.g. osteoarthritis). Other sleep problems are sleep apnoea and involuntary leg movements at night experienced by 20–25% of older people which cause frequent arousal (Münch et al. 2005, Wolkove et al. 2007, Ancoli-Israel 2009, Eggermont et al. 2010).

Medications such as anticholinerase inhibitors, Beta-blockers, decongestants, corticosteroids, diuretics, dopamine agonists, and SSRIs all contribute to insomnia (Münch et al. 2005, Ancoli-Israel 2009). Prescription of hypnotic medication (e.g. benzodiazepines) is also problematic in older people. These have only a short-term effect on sleep, but have had a historical tendency to be prescribed repeatedly and long term without reassessment. Because of reduced renal function (see Chapter 7) medication has a longer half-life within the body (see Chapter 8), with an impact on levels of consciousness throughout the day – with the possible impairment of judgement and reaction times. Reduction of benzodiazepines can also induce withdrawal insomnia. Current advice is not to prescribe hypnotics to older people because of their risk of confusion and ataxia and consequential falls or injury (British National Formulary 2011). Non-medication techniques should therefore be pursued – including an increase in the daily exposure to daylight, increase in exercise and high carbohydrate meals (Wolfson and Katzman 1992). The opportunity to follow such advice is heavily dependant on individual contextual factors – especially for those older people in long-term residential care.

It is important to consider the consequences of sleep disturbances such as poor general health, a decrease in physical functioning, falls, cognitive impairment, fatigue and an increase in mortality (Ancoli-Israel 2009, Hawker et al. 2010) as these will have an impact on the older person's ability to positively and safely participate in their chosen occupations.

Orientation

Orientation to time of day, date and place or season is commonly monitored within cognitive functional assessments of older people. Orientation requires many functions including attention, memory and retention of new information and is influenced by educational levels (Sweet 1999). Disorientation is a symptom of many pathological processes in older people such as depression, Alzheimer's disease, and stroke. Many of us become disorientated (in its true sense) by getting lost or forgetting today's date; however, most people have strategies to resolve this (looking at a watch, a map or diary) but this becomes problematic when an individual is consistently disorientated in time, place or person, impacting upon occupational performance, sense of control and self-esteem.

Intellect

There is much debate whether intellectual ability declines as part of normal ageing or is preserved throughout the lifespan (Goldman and Coté 1991). Definitions of intelligence vary, and an individual's intellectual ability can only be determined by assessment of behaviour. Intellectual functions have been described in terms of crystallised and fluid intelligence, with crystallised intelligence being experience and knowledge of learned information and facts (numeracy, vocabulary). Fluid intelligence involves the perception of complex relationships, reasoning, problem solving and adaptation to new situations, and it is this aspect that is said to decline with age with crystallised intelligence remaining intact (Salthouse et al. 2008). Rabbitt (1997) and Beier and Ackerman (2005) identified that even though older people may not perform so well on tasks requiring quick problem-solving skills (fluid intelligence), they have perfected better problem-solving strategies over a longer period of time, because they can utilise past experience and information to help them. In many cultures, such strategies demonstrate wisdom; a quality that is valued and aspired to (Jeste and Harris 2010).

Energy, motivation, personality and temperament

Not all global functions dramatically change as part of normal ageing. Where changes occur in energy and drive (motivation), personality and temperament, these are likely to be symptoms of pathological processes. These functions come under frontal lobe control and, more specifically, the prefrontal cortex. Damage to this area can range from poor motivation as a key symptom in depression and minor impairments such as irritability, reduced motivation and quick loss of temper to a complete change in personality and loss of social inhibition. Such changes are known as 'frontal lobe syndrome' and occur in stroke, prolonged alcoholism, Korsakoff's syndrome and Alzheimer's disease (Woodruff-Pak 1997).

Specific mental functions

In more recent years, the term 'age-related cognitive decline' has evolved to acknowledge normal cognitive ageing. Cognitive functions most obviously affected by ageing are the specific functions of attention, memory, executive functions and speed of processing, which contribute to effective learning and successful performance of everyday activity. However, how this is established is debated, as it is suggested that this is subjective and dependant upon an individual's previous cognitive performance and intelligence (Jones and Ferris 1999, Deary et al. 2009).

Attention

The ICF defines attention as 'specific mental functions of focusing on an external stimulus or internal experience for the required period of time' (WHO 2001, p. 53). Attention and memory are inextricably linked, with a dysfunction in either causing problems in occupational performance. Attention is not one concept but consists of different types of attention, which will be discussed here. It is contested whether there are age-related changes to specific mental functions such as attention. However, Grady (2008) suggests that there are changes to areas of the brain recruited to achieve the same outcome as a younger person, and hypothesises that older people over-recruit the frontal and parietal regions in tasks requiring great attentional demands. However, it is debated whether this is a form of neural plasticity, to compensate for altered functions in other regions of the brain, or neural inefficiency (Grady 2008).

Sustained attention (or vigilance as it is sometimes known) is the maintenance of abilities to focus attention over a period of time (for example in formal assessment). Perry and Hodges (1999) suggest that the most likely site for sustained attention is in the fronto-parietal cortex. This tends to be assessed subjectively in the clinical setting, as few appropriate tools have been devised. Sustained attention requires an adequate level of arousal and sensitivity to different inputs and can be affected in many tasks, especially as they become more complex (Baddeley et al. 1999). This is also said to be problematic in moderate Alzheimer's disease and it is contested whether this is affected in earlier stages (Baddeley et al. 1999, Perry and Hodges 1999). In depression, individuals such as Mr James have a shorter span of sustained attention, with reduced concentration a common complaint (Butters et al. 2000).

Selective attention involves focusing on a single relevant stimulus at one time, ignoring other irrelevant or distracting stimuli. The areas of the cerebral cortex said to be responsible for selective attention are the posterior parietal cortex and basal ganglia (Perry and Hodges 1999). This requires inhibitory processes to sift out irrelevant stimuli; however, cognitive research identifies that cognitive inhibition deteriorates with old age so that older people have more difficulty in suppressing extraneous information (Woodruff-Pak 1997). This is even more noticeable with people with learning disability and also in Alzheimer's disease and depression. Butters et al. (2000) suggest that the problem with selective attention for depressed clients occurs because cognitive resources are taken up by negative thoughts, which improve with medication. In Alzheimer's disease it is thought that clients have difficulty disengaging and differentiating between stimuli (Perry and Hodges 1999).

Divided attention is the sharing of attention by focusing on more than one relevant stimulus or process at a time. The possible sites responsible for this are the prefrontal cortex and anterior cingulate gyrus (Perry and Hodges 1999). The inability to carry out divided tasks is said to be a problem of the central executive (see following section) and problems with this are well documented with clients with Alzheimer's disease (Baddeley et al. 1991,

Camicoli et al. 1997). Dual tasking is discussed in Chapter 8; it is also considered to be problematic in normal older people but could be considered to be suggestive of underlying pathology (Rabbitt 1997, Woodruff-Pak 1997). The study of divided attention (and dual tasking) is of particular interest for practice as it is common in everyday activity for an individual to be carrying out two tasks at one time, especially a motor task and a visual or cognitive task.

It is therefore important to provide clients with suitable environments for them to attend to or focus on the required task or stimulus. Ensuring that an older person is comfortable, and not distracted by pain, noise or visual stimuli during assessment and intervention, facilitates learning and performance especially of new or complex tasks. An awareness of an older person's ability in selective, sustained and divided attention must be taken into account during occupational performance.

Memory

Memory involves 'the registration, retention and retrieval of information' (Jones and Ferris 1999, p. 212). Although memory loss is perhaps the key concern relating to ageing because of its association with dementia, a linear decline of memory loss with normal ageing is generally accepted, and is known as age-associated memory impairment (Jones and Ferris 1999).

Formation of memory traces requires motivation, arousal, perception and attention. Memory and learning are closely linked with the successful storage of learned skills retrieved from memory and tested through observation of behaviour and performance. The mechanisms of memory are not fully understood but, like attention, it is considered that there are different types of memory, with different functions. Many older people report memory problems which may not be evident from testing and memory deficits do not only occur as part of normal ageing (see Table 6.1).

The three types of memory considered in this section and presented in Table 6.1 are short-term memory, working memory and long-term memory (declarative and procedural).

Declarative memory is a more explicit memory system that relates to recall of factual knowledge and is subdivided into episodic and semantic memory (see Table 6.1). The other long-term memory type is known as procedural memory and is a more implicit memory of how to carry out tasks and activities such as walking, talking and eating. Short-term memory involves the temporary storage of information and experiences within the previous few minutes, working memory involves the temporary storage of verbal and nonverbal information necessary for learning, reasoning and comprehension. It also has a central executive system, which is responsible for control of attention. The concept of a working memory as part of an attentional system was proposed by Baddeley and Hitch in 1974, and has been said to be the 'most significant achievement of human mental evolution' (Goldman-Rakic 1992, p. 73). Working memory consists of the central executive with slave or sub-systems for short-term memories known as the visuo-spatial sketchpad (for visual images) and the phonological loop (for speech-based input). The concept of a working memory replaced the idea of a single short-term memory store. The central executive is said to have access to long-term memory and is said to work as a supervisory attentional system (SAS) as proposed by Norman and Shallice (1980), coordinating

Table 6.1 Concepts of memory, their function, location and changes with ageing and pathological processes.

Memory type	Function	Area of CNS	Normal ageing	Pathological processes
Short-term memory	Temporary storage of events and information within the past few minutes	Hippocampus, and medial temporal lobe	Some changes with ageing	Noticeable changes in Alzheimer's disease and depression
Long-term memory 1. Declarative (explicit) memory consisting of	Directly accessible to conscious recollection			
Episodic memory	Personal experiences, context bound to time and place	Hippocampus of medial temporal lobe, diencephalon	Occurs as part of normal ageing	Korsakoff's syndrome, depression
Semantic memory	Cumulative knowledge of the world, concepts, language	Frontal lobe	More stable and resistant to change	Dementias
2. Procedural (implicit) memory	Learned skills or cognitive operations	Different areas, e.g. motor cortex, cerebellum, etc.	More stable and resistant to change	Occurs in TBI, CVA, multi-infarct dementia
Prospective memory	Manipulates and organises memory, rather than acquisition and storage	Medial temporal lobe	Affected in older age	Occurs in depression, dementias.
Working memory	A workspace for short-term memories, with a central executive and sub systems	Prefrontal cortex	Ageing effects occur	Problems in dementias, Parkinson's disease, depression

(Squire 2004, Shimamura 1990, Katzman and Terry 1992, Woodruff-Pak 1997, Stevens and Ripich 1999) information from different sources. The SAS is said to be able to override ongoing activities such as in dual tasking (to stop walking while talking,) when the SAS is at full capacity. SAS function is said to decline as a result of frontal lobe damage or deterioration (Baddeley et al. 1991). Working memory relies on the interaction of the prefrontal cortex and the hippocampus, with the prefrontal cortex retrieving facts, events and rules from elsewhere in the brain as well as regulating motor behaviour by initiating, programming, facilitating and cancelling commands to brain structures and the hippocampus consolidating new associations and learned memory (Goldman-Rakic 1992). As already discussed, these areas of the brain are most susceptible to atrophy in normal ageing, and working memory and attention are said to be the most vulnerable, especially with the processing of incoming information and with consequential task performance (Fabiani 2012).

Psychomotor functions and speed of processing

Speed of nerve conduction has been discussed in relation to the PNS; however, this is said to impact on slowing of simple motor tasks by a lesser degree than by a reduction in central processing. Performance on timed tasks (reaction time – RT) is said to peak at age 20 and declines thereafter, with Christensen (2001) suggesting that speed of processing drops by 20% at 40 years and by 40–60% at 80 years. Slowing of motor tasks such as writing and sport is said to be relative to previous ability rather than chronological age. Complexity of tasks (discussed in Chapter 8) also impacts on the speed of processing, with an increase in complexity causing an increase in time in older age groups to avoid error (Rabbitt 1997, Endrass et al. 2012). Speed of processing also affects cognitive tasks. It was thought that those individuals with higher intelligence and educational experience performed better than age-equivalents; however, Christensen et al. (1997) demonstrated that RT tasks were the same for both groups but the higher intelligence group did better than age-equivalents on verbal tasks of crystallised intelligence. Such a decline in cognitive speed is also associated with white matter changes in the frontal lobe (Christensen 2001, Deary et al. 2009).

Increase in reaction time above that expected of a normal older person is seen both in depression (Butters et al. 2000) and in Alzheimer's disease (Perry and Hodges 1999) and is seen to be a problem of central processing rather than nerve conduction.

Executive functions

The ICF defines executive functions as higher-level cognitive function (WHO 2001, p. 57) and is seen as the most highly-developed group of functions in humans – involving planning, abstract thought, decision making, cognitive flexibility and the use of appropriate behaviours (Woodruff-Pak 1997). These functions are those that are said to account for most of cognitive decline in older people (Salthouse et al. 2003, Deary et al. 2009) and are also the most noticeable in clients with Alzheimer's disease, learning disability, stroke and Parkinson's disease (Bellelli et al. 2002). The function of spontaneous flexibility such as generation of ideas and reactive flexibility to new ideas and situations (known as switching set) are especially impaired in older age (Woodruff-Pak 1997). Such mental inflexibility is said to be due to depletion of dopamine levels in the CNS as part of ageing and particularly Parkinson's disease.

Other aspects of executive functions are termed as prospective memory – involving planning, organisation and self-monitoring. Many older adults are said to perform badly on tasks such as remembering future events such as birthdays, appointments or taking medications (Shimamura 1990). The use of external cues such as diaries, calendars and 'post-it' notes are important to compensate for prospective memory loss. Other problems with self-monitoring are socially inappropriate comments, impulsive behaviour and keeping track of conversations – leading to repetition of stories and conversations.

Assessments of executive functions are carried out widely with impairments in this area and are said to be key to a diagnosis of Alzheimer's disease, where people complain of problems with everyday tasks such as organising shopping lists (like Darragh in Chapter 5) (Perry and Holmes 1999). However, they are criticised for their lack of ecological validity in their relationship to real-world tasks (Morris et al. 2000) and also for their specificity (Salthouse et al. 2003).

Emotion

Emotional wellbeing and stability are said to occur into very old age (Scheibe and Carstensen 2010). However, as can be seen in Chapter 5, depression is common in older people and characterised by the negative emotions of sadness, helplessness and loss. A sense of wellbeing is important in maintaining occupational performance (Borell et al. 2001), with the voluntary giving-up of independence (termed 'learned helplessness') being a direct link with poorer cognitive functioning and depression. Other emotional changes seen are those in Alzheimer's disease such as inappropriate response and emotional disturbances due to impaired executive functioning.

Perception

Perceptual problems are more commonly associated with older people with stroke or TBI. However, some changes in perceptual ability do occur with normal ageing. Perception of colour, depth and distance of field all deteriorate with age, alongside a reduction in lens accommodation and retinal illumination (Fozzard et al. 1977). Su et al. (1995) also identified deterioration in figure ground, visual memory and spatial relationships. Grady (2008) suggested that older people have higher prefrontal activity in visual perceptive tasks – placing greater emphasis on attentional control to compensate for visual cortex functioning and processing.

Like many other aspects of occupational; therapy, intervention strategies for adults with perceptual problems do not have a strong evidence base. However, the use of either a remedial approach or adaptive approach described by Zoltan (1996) will depend heavily on the older person's attentional ability and their memory in determining their capacity for learning and retaining new skills.

Language

Many changes occur in the structures responsible for processing cognition and language. These changes result in age-related deficits in memory alongside other aspects of cognition, and linguistic skills. Cognition and linguistic skills form the scaffolding upon which language and communication can function. If these are affected, there is usually some negative effect on communication.

As already considered above, semantic memory, which is responsible for understanding the meaning of words, remains relatively stable with normal ageing. Therefore understanding of language remains constant; however, word retrieval and production (including spelling) are more vulnerable to age-related decline (Burke and MacKay 1997).

Even though the changes in communication skills are relatively small in normal older people, changes in cognition and also hearing acuity will impact on the older person's ability to hold and maintain a conversation. Other neurological diseases, such as stroke, Parkinson's disease and dementia, common in older age will cause problems with communication skills. Indeed, Stevens and Ripich (1999) suggest that older people with mild to moderate Alzheimer's disease demonstrate difficulties with communication and meaning of words, and with progression of their dementia show difficulties with syntax, then production of sound and eventually exhibit mutism in end-stage dementia.

Sensory systems' structure and function

Sensory modalities change as part of normal ageing; with an increase in sensory thresholds with ageing means that an increase in sensory input is required before sensory awareness occurs (Dugdale 2010). It is important to be aware that alterations to smell and taste affect eating habits and diet in later life, including the difficulty in ascertaining when food is spoiled and therefore increasing the risk of food poisoning. Quality of life is also affected by alteration to the sensations of touch, vibration, sight, temperature, hearing and balance ability as part of normal ageing (Woodruff-Pak 1997).

Touch

Touch is not only affected by poor circulation causing occlusion of the small capillaries under the surface of the skin, but also by the reduction of touch receptors (Meissner's corpuscles). Reduction in the perception of vibration and pressure also occurs with ageing. Reduction in perception of all of these modalities impacts upon hand function and grip strength, affects postural responses and balance and also increases risk from injury, burns and pressure ulcers (Dugdale 2010, Shumway-Cook and Woollacott 2012).

Pain

The CNS in relation to ageing has been discussed and the peripheral (PNS) sensory receptors detecting mechanical (touch or pressure), thermal (temperature changes) and damage stimuli (producing pain) have also been mentioned. However, one issue that involves both central systems and peripheral systems is that of pain. Pain is an important sensory function which protects the body from possible injury. However, in many cases it can be very distressing to the individual, which could in itself cause significant activity limitation. In some cases, pain responses may be out of proportion to the nature of the stimulus presented to the body and again cause activity limitation.

Pain sensation is transmitted to the CNS via peripheral nerves which, as already discussed, undergo some changes with age. This can lead to a reduction in the transmission frequency and rate of pain-related sensation in older people. However, a study by Gagliese (2009) found no age-related alterations in pain perception. Moreover, pain is often under-reported in older people, not because they feel less pain, but because they fear that more pain might indicate progression of disease (Nishikawa and Ferrell 1993, Ferrell 1996). Because of the diseases that are more common in older age, persistent pain is more prevalent. It is often accepted as part of the ageing process by both older people and medical professionals working with them and, as a consequence, is often left unmanaged. Therefore, because older people may be less likely to voluntarily report pain, professionals working in this area need to be aware of this issue and be proactive in pain management.

Pain in dementia is seen to be a complex issue, with uncertainty of the qualitative experience of pain by older people with dementia. Indeed, it is reported that many older people with dementia are under-prescribed pain relief following fracture or injury as it has been considered that this group of older people do not feel pain with the same intensity or frequency as their cognitively normal counterparts. However, Scherder et al. (2009) concluded that older people with dementia experience pain with the same intensity and frequency, even if this is not reported. These researchers concluded that health professionals must have a greater awareness of differing manifestations of pain, through facial expression, guarding or changes in behaviour when working with this client group.

The eye and visual functions

The eye as a sensory organ is another receptor allowing perception of our environment. However, the visualisation of our environment requires many processes to be meaningful and useful. The eye is anatomically and developmentally closely related to the brain. Information from the eye is transmitted to the brain via the optic nerve. Visual information is then interpreted by the occipital lobe, allowing the brain to form a perception of the visual environment.

> Before reading further it would be useful to review the general structure and function of the eye. In particular, it would be useful to be aware of its anatomy and principal functions.

Deterioration in visual acuity is one of the most common sensory changes occurring with advancing age, with one in five over-75-year-olds having a visual impairment (Philp 2003). Common visual impairments in older age are age-related macular degeneration, cataract, diabetic eye disease and glaucoma (National Ageing Research Institute 2009).

This is often seen when individuals are looking at objects in their immediate 'close' environment. It is also common, as individuals get older, for some deterioration to occur to the corneal layer of the eye. Cell death in this area can cause a decrease in the ability of the cornea to allow light into the eye and cataracts are not uncommon. Other impairments have also been identified, such as spatial discrimination, restriction in upward gaze and the reduction in ability to 'track' (follow) a moving object.

The ear and auditory functions

The ear provides recognition of auditory stimuli and also forms one of the key organs for orientating the body in space, thus contributing to balance. When discussing the anatomy of the ear, we usually refer to three regions: the outer (external) ear, middle ear and inner (internal) ear or labyrinth.

> *Before reading further it would be useful to review the general structure and function of the ear. In particular, it would be useful to be aware of the anatomy and principal functions of external, middle and inner ear.*

The inner ear provides two main functions: hearing and balance information. The ageing process can affect both of these functions. Difficulties in hearing in older people are well documented in the literature and are also a well-known factor to the general public. Indeed, it is said that hearing loss is one of the most common chronic conditions in older age (Dalton et al. 2003) and is commonly associated with reduced sense of wellbeing, poorer quality of life, and social isolation because of the diminished opportunities for communication with others (Dalton et al. 2003, Gopinath et al. 2012).

Hearing loss related to ageing is known as presbycusis and is the most common hearing disorder (Langan 2010, Deafness Research UK 2012). Presbycusis is caused by a combination of intrinsic and extrinsic factors. Intrinsic factors affecting hearing may be related to apoptosis in some of the cells related to the nerve conduction to the brain. They may also relate to cell loss and death in the specialist hair cells (stereocilia), producing an inability of the system to detect sounds at certain frequencies. The blood (vascular) supply to the inner ear may deteriorate with age, which could contribute to loss of neural cells or stereocilia. Thickening of the tympanic membrane, loss of elasticity in the ossicular chains and atrophy of the cochlea all impair hearing (Zoltan 1996). Extrinsic factors, which may contribute to this process, include issues such as exposure to chronic noise (accounting for the largest single reason for hearing impairment in older people), smoking and a high-fat diet (Verschuur et al. 2012). Functionally, this can result in deterioration in hearing at certain frequencies and difficulty in following conversation and speech in unfavourable listening conditions (Langan 2010, Deafness Research UK 2012).

Box 6.3   Balance activity.

- Stand opposite a partner.
- Take it in turns to observe each other for approximately 30–45 seconds in quiet standing, firstly with the eyes open and then with the eyes shut.
- What do you observe?

Balance

Balance is affected as part of the ageing processes occurring in several body structures and functions. Balance mechanisms are reliant upon input from the visual system, the PNS and vestibular structures in the inner ear, along with CNS processing. In a similar way to the cellular deterioration of auditory structures, vestibular structures of the inner ear are susceptible to cellular deterioration. The saccule, utricle and semicircular canals rely on specialist sensory cells, which are similar to stereocilia and indicate the movement of fluid in these structures, providing information regarding the body's position in space. Cell loss takes place in these structures as part of normal ageing, and leads to a decrease in the response time to balance perturbations registered by structures of the inner ear. This is also linked to cellular loss in the cerebellum and higher brain centres involved with balance.

Deterioration in the inner ear structures involved with balance should be considered alongside reduced conduction velocities in the PNS and the reduction in sensitivity of sensory receptors. Joint position receptors (proprioceptors), muscle spindles and skin pressure receptors all need increased stimulus before firing, as individuals get older. This means that body position information from joint positions, muscle length and skin pressure are all slightly reduced. The CNS correlates this information with body position information from the structures of the inner ear and with information from the visual system. These three systems then work together to produce functional balance and correction of balance when perturbations (loss of balance) occur.

Shumway-Cook and Woollacott (2012) identify that the vestibular system provides the reference point for the visual and peripheral sensory systems, and therefore this system is especially important in balance control.

The visual system is said to dominate over the proprioceptive and vestibular systems in quiet standing, when normal subjects are observed to increase their antero-posterior sway (known as postural sway) with the eyes shut. An increase in postural sway is also observed in quiet standing with the eyes open by those people with poor visual acuity, young children and also older people. Balance correction is required in a number of different circumstances in everyday activity. Shumway-Cook and Woollacott (2012) describe two different types of balance control – reactive and proactive – which are dependent upon constant postural adjustments and adaptation, equilibrium, righting and protective reactions. Reactive control of balance is required in both quiet standing and sitting or when standing still on a moving platform such as a bus and reacting to a sudden jolt or perturbation. Proactive control of balance is required where postural adjustments are made in advance of a potentially destabilising situation, such as hanging clothes on a washing line or picking up a heavy shopping basket. In walking, both types of balance control are required – to avoid tripping over an obstacle on the floor or regaining one's balance as a result of a trip. These situations place increased pressure on the balance control systems. Reduction in postural balance occurs gradually with ageing; however, this decline in balance is associated more with levels of physical activity and fitness rather than chronological age (Spirduso et al. 2005). Deterioration in the combined factors producing a reduction in postural balance lead to an increased risk of falls as already described in Chapter 5.

Summary

This chapter has considered those body functions and structures primarily related to the central and peripheral nervous systems. Impairments of these systems, both in normal ageing and also in pathological states such as stroke, Parkinson's disease and dementia, impact not only on motor skills but the more complex and higher cognitive and language functions. Many of these are still not fully understood and it is only more recently, since the more common usage of PET and MRI scanning, that those theoretical concepts about human functioning and the ageing process can be scrutinised.

References

American Occupational Therapy Association (2002) Occupational Therapy Practice Framework: Domain and process. *American Journal of Occupational Therapy* **56(6)**, 609–639.

American Occupational Therapy Association (2008) Occupational Therapy Practice Framework: Domain and process, 2nd ed. *American Journal of Occupational Therapy* **62(6)**, 625–683.

Ancoli-Israel, S. (2009) Sleep and its disorders in ageing populations. *Sleep Medicine* **10**, S7–S11.

Angevaren, M., Aufdemkampe, G., Verhaar, V.A., Aleman, A., Vanhees, L. (2008) Physical activity and enhanced fitness to improve cognitive function in older people without cognitive impairment. *Cochrane Database of Systematic Reviews*, Issue 3. Art.No.: CD005381.

Baddeley, A.D., Bressi, S., Della Salla, S., Logie, R. and Soinnler, H. (1991) The decline of working memory in Alzheimer's disease. *Brain* **114(pt6)**, 2521–2542.

Baddeley, A.D., Cocchini, G., Della Sala, S., Logie, R.H. and Spinnler, H. (1999) Working memory and vigilance: Evidence from normal ageing and Alzheimer's disease. *Brain and Cognition* **41(1)**, 87–108.

Baken, R.J. (2005) The ageing voice: A new hypothesis. *Journal of Voice* **19(3)**, 317–325.

Beier, M.E. and Ackerman, P.L. (2005) Age, ability and the role of prior knowledge in the acquisition of new domain knowledge: Promising results in a real world learning environment. *Psychology and Ageing* **20(2)**, 341–355.

Bellelli, G., Lucchi, E. and Cipriani, G. (2002) Executive dysfunction and depressive symptoms in cerebrovascular disease (letter). *Journal of Neurology, Neurosurgery and Psychiatry* **73(4)**, 460–464.

Borell, L., Lilja, M., Sviden, G.A. and Sadlo, G. (2001) Occupations and signs of reduced hope: An explorative study of older adults with functional impairments. *American Journal of Occupational Therapy* **55(3)**, 311–316.

British National Formulary (2011) BNF No. 61 (March 2011). London: British Medical Association and Royal Pharmaceutical Society of Great Britain.

Buchthal, F., Rosenfalck, A. and Behse, F. (1984) Sensory potentials of normal and diseased nerves. In: Dyck, P.J., Thomas, P.K., Lambert, E.H. and Burge, R. (eds) *Peripheral Neuropathy*. Philadelphia: WB Saunders, pp. 981–1105.

Burke, D.M. and MacKay, D.G. (1997) Memory, language and ageing. *Philosophical Transactions of the Royal Society: B Biological Sciences*, **352**, 1845–1856.

Butters, M.A., Mulsant, B.H., Hagerty, B.M., Therrien, B. and Williams, R.A. (2000) Changes in attention and short processing speed mediate cognitive impairments in geriatric depression. *Psychological Medicine* **30(3)**, 679–691.

Camicoli, R., Howieson, D., Lehman, S. and Kaye, J. (1997) Talking while walking: The effect of a dual task in ageing and Alzheimer's disease. *Neurology* **48(4)**, 955–958.

Christensen, H. (2001) What cognitive changes can be expected with normal ageing? *Australian and New Zealand Journal of Psychiatry* **35(6)**, 768–775.

Christensen, H., Henderson, A.S., Griffiths, K. and Levings, C. (1997) Does ageing inevitably lead to declines in cognitive performance? A longitudinal study of elite academics. *Personality and Individual Differences* **23(1)**, 67–78.

Christensen, H., Low, L.-F. and Anstey, K.J. (2006) Prevalence, risk factors and treatment for substance abuse in older adults. *Current Opinion in Psychiatry* **19**, 587–592.

Cowell, P.E., Tuetsky, B.I., Gur, R.C., Grossman, R.I., Shtasel, D.R. and Gur, R.E. (1994) Sex differences in ageing of the human frontal and temporal lobes. *Journal of Neuroscience* **14(8)**, 4748–4755.

Crome, I.B., Crome, P. and Rao, R. (2011) Addiction and ageing – awareness, assessment and action. *Age and Ageing* **40(6)**, 657–658.

Dalton, D.S., Cruickshanks, K.J., Klein, B.E.K., Klein, R., Wiley, T.L. and Nondahl, D.M. (2003) The impact of hearing loss on quaity of life in older adults. *The Gerontologist* **43(5)**, 661–668.

Deafness Research UK (2012) Age-related hearing loss. Accessed 16.07.2012. Available at: http://www.deafnessresearch.org.uk/content/your-hearing/main-types-of-hearing-loss/age-related-hearing-loss/

Deary, I.J., Corley, J., Gow, A.J., Harris, S.E., Houlihan, L.M., Marioni, R.E., Penke, L., Rafnsson, S.B. and Starr, J.M. (2009) Age-associated cognitive decline. *British Medical Bulletin* **92**, 135–152.

Dorfman, L.J. and Bosley, T.M. (1979) Age related changes in peripheral and central nerve conduction in man. *Neurology* **29(1)**, 38–44.

Dugdale, D.C. (2010) Aging changes in the senses. Medline Plus. Accessed 20.05.12. Available at: http://www.nlm.nih.gov/medlineplus/ency/article/004013.htm

Eggermont, L.H.P., Blankevoort, C.G. and Scherder, E.J.A. (2010) Waking and night-time restlessness in mild-to-moderate dementia: A randomised control trial. *Age and Ageing* **39(6)**, 746–749.

Endrass, T., Schreiber, M. and Kathmann, N. (2012) Speeding up older adults: Age-effects on error processing in speed and accuracy conditions. *Biological Psychology* **89**, 426–432.

Fabiani, M. (2012) It was the best of times, it was the worst of times: A psychologist's view of cognitive ageing. *Psychophysiology* **49**, 283–304.

Ferrell, B.A. (1996) Overview of aging and pain. In: Ferrell, B.R. and Ferrell, B.A. (eds) *Pain in the Elderly*. Seattle: IASP Press, pp. 1–10.

Fillenbaum, G.G., Landerman, L.R., Blazer, D.G., Saunders, A.M., Harris, T.B. and Launer, L.J., (2001) The relationship of APOE genotype to cognitive functioning in older African-American and Caucasian community residents. *Journal of the American Geriatrics Society* **49(9)**, 1148–1155.

Forette, F. and Rockwood, K. (1999) Therapeutic intervention in dementia. In: Wilcock, G.K., Bucks, R.S. and Rockwood, K. (eds) *Diagnosis and Management of Dementia: A manual for memory disorders teams*. Oxford: Oxford University Press, pp. 294–310.

Foresight Mental Capacity and Wellbeing Project (2008) *Final Project Report*. London: The Government Office for Science.

Fozzard, J., Wolf, E., Bell, B., McFarland, R. and Podolsky, S. (1977) Visual perception and communication. In: Birren, J. and Schaie, K. (eds) *Handbook of Psychology of Aging*. New York: Van Nostrand Reinhold Co.

Gagliese, L. (2009) Pain and aging: The emergence of a new subfield of pain research. *The Journal of Pain* **10(4)**, 343–353.

Gilhooly, M., Phillips, L., Gilhooly, K. and Hanlon, P. (2003) Quality of life and real life cognitive functioning. Economic Social Research Council Growing Older Programme. Accessed 06/05/2012. Available at: http://www.shef.ac.uk/uni/projects/gop/MaryGilQOL_F15.pdf

Goldman, J. and Coté, L. (1991) Ageing of the brain: Dementia of the Alzheimer's type. In: Kandel, E.R., Schwartz, J.H. and Jessell, T.M. (eds) *Principles of Neural Science*, 3rd edition. Connecticut: Prentice-Hall International Inc., pp. 974–982.

Goldman-Rakic, P.S. (1992) Working memory and the mind. *Scientific American* **9**, 73–79.

Gopinath, B., Schneider, J., McMahon, C.M., Teber, E., Leeder, S.R. and Mitchell, P. (2012) Severity of age-related hearing loss is associated with impaired activities of daily living. *Age and Ageing* **41(2)**, 195–200.

Grady, C.L. (2008) Cognitive neuroscience of aging. *Annals of New York Academy of Sciences* **1124**, 127–144.

Hastings, M. (1998) The brain, circadian rhythms, and clock genes. *BMJ* **317**, 1704–1707.

Hawker, G.A., French, M.R., Waugh, E.J., Gignac, M.A.M., Cheung, C. and Murray, B.J. (2010) The multidimensionality of sleep quality and its relationship to fatigue in older adults with painful osteoarthritis. *Osteoarthritis and Cartilage* **18**, 1365–1371.

Hayden, K.M., Reed, B.R., Manly, J.J., Tommet, D., Pietrzak, R.H., Chelune, G.J., Yang, F.M., Revell, A.J., Bennett, D.A. and Jones, R.N. (2011) Cognitive decline in the elderly: An analysis of population heterogeneity. *Age and Ageing* **40(6)**, 684–689.

Holland, A.J. (2000). Ageing and learning disability. *British Journal of Psychiatry* **176**, 26–31.

Jeste, D.V. and Harris, J.C. (2010) Wisdom: A neuroscience perspective. *Journal of the American Medical Association* **304(14)**, 1602–1603.

Joaquin, A.M. and Gollapudi, S. (2001) Functional decline in aging and disease: A role for apoptosis. *Journal of the American Geriatrics Society* **49(9)**, 1234–1240.

Jones, R.W. and Ferris, S.H. (1999) Age-related memory and cognitive decline. In: Wilcock, G.K., Bucks, R.S. and Rockwood, K. (eds) *Diagnosis and Management of Dementia: A manual for memory disorders teams*. Oxford: Oxford University Press, 211–230.

Katzman, R. and Terry, R. (1992) Normal ageing of the nerious system. In: Katzman, R. and Rowe, J.W. (eds.) *Principles of Geriatric Neurology*. Philadelphia: FA Davis Company, pp. 18–58.

Kilpatrick, C.J. and Lowe, A.J. (2002) Management of epilepsy in older people. *Journal of Pharmacy Practice and Research* **32(2)**, 110–114.

Kim, M., Beversdorff, D.Q. and Heilman, K.M. (2000) Arousal response with aging: Pupillographic study. *Journal of the International Neuropsychological Society* **6(3)**, 348–350.

Langan, M. (2010) Age-related hearing loss. Medline Plus. Accessed 16/07/2012. Available at: http://www.nlm.nih.gov/medlineplus/ency/article/001045.htm

Law, M. and Baum, C. (2001) Measurement in occupational therapy, In: Law, M., Baum, C. and Dunn, W. (eds) *Measuring Occupational Performance: Supporting best practice in occupational therapy*. Thorofare: Slack Incorporated, pp. 3–19.

Linville, S.E. (2004) The aging voice. The ASHA leader. Accessed 16/07/2012. Available at: http://www.asha.org/Publications/leader/2004/041019/041019e.htm

Lipsitz, L.A. and Jonsson, P.V. (1992) Transient loss of consciousness. In: Katzman, R. and Rowe, J.W. (eds) *Principles of Geriatric Neurology*. Philadelphia: FA Davis Company, pp. 300–313.

Llewellyn, D.J., Lang, I.A., Langa, K.M. and Huppert, F.A. (2008) Cognitive function and psychological well-being: Findings from a population-based cohort. *Age and Ageing* **37(6)**, 685–689.

Maki, P. and Resnick, S. (2000) Longitudinal effects of oestrogen replacement therapy on PET cerebral blood flow and cognition. *Neurobiology and Aging* **21(2)**, 373–383.

Mattson, M.P., Maudsley, S. and Bronwen, M. (2004) A neural signaling triumvirate that influences ageing and age-related disease: Insulin/IGF-1, BDNF and serotonin. *Ageing Research Reviews* **3**, 445–464.

Middleton, L.E., Mitnitski, A., Fallah, N., Kirkland, S.A. and Rockwood, K. (2008) Changes in cognition and mortality in relation to exercise in late life: A population based study. *PLoS ONE* **3(9)**, e3124.

Morris, R.G., Worsley, C. and Matthews, D. (2000) Neuropsychological assessment in older people: Old principles and new directions. *Advances of Psychiatric Treatment* **6(5)**, 362–372.

Münch, M., Knoblauch, V., Blatter, K., Schröder, C., Schnitzler, C., Kräuchi, K., Wirz-Justice, A. and Cajochen, C. (2005) Age-related attenuation of the evening circadian arousal signal in humans. *Neurobiology of Ageing* **26**, 1307–1319.

Murdoch, E. (1998) *Dysarthria: A physiological approach to assessment and treatment*. Cheltenham: Stanley Thornes.

National Ageing Research Institute (2009) Tips on healthy ageing: Vision. Accessed 13/04/2012. Available at: http://www.mednwh.unimelb.edu.au/tips_on_ageing/vision_tips.htm

Nishikawa, S.T. and Ferrell, B.A. (1993) Pain assessment in the elderly. *Clinical Geriatric Issues in Long Term Care* **1**, 15–28.

Norman, D.A. and Shallice, T. (1980) Attention and Action: Willed and automatic control of behaviour. GHIP Report 99. San Diego: University of California.

O'Sullivan, M. (2009) Patterns of brain atrophy on magnetic resonance imaging and the boundary between ageing and Alzheimer's disease. *Reviews in Clinical Gerontology* **19**, 295–307.

Op den Velde, W. (1976) Some cerebral proteins and enzyme systems in Alzheimer's presenile and senile dementia. *Journal of the American Geriatrics Society* **24(1)**, 12–16.

van Paasschen, J., Clare, L., Woods, R.T. and Linden, D.E.J. (2009) Can we change brain functioning with cognition-focused interventions in Alzheimer's disease? The role of functional neuroimaging. *Restorative Neurology & Neuroscience* **27**, 473–491.

Parhad, I.M., Scott, J.N., Cellars, L.A., Bains, J.S., Kerkoski, C.A. and Clark, A.W. (1995) Axonal atrophy in aging is associated with a decline in neurofilament gene expression. *Journal of Neuroscience Research* **41(3)**, 355–366.

Perry, I. (1995) Prospective study of serum total homocysteine concentration and risk of stroke in middle-aged British men. *Lancet* **346**, 1395–1398.

Perry, R.J. and Hodges, J.R. (1999) Attention and executive deficits in Alzheimer's disease: A critical review. *Brain* **122(pt3)**, 383–404.

Philp, I. (2003) *Improving the Way Health and Social Care Organisations Provide Services for Older People with Sight Problems*. London: RNIB.

Pruessner, J.C., Li, L.M. and Serles, W. (2000) Volumetry of hippocampus and amygdala with high-resolution MRI and three-dimensional analysis software: Minimizing the discrepancies between laboratories. *Cerebral Cortex* **10**, 433–442.

Rabbitt, P. (1997) Ageing and human skill: A 40th anniversary. *Ergonomics* **40(10)**, 962–981.

Raz, N. (1996) Neuroanatomy of the aging brain: Evidence from structural MRI. In: Bigler, E. (ed.) *Neuroimaging. II Clinical Applications*. New York: Academic Press, pp. 153–182.

Raz, N. (2000) Aging of the brain and its influence on cognitive performance: Integration of structural and functional findings. In: Craik, F., Salthouse, T. (eds) *The Handbook of Aging and Cognition*. New Jersey: Lawrence Erlbaum Associates, pp. 1–90.

Raz, N., Gunning, F.M., Head, D., Dupuis, J.H., McQuain, J., Briggs, S.D., Loken, W.J., Thornton, A.E. and Acker, J.D. (1997) Selective aging of human cerebral cortex observation in vivo: Differential vulnerability of the prefrontal grey matter. *Cerebral Cortex* **7(3)**, 268–282.

Richards, M., Kuh, D. and Hardy, R. (1999) Lifetime cognitive function and timing of the natural menopause. *Neurology* **53(2)**, 308–314.

Robertson, J. and Thompson, S. (1987) *Working with Dysarthric Clients: A practical guide to therapy for dysarthria*. Austin, Texas: Pro Ed.

Royal College of Psychiatrists (2011) *Our Invisible Addicts*. London: Royal College of Psychiatrists.

Salthouse, T.A., Atkinson, T.M. and Berish, D.E. (2003) Executive functioning as a potential mediator of age-related cognitive decline in normal adults. *Journal of Experimental Psychology* **132(4)**, 566–594.

Salthouse, T.A., Pink, J.E. and Tucker-Drob, E.M. (2008) Contextual analysis of fluid intelligence. *Intelligence* **36**, 464–486.

Savory, J., Rao, J.K., Huang, Y., Letada, P.R. and Herman, M.M. (1999) Age-related hippocampal changes in Bcl-2 Bax ratio, oxidative stress, redox-active and apoptosis associated with aluminium-induced neurodegeneration: Increased susceptibility with ageing. *Neurotoxicology* **20(5)**, 805–817.

Scheibe, S. and Carstensen, L.L. (2010) Emotional aging: Recent findings and future trends. *Journal of Gerontology: Psychological Sciences* **65B(2)**, 135–144.

Scherder, E., Herr, K., Pickering, G., Gibson, S., Benedetti, F. and Lautenbacher, S. (2009) Pain in dementia. *Pain* **145**, 276–278.

Schuurmans, M.J., Duursma, S.A. and Shortridge-Baggett, L.M. (2001) Early recognition of delirium: A review of the literature. *Journal of Clinical Nursing* **10(6)**, 721–729.

Selkoe, D.J. (1992) Ageing brain, ageing mind. *Scientific American* **267(3)**, 134–142.

Selhub, J., Jacques, P.F., Bostom, A.G., D'Agostino, R.B., Wilson, P.W., Belanger, A.J., O'Leary, D.H., Wolf, P.A., Schaefer, E.J. and Rosenberg, I.H. (1995) Association between plasma homocysteine concentrations and extra cranial carotid-artery stenosis. *New England Journal of Medicine* **332(5)**, 286–291.

Selwood, A. and Orrell, M. (2004) Long term cognitive dysfunction in older people after non-cardiac surgery. *BMJ* **328**, 120–121.

Shimamura, A.P. (1990) Aging and memory disorders: A neuropsychological analysis. In: Howe, M.L., Stones, M.J. and Brainerd, C.J. (eds) *Cognitive and Behavioural Performance Factors in Atypical Ageing*. New York: Springer, pp. 37–65.

Shumway-Cook, A. and Woollacott, M.H. (2012) *Motor Control: Translating research into clinical practice*, 4th edition. Baltimore: Lippincott, Williams & Wilkins.

Sims, N., Bowen, D. and Smith, C. (1980) Glucose metabolism and acetylcholine synthesis in relation to neuronal activity in Alzheimer's disease. *Lancet* **1**, 333–336.

Sofroniew, M.V. (1997) Cellular recovery. In: Greenwood, R., Barnes, M.P., McMillan, T.M. and Ward, C.D. (1997) *Neurological Rehabilitation*. Hove: Psychology Press, pp. 67–84.

Spirduso, W., Francis, K. and MacRae, P. (2005) *Physical Dimensions of Aging*. Champaign, IL: Human Kinetics.

Stevens, S. and Ripich, D. (1999) The role of the speech and language therapist. In: Wilcock, G.K., Bucks, R.S. and Rockwood, K. (eds) *Diagnosis and Management of Dementia: A manual for memory disorders teams*. Oxford: Oxford University Press, pp. 137–157.

Su, C.Y., Chien, T.H., Cheng, K.F. and Lin, T.Y. (1995) Performance of older adults with and without cerebrovascular accident on the test of visual perceptual skills. *American Journal of Occupational Therapy* **49(6)**, 491–499.

Sumic, A., Michael, Y.L., Carlson, N.E., Howieson, D.B. and Kaye, J.A. (2007) Physical activity and the risk of dementia in the oldest old. *Journal of Aging and Health* **19(2)**, 242–259.

Sweet, J.J. (1999) Normative clinical relationships between orientation and memory: Age as an important moderator variable. *The Clinical Neuropsychologist* **13(4)**, 495–508.

Troller, J.N. and Valenzuela, M.J. (2001) Brain ageing in the new millennium. *Australian and New Zealand Journal of Psychiatry* **35(6)**, 788–805.

Valenzuela, M.J., Sachdev, P.S., Wen, W., Shnier, R., Brodaty, H. and Gillies, D. (2000) Dual voxel proton magnetic resonance spectroscopy in the healthy elderly: Subcortico-frontal axonal N-acetylaspartate levels are correlated with fluid cognitive abilities independent of structural brain changes. *Neuroimage* **12(6)**, 747–756.

Vaughan, D.W. (1992) Effects of advancing age on peripheral nerve regeneration. *Journal of Comparative Neurology* **323(2)**, 219–237.

Verdu, E., Buti, M. and Navarro, X. (1995) The effect of aging on efferent nerve fibre regeneration in mice. *Brain Research* **696(1–2)**, 76–82.

Verdu, E., Celballos, D., Vilches, J.J. and Xavier, N. (2000) Influence of aging on peripheral nerve function and regeneration. *Journal of the Peripheral Nervous System* **5(4)**, 191–208.

Verghese, J., Lipton, R.B., Katz, M.J., Hall, C.B., Derby, C.A., Kuslansky, G., Ambrose, A.F., Sliwinski, M. and Buschke, H. (2003) Leisure activities and the risk of dementia in the elderly. *New England Journal of Medicine* **348(25)**, 2508–2516.

Verschuur, C.A., Dowell, A., Syddall, H.E., Ntani, G., Simmonds, S.J., Baylis, D., Walsh, B., Cooper, C. and Lord, J.M. (2012) Markers of inflammatory status are associated with hearing threshold in older people: Findings from the Hertfordshire Ageing Study. *Age and Ageing* **41**, 92–97.

Volkow, N. (1996) Measuring age-related changes in DA D2 receptors with [11C] raclopride and with [18F] N-methylspiroperidol. *Psychiatry Research* **67(1)**, 11–16.

Volkow, N., Gur, R. and Wang, G. J. (1998) Association between decline in brain dopamine activity with age and cognitive and motor impairment in healthy individuals. *American Journal of Psychiatry* **155(3)**, 344–349.

Volloch, V., Mosser, D.D., Massie, B. and Sherman, M.Y. (1998) Reduced thermotolerance in aged cells results from a loss of an hsp72-mediated control of JNK signalling pathway. *Cell Stress Chaperones* **3(4)**, 265–271.

Wolkove, N., Elkholy, O., Baltsan, M. and Palayew, M. (2007) Sleep and aging: 1. Sleep disorders commonly found in older people. *Canadian Medical Association Journal* **176(9)**, 1299–1304.

Wolfson, L. and Katzman, R (1992) The neurologic consultation at 80 II: Some specific disorders observed in the elderly. In: Katzman, R. and Rowe, J.W. (eds) *Principles of Geriatric Neurology*. Philadelphia: FA Davis Company, pp. 339–355.

Woodruff-Pak, D.S. (1997) *The Neuropsychology of Aging*. Malden, USA: Blackwell Publishing.

World Health Organization (2001) *The International Classification of Functioning Disability and Health*. Geneva: World Health Organization.

Wu, L.-T. and Blazer, D.G. (2011) Illicit and nonmedical drug use among older adults: A review. *Journal of Aging and Health* **23(3)**, 481–504.

Ylikoski, R., Ylikoski, A., Erkinjuntti, T., Sulkava, R., Raininko, R. and Tilvis, R. (1993) White matter changes in healthy elderly persons correlate with attention and speed of metal processing. *Archives of Neurology* **50(8)**, 818–824.

Ylikoski, A., Erkinjuntti, T., Raininko, R., Sarna, S., Sulkava, R. and Tilvis, R. (1995) White matter hyper-intensities on MRI in the neurologically non-diseased elderly: Analysis of cohorts of consecutive subjects aged 55–85 years living at home. *Stroke* **26(7)**, 1171–1177.

Zoltan, B. (1996) *Vision, Perception and Cognition: A manual for the evaluation and treatment of the neurologically impaired adult*, 3rd ed. New Jersey: Slack Inc.

Chapter 7

The ageing body – body functions and structures: Part 2

Linda Gnanasekaran

Ageing is an inevitable consequence of the passage of time interacting with biology. The ageing process is characterised by change, largely decremental, in the anatomical structures and physiological functions of the body. These changes are most frequently viewed as negative, seeming to manifest as loss – of capacity or potential for extremes of human endeavour, of physical attractiveness, and of health. A young person may perceive the behaviours and lifestyle of an older person to result from impairments of function, giving rise to activity limitations and participation restrictions. For older people, however, behaviour and lifestyle differences may represent adaptive changes, forming part of a process of accommodation of habits, activities and roles to the gradually changing capacities and functions of the body. Old age is the only life stage in which a decline in homeostatic functioning is both normal and inevitable, although rate, timescale and onset of decline will vary enormously between individuals (see Chapter 2 and also Victor (2010), for a discussion of factors related to ageing and health). For example, a person who has spent his adult life engaged in active outdoor pursuits may show accelerated ageing of exposed skin, but might maintain a higher level of cardiovascular and musculoskeletal fitness compared to a more sedentary person of the same age. The pattern and nature of this decline will be influenced by personal and contextual factors (health, gender, nutrition, education, lifestyle, occupation, disability, etc.). This increased vulnerability to health threats, and potential decline into frailty, are risks that all people face in later life. But whilst physiological change is generally decremental, it need not limit a person's activities and abilities, and does not make disability inevitable.

All body systems are essential for homeostasis. Those which impact primarily upon occupational performance are those systems that directly affect the interaction of the person with his/her physical and social environments, i.e. the cardiovascular, respiratory, neuromuscular and musculoskeletal. Less direct in their role and impact are those systems that support homeostasis, maintain biological integrity and mediate autonomic processes, i.e. the endocrine, immune, digestive, reproductive, excretory and integumentary systems.

Occupational Therapy and Older People, Second Edition. Edited by Anita Atwal and Anne McIntyre.
© 2013 Blackwell Publishing Ltd. Published 2013 by Blackwell Publishing Ltd.

For this chapter, a basic knowledge of anatomy and physiology of the body systems is assumed. The reader is therefore recommended to consult one of the many anatomy and physiology texts available for students of the health professions.

Two key concepts form the focus of discussion in this chapter: systems integration and homeostatic resiliance. An understanding of both concepts, and their implications for health and wellbeing with advancing age, is essential to any health or social care practitioner working with older people and their support networks. Such an understanding is founded on knowledge of age-related physiological changes that affect body structures and functions.

By the end of this chapter, the reader will have gained knowledge and understanding of:

- Age-related changes that occur in the major body systems
- The functional effects of these changes upon physical capacity and performance
- The threats and challenges to homeostasis that arise as a result of age-related change
- The impact of changes across systems and their compounding effect in the development of common pathologies and syndromes of ill-health
- How this knowledge and understanding informs occupational therapy.

Age-related changes in any one system have the potential to influence functioning in other systems, and alter the body's response to illness or injury. Even a healthy older person will be more vulnerable to complications, take longer to recover, and be more likely to experience irreversible or treatment-resistant changes to body structure or function that reduce functional capacity and performance, compared to younger adults. For example, a flesh wound to the leg will take longer to heal due to changes in metabolic activity in the tissues, reduced cardiovascular efficiency, and reduced immune responses. Hence, changes in four body systems (integumentary, endocrine, cardiovascular and immune) are impacting upon recovery time and healing, not just one. Such knowledge and understanding is important to ensure that approaches to, and methods of, intervention with this client group are appropriate, effective and not likely to compound or accelerate existing problems.

Key physiological changes to body systems (structures and functions)

Table 7.1 lists the major body systems, with their composite structures and functions. As in Chapter 6, the descriptions of these systems follow the framework of the ICF (WHO 2001) and those considered are listed in Box 7.1.

Column 2 of Table 7.1 describes the key age-related changes that affect these systems. The list is not exhaustive but serves as a useful summary and reference source. The reader is encouraged to refer back to the table as aspects of functional and structural change are discussed through the rest of the chapter.

Box 7.1

- Structures and functions of the Integumentary system.
- Structures and functions of the cardiovascular, respiratory and Immune system.
- Structures and functions of the neuromusculoskeletal system.
- Structures and functions of the digestive, metabolic and endocrine system.
- Structures and functions of the Ggenitourinary and reproductive systems.

Table 7.1   Normal age related changes to body structures and functions.

Body system: principal structures and functions	Age-related changes
Integumentary system *Epidermis, dermis, nails, hair, sweat glands, hair follicles, subcutaneous adipose tissue* Largest organ of the body. A physical barrier against the external environment, medium for sensory information about the effects of the external **physical environment** upon the body. Protects underlying structures, regulates temperature, provides insulation and shock absorption, water proofing, secretion of waste, synthesis of vitamin D, production of chemicals to prevent infection, and protection against harmful light waves.	• Collagen fibres in the dermis progressively stiffen and break apart. They reduce in number, becoming tangled and disorganized. • Elastic fibres lose elasticity and clump together. • Fewer of both types of fibre are produced, so that degeneration exceeds new production. • Langerhans cells decrease in number and immune responsiveness decreases (see the *Immune system*). • Sebaceous and sweat glands reduce in number and productiveness. Skin therefore becomes drier, more liable to break, and less able to perform its cooling function. • Keratinocyte production slows, skin becomes thinner. • Melanocytes reduce; hair loses pigmentation and skin develops uneven pigmentation. • The adipose layer becomes thinner. • Walls of blood vessels stiffen and become less permeable. • Growth of hair and nails slows.
Cardiovascular system *The heart, blood vessels and blood* Transport system through which all cells, tissues and organs receive the substances essential to their survival, growth and function. Ensures maintenance of optimal fluid environment within the body for all metabolic processes. A communication system by which chemical messengers travel from their point of production to their target tissues, to alter activity within those tissues.	*The heart*: • Fibrotic change in conducting fibres slows the rate of cardiac impulses and can give rise to irregularities. • The myocardium becomes less elastic and more fibrous. Contraction is less efficient with reduced stroke volume and less response variability. The mass and volume of muscle fibres decrease. • Valves become stiffer and less pliable. *Blood vessels*: • Decrease in elasticity, increased stiffness and rigidity, loss of distensibility. • The reservoir capacity of the venous system decreases. • Arterial BP increases. • Lowered responsiveness of smooth muscle to neural and hormonal influences. *Blood*: • Decreased production of erythrocytes; reduced oxygen-carrying capacity. • Lowered white cell count (see *Immune system* below) – poorer immune response. • Increased systemic BP impacts upon diffusion and bulk flow into and out of capillaries.

Table 7.1 *(cont'd)*

Body system: principal structures and functions	Age-related changes
Respiratory system *Upper and lower respiratory tracts, thoracic cage and muscles of respiration* External respiration: gaseous exchange between the atmosphere and the blood. Blood gas homeostasis.	• Smaller airways become less elastic. • Alveoli become more fibrous and less elastic – degree of recoil on expiration reduces, and residual air volume (the air left in the lungs at the end of expiration) increases. • Alveolar surface areas, and the pulmonary capillary bed, are thought to decline (Bonder and Dal Bello-Haas 2009). Changes to the musculoskeletal system (joint stiffness, muscle fibre atrophy, calcification of costal cartilages) reduce the amount of movement of the chest wall during breathing. • Loss of abdominal muscle strength makes coughing less effective. • Reduction of sensorineural effectiveness may reduce strength of protective reflex responses, and lead to less efficient adjustment of breathing patterns in response to blood gas changes.
Immune system *Lymph, lymphatic vessels and lymph nodes, thymus gland, red bone marrow and spleen. Anti-microbial proteins, natural killer cells and phagocytes.* Protects the body against foreign substances (pathogens), through non-specific and specific immune mechanisms. Nasal mucosa and cilia, tears, saliva, digestive juices and the skin form first lines of defence. Cell and antibody mediated responses act on specific pathogens. Inflammation is a general response to tissue damage. Fever (pyrexia) is a response to the presence of certain toxins in the body, which can have the effect of inhibiting viral or bacterial activity.	*Primary changes within the immune system include*: • Atrophy of the thymus gland (commences at puberty and continues into old age). • Falling concentrations of T-cells and reduced responsiveness to antigens. • Reduced responsiveness of B-cells and impaired antibody production. • Increased risk of autoimmune responses (B-cell response to self-antigen not so effectively eliminated). • Altered inflammatory response, and longer wound healing time. (Kirkwood and Ritter 1997, Horan and Ashcroft 1997) *Secondary factors*: • Changes to the integumentary, cardiovascular and respiratory systems allow pathogens to breach innate primary defences more easily, so challenges to the system increase just as its efficiency is decreasing.
Neuromusculoskeletal system *Lower motor neurons (LMNs), skeletal muscle, bones joints* *Functional role*: Enables posture, voluntary movement and communication (speech, gesture, expression).	• Numbers of LMNs may decline with age. Fewer functional motor units, which increase in size as surviving axons innervate nearby muscle fibres that have lost their original innervations. An individual LMN may control more muscle fibres (Kevorkian and Morley 1998).

(Continued)

Table 7.1   *(cont'd)*

Body system: principal structures and functions	Age-related changes
Homeostatic role: Bone: important mineral store and acts as a buffer against fluctuating blood levels of calcium. Muscle: generates heat, assists blood circulation and lymph drainage, and in circumstances of nutritional deficit provides energy and protein to the body. Forces generated by muscle contraction stimulate bone growth	• Overall number of skeletal muscle fibres reduce, (sarcopaenia) and older muscle fibres may be weaker for their given size. • Relative proportions of muscle fibre types within any given muscle may alter, with a decline in the proportion of Type II fibres (slow twitch, aerobic, fatigue resistant). This may change the contraction characteristics and lower the fatigue resistance of the muscle (Kevorkian and Morley 1998). • Progressive loss of fast-twitch anaerobic muscle fibres. • Thickening and stiffening of synovial joint capsules. • Decreased bone tissue density due to hormonal change (see *Endocrine system* above) and digestive system changes (see below) causing mineral loss.
Digestive system *Mouth, tongue, salivary glands, teeth, oesophagus, stomach, small and large intestines, pancreas, liver, gall bladder* Nutrients and water are taken into the body as food and drink through the mouth. Involves chewing and manipulating in the mouth, salivation, swallowing, digestion, assimilation of nutrients in the body, and excretion of waste by defecation	• Loss of teeth may affect range of foods eaten due to poor mastication. • Reduced salivation. • Reduced absorbtion of some nutrients, e.g. calcium. • Slower transit time through digestive system.
Endocrine system *Organs such as the Pineal gland, hypothalamus, pituitary glands, thyroid and parathyroid glands, pancreas, adrenal gland, ovaries and testes, and the hormones they produce* Endocrine organs produce hormones and secrete these into the bloodstream. Hormones have a wide range of actions on body tissues that support homeostasis, metabolism, growth, maturation, reproduction and life-preserving responses	Some hormonal changes that occur include: • Decrease in insulin production and development of insulin resistance. • Reduction in production of testosterone and oestrogen contributes to declines in cognitive function, muscle mass and bone mineral density, as well as decline and loss of fertility. • Decline in vitamin D production due to poor nutritional uptake and poor exposure to sunlight. • (Drake et al. 2000, Morley 2003) • Reduced thyroid hormone production (lower metabolic rate). • Reduced calcitonin, increased parathyroid production (increased resorption of bone).

Table 7.1   *(cont'd)*

Body system: principal structures and functions	Age-related changes
Genito-urinary system *Kidneys, ureters, bladder and urethra.* *Organs of sexual reproduction* Fluid homeostasis, excretion of water soluble waste products and chemicals. Sexual functions.	• Kidney function declines, affecting fluid homeostasis and drug clearance times. • Bladder capacity and contractility declines. • Decline in oestrogen levels, contributing to atrophy of the uterus, loss of vaginal elasticity and reduced lubrication. • Decline in testosterone levels contributing to gradual decline in sexual functioning.

The integumentary system

Arguably the most visible signs of ageing are manifest in changes to the skin and one of its accessory structures, hair. The skin is the largest organ of the body, its principle functions being as a physical barrier against the external environment, and an essential medium for sensory information about the effects of the external physical environment upon the body. It protects underlying structures, regulates temperature, provides insulation and shock absorption, water proofing, secretion of waste, synthesis of vitamin D, production of chemicals to prevent infection, and protection against harmful light waves (Tortora and Derrickson 2009).

The appearance and texture of integumentary tissues provide a visible signal to the self and others, not only of the health status of the tissue but often of the physical health and psychological state of the individual as a whole. The rich supply of blood vessels to the skin means that states of emotional arousal, triggering autonomic nervous system activity, rapidly produce significant circulatory change with consequent change to skin colouration. States of ill-health (e.g. hypothermia, anaemia or hypotension) result in reduced blood flow to the skin, to preserve core body temperature or maintain adequate circulatory supply to essential organs such as the heart and brain. Hence the skin can suffer as a secondary consequence of diseases of other organs/systems, and can convey signs of health status to the careful observer.

The skin generally becomes thinner, drier and less elastic with age; therefore it is more easily damaged. Shock-absorbing and cushioning properties are reduced. Temperature regulating (insulating and cooling) properties are reduced, which in turn makes it harder to keep cool and older adults could be at risk of developing heat strokes.

Reduced secretions mean that the skin is less hostile to microbes, and bacteria might more easily enter the skin and, hence, the bloodstream. Wound healing is four times slower and there is a greater susceptibility to sun damage and to neoplasms.

Effects of changes in other body systems

Age-related changes to almost all other body systems can impact upon the health and integrity of the skin, and therefore also affect how it ages. For example:

• Vascular and cardiac competence determines the effectiveness of the transport of nutrients and waste to and from the skin, and its oxygenation. As it is also the transport medium for immune and inflammatory agents and responses, the cardiovascular system may determine the resistance of the skin to infection and its healing.

- Nutritional intake and hydration will impact the skin; protein and calcium are essential for healing of injuries and maintainance of collagen, water for maintaining circulation and fluid levels in all tissues. Inadequate calorie intake will lead to weight loss and increase the loss of subcutaneous adipose tissue, hence loss of insulation and protection.

Pathologies of the system

Primary disorders and diseases of the skin include infections (e.g. impetigo), allergies (e.g. hives), neoplasms (e.g. warts, cancers), and traumatic damage such as cuts and burns. The older adult is as much at risk of these disorders as at any other age, but susceptibility to some may increase as a direct result of longevity (cumulative total exposure to sunlight increases the risk of malignant melanoma), and of the declining strength and resilience of the skin (increasing age is again positively correlated with risk of developing decubitus ulcers if subjected to prolonged pressure). Skin breakdown may also occur as a result of diseases of other systems (infectious organisms might take hold and result in serious damage or even death if the circulatory or immune systems are compromised and cannot effectively combat the invasion, as in diabetes or AIDS, and the infection becomes systemic). Pre-existing conditions such as heart failure or respiratory disease will seriously compromise the blood supply to, and healing capabilities of, skin, over and above age related changes. The lower limbs will be particularly prone to skin breakdown in the presence of oedema or impaired arterial supply. Finally, side effects of medication could have long-term and permanent effects upon the skin, such as corticosteroids (collagen breakdown and thinning of the skin), or photosensitivity reactions.

Therefore, the skin can be a primary target of disease or damage, or suffer significant secondary effects of disease in other body systems. Overall, age-related changes reduce the effectiveness of the skin across all of its functions, and therefore throughout the occupational therapy process the structural and functional integrity of this organ/system could be both a target of intervention and an important secondary consideration.

Considerations in practice

Prevention

Because most skin changes are related to sun exposure, prevention is a lifelong process. Basic precautions include:

- Preventing sunburn if at all possible.
- Use of a good quality sunscreen when outdoors, even in the winter
- Wearing protective clothing and hats as necessary.

Good nutrition and adequate fluids are also helpful. Dehydration increases the risk of skin injury. Sometimes minor nutritional deficiencies can cause rashes, skin lesions and other skin changes, even if no other symptoms are apparent.

Skin should be kept moist with lotions or other moisturisers. Soaps that are heavily perfumed should be avoided. Bath oils are not recommended because they can cause people to slip and fall. Moist skin is more comfortable and will heal more quickly.

Assessment and intervention

Examination of the skin should form a routine part of any physical assessment – its colour, texture, moistness, temperature and blood supply, any signs of damage or infection, known sensitivities (e.g. to plasters) or allergens. Knowledge of medication is also important to be aware of signs of possible adverse reactions, or to know to take precautions against interactions of drugs with, for example, exposure to sunlight.

Pressure risk assessment, together with a visual assessment of known pressure risk areas of the body, could do much to prevent unnecessary and avoidable decubitus ulcer formation. Once such an ulcer develops, it renders an individual vulnerable to infection, as well as being a source of pain and disability and taking weeks or months to heal.

In some cases, the skin is a primary focus of intervention, such as in the treatment of burns. In others, knowledge of its structure, functions, and the changes that occur with advancing age will lead to modifications of planned treatment, or adjustment of certain parameters of intervention. The poorer thermal regulating properties of older skin could mean increasing the room temperature during treatment sessions to minimize heat loss, or taking care to reduce sun exposure during outdoor activities.

Trauma to the skin is more likely to lead to bruising, and will be more painful if the adipose layer is minimal. Reduced or delayed sensory processing from cutaneous receptors, and/or slowed motor response times further add to the risks of sustaining damage to the skin from activities such as cooking, gardening or sewing. Similarly, the wearing of a prosthesis or orthosis might result in skin breakdown more easily in an older person whose skin is less elastic, less resilient and less padded.

Where pre-existing conditions severely compromise the integrity of the integumentary system, the affected individual must learn and incorporate skin care into daily life and routines. Visual checking, good skin hygiene, avoidance of extremes of temperature, protecting the limbs from knocks and cuts, and aiding fluid circulation through exercise and limb elevation, will all aid good integumentary health in such cases.

Finally, it is important to bear in mind that skin also has a communication function. Most obviously, it can indicate emotional state (blushing or pallor) but the appearance of unexplained tissue trauma or bruising might indicate that an older person is, for example, experiencing falls but not wanting to admit to it, may be subject to physical abuse, or may be self-harming. Any skin damage for which a cause has not been identified must be investigated carefully and sensitively.

The cardiovascular system

The cardiovascular system – heart, blood vessels and blood – is the transport system through which all cells, tissues and organs and systems of the body receive the substances essential to their survival, growth and function, and which ensures the maintenance of an optimal fluid environment within the body for all metabolic processes. It is also a communication system by which chemical messengers travel from their point of production to their target tissues, to alter activity within those tissues. It is the medium of transport and environment of activity of many immune processes. The behaviour of the cardiovascular system therefore impacts upon and can modify the activity of every other tissue/organ/system within the body, and any change within it will have consequences for the health and functioning of the organism as a whole.

Ageing affects all components of the system, as detailed in Table 7.1, but as with many body structures and functions, the cardiovascular system has considerable reserve capacity. In normal health, ageing *per se* has negligible impact upon its efficiency and effectiveness. Of more significance is the incidence and prevalence of pathological change, which is highly correlated with increasing age and certain lifestyle factors. It is the interrelationship of age-related change and pathology which raises significant concerns for functioning and cardiovascular health.

Reduction in cardiovascular efficiency affects all body systems, in that there will be a reduction in oxygen and nutrient supply, of waste clearance, and lessened ability to respond to sudden changes in demand from tissues. Thermostatic regulation may be less effective. Wound healing and tissue repair may be slowed, with poorer immune responses to infections. Fluid volume adjustments in response to position change relative to gravity (orthostatic adjustment) may be slower.

Effects of changes in other body systems

Changes in other systems can have a compounding or cumulative effect. Changes to the musculosketal and respiratory systems impact upon the effectiveness of cardiovascular function because of the assistive role of skeletal muscle action in circulation of the blood (Tortora and Derrickson 2009). Reduced muscle bulk and contraction force leads to reduced effectiveness of the skeletal muscle pump, whereby contracting muscle (for example, in the legs) squeezes veins and assists venous return. Inhalation creates a negative pressure gradient in the thoracic cavity, and this increases venous return to the heart, and so reduced depth of breathing as the rib cage stiffens, muscles weaken, and vital capacity of the lungs decreases. As discussed below, chronic respiratory disease with extensive damage to lung tissue will impair pulmonary blood flow, and therefore cause a backlog of blood in the right heart, which in time will distend and damage the right ventricle leading to right heart failure. Diabetes is a disease of the endocrine system, but the resultant disorder of blood glucose regulation leads over time to damage to the circulatory system, and people with diabetes are at greatly increased risk of cardiovascular disorders such as coronary heart disease, stroke, and peripheral vascular disease.

Pathologies of the system

Blood pressure rises with age, particularly in Western and more technologically-developed societies. Whilst hypertension is a pathological condition, its prevalence in the United Kingdom is so high that its development in an individual could almost be considered a normal aspect of ageing. However, it must always be treated where it exists because of its known causative relationship to other pathologies (NHS Choices 2011). Aside from hypertension caused by a known disease such as renal failure or aortic stenosis (termed secondary hypertension), the majority of cases are of 'primary' or 'essential' hypertension, so-called because there is no clearly identifiable cause. Table 7.2 gives the prevalence of hypertension in people aged 45 years and over, in England.

Table 7.2   Prevalence of hypertension* by sex and age, in the adult population aged 45 years and over. England, 2008. (*Source*: British Heart Foundation 2010).

	45–54 yrs %	55–64 yrs %	65–74 yrs %	75yrs + %
Men	33	52	62	68
Women	25	41	62	73

*Hypertension is defined as systolic blood pressure of 140 mmHg or over, or diastolic blood pressure of 90 mmHg or over.

Table 7.3   Percentages of all deaths caused by cardiovascular diseases in people aged 65 years and over, England, 2008. (*Source*: British Heart Foundation 2010).

Cause of death	65–74 yrs %	75 yrs + %	Total 65 yrs and older %
Coronary heart disease	16.6	15.7	15.9
Stroke	5.7	8.9	8.2
Other diseases of the circulatory system	7.0	12.4	11.3
Deaths from cardiovascular diseases as a percentage of all deaths	29.3	37	35.4

Cardiovascular diseases (CVD) are amongst the most prevalent disorders affecting older age groups in Western societies and are the main cause of death in the United Kingdom, accounting for 1 in 3 of all deaths (British Heart Foundation 2010). Table 7.3 gives a breakdown of mortality figures by cause. The underlying pathological changes involved in the causation of most cardiovascular and circulatory disorders (aside from known pathologies such as diabetes and renal disease) are hypertension and atherosclerosis. In turn, the most common risk factors for the development of these pathological changes are generally accepted to be one or more of smoking, poor diet (high salt intake, high fat intake, weight gain and obesity), physical inactivity and alcohol consumption. These factors are all considered modifiable, whereas factors such as genetic inheritance or pre-exising pathologies are not. The effects are cumulative such that the more risk factors a person has, the more their risk of CVD increases.

The risk of cardiovascular disease can be reduced with attention to known modifiable factors, and those with diagnosed and established pathology are invariably advised to make important lifestyle adjustments which will help to slow or halt progression of the disease (e.g. lose weight, stop smoking, increase exercise, make dietary changes). This is not always easily done, if one considers that older people frequently have other conditions (e.g. osteoarthritis) or limitations (e.g. financial) which prevent them from taking action, or are being asked to change habits that have been with them throughout adult life, or are a source of pleasure, and are very difficult to forgo or change.

Considerations in practice

The prevalence of cardiovascular disorders in the older population means that all therapists will work with older people with some cardiovascular pathology, whether or not that is the reason for their presenting difficulties. Even if working with individuals who have no apparent or clinically diagnosed pathology, initial assessment should include levels of physical activity, diet, and lifestyle factors that may have a bearing on cardiovascular health. Tolerance for exercise and exertion, and the person's capacity to meet and recover from physically demanding tasks, should be ascertained. Many people will be functioning within narrowed margins of cardiovascular responsiveness and capacity. Periods of ill health, or hospitalisation for surgery or treatment of other conditions, will impact upon a system that may not have been challenged for some time, and compound the degree of deconditioning that occurs. It is therefore important for this to be identified and taken into account when planning rehabilitation or other interventions. A combination of interview, screening for symptoms and signs of cardiovascular limitation or distress, and observation of ADLs, will provide early indications if function is compromised. Activity–rest balance, diet, sleep quality and quantity, and habits such as smoking or drinking should be explored. Episodes of breathlessness, excessive fatigue, dizziness or fainting, complaints of feeling unwell or weak, of chest or arm pain, skin colour changes, or any other indications of cardiovascular dysfunction should be investigated and must not be disregarded.

In addition to assessment, the therapist must incorporate risk management and precautionary measures into therapeutic interventions. Some activities and tasks may be contraindicated. The reader is referred to Chapter 5 and other therapy texts for information about cardiac rehabilitation (Trombly and Radomski 2002, Crepeau et al. 2009) but the following are some considerations in relation to age-related aspects of cardiovascular function and occupational interventions:

- Awareness of delayed or impaired orthostatic adjustment: careful preparation for transfers or other major positional changes need to be made with education of client and carer for prevention and management of the effects of postural hypotension.
- Knowledge of psychological and physical stress responses including the impact of sympathetic arousal on the cardiovascular system (increased cardiac output, vasoconstriction, increased BP and increased venous return).
- Avoidance of anxiety and distress.
- Provision of timely and appropriate information and reassurance.
- Techniques to aid relaxation and restful sleep may be beneficial as these promote parasympathetic activity and reduce sympathetic activity.
- Attention to environmental stressors: extremes of temperature, or sudden changes triggering peripheral circulatory adjustments (vasoconstriction or dilation) impacting upon blood pressure and blood supply to peripheral tissues. The heart will be less efficient in its response to altered demand.
- Other factors, for example:
  ○ Acute emotional distress can trigger cardiac arrhythmias.
  ○ Medications carry the risk of cardiovascular side effects, including iatrogenic cardiovascular problems.
- The development or continuation of habits (e.g. tobacco smoking, excessive drinking, poor diet) known to contribute to development of CVD.

The respiratory system

The respiratory system provides the structures and mechanisms by which gaseous exchange occurs between the atmosphere and the blood. Blood gas homeostasis is essential to the functioning of all body structures and systems including, critically, the control of blood pH, and so the functioning of the respiratory system is closely bound up with that of the cardiovascular system, which must deliver blood to the lungs, and then transport it around the body.

The respiratory system is conventionally described as having two structural divisions – the upper respiratory tract (URT), consisting of nose, pharynx and associated structures (as discussed in Chapter 6), and the lower respiratory tract (LRT), comprising the larynx, trachea, bronchi and lungs (Tortora and Grabowski 2009). This description belies the reliance of these structures upon other body systems for their functioning. The ICF (WHO 2001) more accurately includes the thoracic cage, intercostal muscles, diaphragm, and accessory muscles, which cause lung expansion (inspiration), assist their deflation (expiration) and are responsible for forced expiration. Functionally, the structures are divided into two zones – the conducting zone and the respiratory zone (Tortora and Grabowski, 2009) but this categorisation does not include the musculoskeletal components.

Ageing affects the respiratory system through changes in the tissues of the airways, lung parenchyma, musculoskeletal components (rib cage, thoracic muscles, abdominal muscles) and nervous system components. Cardiovascular decline or pathology also impact upon efficiency of gaseous exchange, and may accelerate lung deterioration, as discussed below.

The trachea and bronchii undergo little change with ageing, but the smaller airways become less elastic. The alveoli become more fibrous and less elastic, so the degree of recoil on expiration reduces, and residual air volume (the air left in the lungs at the end of expiration) increases. Both the alveolar surface areas and the pulmonary capillary bed are thought to decline (Bonder and Dal Bello-Haas 2009). Changes to the musculoskeletal system (joint stiffness, muscle fibre atrophy, calcification of costal cartilages) reduce the amount of movement of the chest wall during breathing. Loss of abdominal muscle strength makes coughing less effective. The net consequence of ageing is a decline in efficiency. The lungs deflate less well and the chest wall and diaphragm move less (both in inspiration and exhalation), so overall airflow decreases. With a greater residual volume of air in the lungs, coupled with decreased alveolar surface and capillary density, gaseous exchange is less efficient.

For a person in good health, the impact of these changes could be minimal. Respiration can vary by rate as well as volume, so a slightly increased breathing rate may compensate for reduced volume. Inactivity or restricted mobility will compound ageing, so maintenance of activity and exercise becomes important for keeping up respiratory muscle strength and joint range of movement, hence countering the decreased elasticity of the lungs. Physical activity is also important for cardiovascular fitness, which in turn will help maintain pulmonary efficiency.

There will be an increased vulnerability to pathogens; the ciliary action of the epithelium that lines the conducting zone decreases with age, and the alveolar macrophages become less active, therefore non-specific resistance to disease decreases. Ageing of the immune system means less effective specific immune responses, so infections are more likely to occur, and with greater severity. Again, lack of physical activity could compound this situation. Stagnant air and moisture remain in the alveoli, because of greater residual volume, creating ideal conditions for bacterial growth. Heart failure, causing pulmonary congestion, has a similar effect. Hence, an important precaution for older people and those with respiratory or cardiac disease is to receive influenza vaccinations each winter to protect against possible complications.

Effects of changes in other body systems

Because some structures considered intrinsic to the respiratory system are also part of other systems (i.e. the rib cage, muscles of respiration, and immune components), changes to these other systems have already been considered immediately above.

Reduction of sensorineural effectiveness could further reduce the strength of protective reflex responses, and lead to less efficient adjustment of breathing patterns in response to blood gas changes. Cardiovascular disease, atherosclerosis of the aorta and carotid vessels, or impaired brainstem blood supply could contribute to this.

Pathologies of the system

The healthy and active older adult should demonstrate little observable difference in pulmonary function to a younger adult. Persistent cough, excessive production of mucous or bloodstained sputum, wheezing, breathlessness at rest or with mild exertion, or pain, will be as abnormal in healthy old age as at younger ages, and should be investigated. Where pulmonary or cardiovascular disease is present, respiratory function will be impaired, and this must be taken into account.

The greatest threat to respiratory health continues to be environmental, from the contents of the air we inhale. Active (i.e. deliberate) and passive inhalation of tobacco smoke, exposure to irritant particles and substances in the workplace (e.g. cotton mills, sawmills, bakeries, coalmines), exposure to noxious gases (e.g. from mistakes made in chlorine treatment of swimming pools) and general atmospheric pollutants have a cumulatively damaging effect upon the protective mechanisms of the airways, and the delicate lung parenchyma. This damage may lead to chronic obstructive pulmonary diseases (COPD) such as bronchitis and emphysema.

The symptoms (e.g. coughing, dyspnoea) of chronic and advanced respiratory diseases are distressing and physically exhausting in themselves. The extra mechanical work demanded of musculoskeletal structures to effectively inflate and deflate diseased lungs, that are themselves stiffer and less effective, increases the energy demands of breathing. Expiration tends to be prolonged with rapid shallow breaths to minimise the metabolic costs to the muscles. Hypoxia and hypercarbia alter the chemical and pH balance of the blood, affecting metabolism in all cells. Individuals will have limited capacity and tolerance for activity, experience fatigue, and might experience mood disturbances. Depression and anxiety have been found to be common in those with chronic and severe respiratory disease and medication to assist with this is thought to be under-used (Scullion and Holmes 2011, Swigris et al. 2008). Cardiac dysfunction could also be present; right ventricular afterload increases, and this, coupled with myocardial hypoxia and cardiac deconditioning, might contribute to the development of heart failure. Even eating a meal might be difficult, as it will interfere with breathing rhythm, and the metabolic requirements of digestion will increase oxygen demand. Certainly, weight loss is common in advanced respiratory disease as appetite reduces and ability to eat becomes becomes more difficult (Scullion and Holmes 2011).

Considerations in practice

Because of the close functional coupling of the respiratory and cardiovascular systems, many of the practice considerations discussed above for the cardiovascular system equally pertain to the respiratory system. Additionally:

- The sympathetic responses to stress of the autonomic system lead to dilation of airways, increase the metabolic activity of key organs and increase the demand for oxygen, and so knowledge of the physiological stress response, and its triggers, is important.
- Ability to vary respiration will be limited with longer adjustment time needed as the physical demands of an activity change. Recovery after exertion will take longer. This should be taken into account in activity planning.
- Promoting and encouraging good posture and optimal physical activity (within the person's limitations) will aid maintainance of respiratory, as well as cardiovascular, fitness, and so should always be incorporated into interventions.
- Increased vulnerability to infections, and decreased effectiveness of immune and protective responses, make infection control an important consideration. Health professionals must be careful to observe good hygiene practices and avoid infecting others if they have respiratory infections themselves.
- Early detection and treatment of acute respiratory illness is essential to avoid possible complications, so health professionals must act swiftly to encourage and support access to medical treatment, and encourage take-up of preventative services such as 'flu immunization.
- Medications used to treat inflammatory diseases of the system, i.e. steroids, can have significant side effects, especially if used long-term. These include thinning of the skin, osteoporosis, muscle wastage and weight gain. These effects need to be understood by the health professional as they carry implications for the suitability of some activities used for assessment or intervention and may require precautions to be taken, or even lead to an activity being contraindicated.

The immune system

The immune system is concerned with protecting the body against foreign substances (pathogens), through the action of non-specific and specific immune mechanisms. This involves cell and antibody mediated responses, the functions of lymph, lymphatic vessels and lymph nodes (Tortora and Derrickson 2009).

Other innate and non-specific defenses operate as a first line of defence to protect the body and/or remove pathogens, for example the nasal mucosa and cilia, and the skin. These are not components of the immune system and are identified in this chapter as parts of the systems to which they belong (e.g. respiratory system, integumentary system).

Non-specific immune mechanisms include anti-microbial proteins, natural killer cells and phagocytes. These are carried in the blood, and are capable of diffusing into tissues.

Inflammation is a general response to tissue damage, and fever (pyrexia) is a response to the presence of certain toxins in the body, which can have the effect of inhibiting viral or bacterial activity (Tortora and Derrickson 2009).

Specific resistance involves the production of cells and antibodies able to recognise and destroy specific antigens. This requires mechanisms to monitor and detect the presence of antigens, respond rapidly to them, and leave 'memory' cells in the system that can rapidly reactivate resistance should the same pathogen present in the future.

Age-related changes to the immune system (immunosenescence) can be considered as primary, affecting the immune tissues and organs directly, or secondary, occurring in other systems but impacting upon immune functioning.

Primary changes within the immune system include atrophy of the thymus gland (commencing at puberty), falling concentrations of T-cells, reduced responsiveness to antigens, and reduced responsiveness of B-cells with impaired antibody production. There is an increased risk of autoimmune responses (B-cell response to self-antigen not so effectively eliminated). The acute inflammatory response is reduced, and wound healing takes longer. Paradoxically, chronic inflammatory mechanisms that are implicated in chronic diseases such as atherosclerosis, cancer and osteoporosis are heightened with advancing age (Graham et al. 2006; Weiskopf et al. 2009).

As with other body systems, there are wide individual variations in immune system effectiveness and rate of decline. Nutrition, cardiovascular and musculoskeletal health, heredity, environment and stress will impact upon immune function. In general, ageing, especially interacting with stress, will compromise the homeostatic function and general competence of the immune system (Graham et al. 2006; Lovallo 2005).

With increasing age, immunisation becomes less effective. However, vaccination against influenza, for example, is advised for older people in order to boost their protection against such viruses which carry a much higher risk of complications such as chest infections and increased cardiac workload.

However, the immune system presents one example where ageing can confer benefit to the individual. Reduced levels of T and B lymphocytes can weaken allergic responses (to harmless substances) and also reduce the likelihood of organ or tissue rejection following transplantation. Older people also show increased numbers of memory B cells, related to their prior exposure to antigens over time, and so may be resistant to diseases that younger people are vulnerable to. The recent outbreaks of H1N1 influenza have seen a greater incidence of severe illness in younger age groups than in the older, thought to arise from their greater immune responsiveness. With age, there is undoubtedly an increase in the incidence of infections, autoimmune disorders and neoplasms. Adaptive responses to physical stressors such as temperature extremes, exercise and fluid balance disturbance take longer, and recovery to a homeostatic baseline also takes longer to achieve (Herbert 1991).

Effects of changes in other body systems

Secondary changes affect systems involved in first-line defence, and systems which support immune function. Ageing of the skin and other barriers allows pathogens to breach these defences more easily, so increasing the number of challenges to both the non-specific and specific immune mechanisms at a time when these mechanisms are themselves becoming less efficient. Changes to haemodynamics (blood pressure, flow, resistance, etc) because of ageing of the cardiovascular system will affect the circulation of lymphocytes and platelets, and the movement of fluid, cells and particles between capillaries, interstitial spaces and lymphatic vessels.

Crucially, stressful events are commonplace in old age, whether illness and hospitalisation, bereavement or isolation, financial or housing worries, or caring for a disabled relative. Stress evokes activation of sympathetic neuro-endocrine responses. Suppressed immune function is associated with sustained stress levels of cortisol circulating in the bloodstream, and also with exposure to negative emotional experiences (distress) and chronic or recurrent stressful events. It also results in lowered resistance to new infections and likely reactivation of latent viruses such as varicella zoster, causing shingles (Lovallo 2005).

A study of older people caring for spouses with Alzheimer's disease found a correlation between degree of distress, low social support, and levels of cellular immunity. The same group experienced more respiratory tract infections and slower wound healing than older non-carers (Kiecolt-Glaser et al. 1995). (For a fuller discussion of the relationship between immune function and stress, see Lovallo 2005, and Graham et al. 2006).

Pathology in other systems can impact upon immune function, perhaps most significantly the cardiovascular system. Right heart failure, for example, will cause congestion of the venous system, forcing excess fluid to leak from capillaries into tissues (most notably in the legs and feet due to gravity), causing oedema. This impairment of circulation and excess interstitial fluid makes normal diffusion of substances in and out of cells difficult, and slows immune reactions in areas of damage or infection. Pathogens that may enter through damaged skin cannot be contained or destroyed effectively, and ulcers might develop on the legs. Lymphatic vessels cannot drain fluid away efficiently because they too ultimately drain back in to the great veins, which are congested.

Pathologies of the system

There are five basic types of pathological dysfunction that affect the immune system: allergic reactions, autoimmune responses (loss of self-tolerance), viral infections that specifically target immune tissues (e.g. the Human Immunodeficiency Virus; HIV), cancers of the lymphatic tissues and, more rarely, primary immunodeficiency due to genetic disorder (Tortora and Derrickson 2009).

Despite some of the beneficial aspects of immunosenescence mentioned above, a reduced ability to fight off infections and decreased immune surveillance make the older person more vulnerable to development and growth of tumourous tissue, and more severely affected by some viruses and bacteria, with longer recovery periods and increased susceptibility to secondary complications.

With age, the efficiency with which self-reactive T- and B-cells are inactivated becomes less, with a greater risk of autoimmune responses developing. However, T- and B-cells become less responsive with ageing, so there may be some mutual cancelling out. In some autoimmune diseases there is a reduction in disease activity in later life (rheumatoid arthritis, for example) and inflammatory activity may subside.

Immune suppression may be a deliberate aim of drug treatment (for organ/tissue grafting, for example) or the result of disease, most typically infection with the HIV leading to acquired immune deficiency syndrome (AIDS). With the basic mechanisms of immune surveillance and responsiveness suppressed, the organism becomes vulnerable to a wide range of opportunistic infections and neoplastic growth. However, improvements in medical treatments, particularly for HIV and AIDS, mean that people with access to the most recent drug treatments are more likely to survive into older age with functioning immunity, and so opportunistic infections may be less of a threat (Tortora and Derrickson 2009).

Considerations in practice

Immune status and immune function are not primary targets of occupational assessment or interventions, but are factors that require consideration with any older person, and particularly where immunity is known to be compromised or abnormal in some way. Therefore, the occupational therapy process should be dictated by good professional standards of care and practice, and knowledge of and adherence to health and safety guidelines and requirements, to support immune function.

Where a person has an identified pathology such as HIV/AIDS, is a known carrier of a virus harmful to others (e.g. hepatitis) or is on immuno-suppressing medication, the risks to the individual, the therapist, or others, must be assessed and appropriate protocols and precautions followed. All hospitals and services dealing with such people should have appropriate procedures in place, and therapists must be cognisant with them (see Chapter 4).

Screening and assessment procedures should incorporate information gathering that will identify particular immune considerations, including allergies, cardiac disease and predispositions to particular conditions such as bronchitis.

As identified and discussed above, there are many factors which have a bearing upon immune functioning. So whilst it can be argued that immune function is not a prime consideration for occupational therapy, it must equally be recognised that occupational therapists can do much to help to support or strengthen immune functioning because of the general health effects of occupational therapy interventions. Table 7.4 identifies some common occupational interventions and their indirect benefits to immune system functioning.

Table 7.4 Benefits to immune system functioning of occupational interventions.

Occupational intervention	Immune system benefit
Relaxation training/stress management	Reduction in blood cortisol levels; immune responsiveness improved
Self-care: washing/bathing	Improved hygiene, skin defences supported, reduced pathogenic threat
Self-care: feeding	Improved nutrition and hydration, supports immune system health and wound healing
Domestic ADL: cooking skills	Improved nutritional intake, as above
Environmental adaptation for access	Easier mobility, increased physical activity: improved blood circulation and muscle action (lymphatic drainage and wound healing)
Wheelchair provision, seating and support systems	Prevention of pressure sores, maintaining circulation. Reduces risk of infection and oedema

The neuromusculoskeletal system

The production of purposeful movement requires sensorineural processing and integration, motor output, a responsive muscle system, and an articulated bony framework for muscle forces to act upon. The central and peripheral nervous systems (CNS and PNS), skeletal muscles, and the skeletal system form the essential component structures for this function.

Movement is immensely variable, from the delicate and subtle movements of facial expressions, to the massive force generated by a weight lifter. Muscle action is the medium through which we express ourselves and communicate (speech, expression, gesture), interact with the environment and meet our needs. All individuals have characteristic movement patterns and habits, and movement and posture also alter with age.

Bone and muscle tissue have important metabolic and homeostatic functions as well as their roles in movement and stability of the body. For example, bone is an important mineral store and acts as a buffer against fluctuating blood levels of calcium. Muscle is an important generator of heat, assists blood circulation and lymph drainage, and in circumstances of nutritional deficit provides a protein source to the body. The forces generated by muscles acting on bone stimulate bone growth, so movement is important for bone density and strength.

In Chapter 6, many aspects of nervous system functioning were discussed, and the reader should bear in mind the content of that chapter whilst considering ageing and the motor system. Large areas of the brain are involved directly or indirectly in movement production. Therefore, general changes in brain structure or function will impact upon motor processes and movement. Deterioration of sensory, integrative, cognitive and perceptual functions will affect reflex responses and the quality and effectiveness of voluntary movements. Deterioration of subcortical and brainstem structures will affect reflexes, tone and postural mechanisms.

It can be very difficult to separate out the neural contribution to decline in movement functions from the musculoskeletal contribution. Movement is a result of CNS output to lower motor neurons (LMNs), their communication with muscle fibres at the neuromuscular junction, and the consequent contractile behaviour of the muscle fibres. Movement quality and quantity derive from the integrity and health of all these structures and processes.

Two models of age-related change have been proposed to account for decline in movement-related functions: one considers the decline as due to primary neuronal loss and neurodegeneration, the second attributes decline to deterioration arising from secondary factors such as pathology, immobility secondary to disability, or environmental and lifestyle factors. Table 7.1 details key changes to the body structures that impact directly upon movement.

Bone tissue is affected both in the mineral component (hardness), and the collagen matrix (tensile strength). Through childhood and youth, mineral deposition exceeds resorption (though influenced by diet and exercise), so bone increases in density and strength. With advancing years, resorption exceeds deposition, so bone density decreases by approximately 1% each year, although varying by age, gender and other factors (Tortora and Derrickson 2009). Protein synthesis also decreases, hence the collagen matrix deteriorates and bones become more brittle. In women, the menopause, with its associated decrease in oestrogen levels, accelerates the process with increased risk of osteoporosis (see Chapter 5). Bone mineral density (BMD) is increased by regular progressive exercise and the skeleton can respond and increase BMD up until the eigth decade, therefore exercise to counteract the 1% loss is worthwhile (Bassey 2001).

Joint structures and tissues include the articulating surfaces of the bones, cartilages, synovial membranes and synovial fluid, joint capsules, ligaments and other connective tissues. With ageing, connective tissues change whereby the joint capsule and ligaments stiffen and lose elasticity and some shortening of fibres occurs. Synovial fluid production decreases and cartilage thins. Osteoarthritis, although a recognised joint pathology, may be at least partially attributable to wear and tear over time. The combination of wear and tear with age-related tissue changes means that virtually all people over the age of 70 have some degree of osteoarthritic change (Tortora and Grabowski 2009).

The organisation, flexibility and capacity of the neuromusculoskeletal system means that throughout life and into old age new motor skills and movement abilities can be developed and learned. However, the general impact of ageing on all the component structures tends towards decline in function, but once again this is immensely variable between individuals and highly dependent upon past and present health status, and (as will be seen later) activity levels. As with our earlier consideration of the immune system, it is perhaps more salient to consider normal age-related changes in relation to risk, vulnerability, and the capacity to withstand stresses – physiological and mechanical in this case.

Functionally, the ageing adult is likely to experience:

- A decline in muscle strength and endurance, with reduced fatigue resistance
- Reduced joint flexibility
- Changes in postural alignment (increased spinal flexion), with concomitant changes to gait, posture and equilibrium adjustments
- Slowed reaction times to sensory stimuli including balance disturbance
- Reduced bone density and tensile strength (prone to fracture)
- Slower tissue healing
- Impaired heat generation and retention due to decreased muscle mass and reduced metabolic activity
- Poorer venous return due to decreased activity.

The loss of soft tissues (muscle and fat) reduces cushioning and this, coupled with bone changes, increases the risk of more severe damage from falls and other impact events. The reduced flexibility of joints renders the soft tissues more prone to strains and sprains, and the avascular nature of ligaments and tendons makes them more prone to rupture under sudden or excessive force, and very slow to heal.

Effects of changes in other body systems

Cardiovascular and respiratory function will affect muscle performance through the efficiency of blood supply, gaseous exchange and waste removal. In turn, decline in skeletal muscle function will impact upon respiratory efficiency and venous return through reduction in inhalatory and exhalatory movements of the thorax, and a decline in skeletal muscle pump action assisting venous return, as discussed earlier.

Endocrine function, physical exercise and nutrition are particularly critical to bone density, as blood calcium concentrations are closely controlled through the interplay of parathyroid hormone (PTH) (calcium resorption from bone) and calcitonin (calcium deposition into bone). Should a dietary deficiency of calcium or deficiency of vitamin D occur, parathyroid hormone levels will rise and calcium will be taken from bone. If physical activity is minimal, this depresses calcitonin production and PTH levels again rise, with consequent loss of calcium from bone (Hunt et al. 2010a, b, Di Pietro 2001).

These factors emphasise the critical interplay of multiple systems in maintaining homeostasis and health, and how changes in different systems compound and accelerate decline in body structures and functions, with significant consequences for health and wellbeing (discussed in more detail in the final section of this chapter, below).

Pathologies of the system

There are numerous primary pathological changes that can affect one or all of the component subsystems (neural, muscular and skeletal) and impact upon movement-related and homeostatic functions. Many, if not all, such pathologies such as stroke, osteoarthritis, or Parkinson's disease, though frequently associated or more common with ageing, are not unique to later life. Our consideration here, then, must be about the interrelationship of these pathologies with ageing and the consequent impact upon the person affected.

A key factor in all pathologies that affect this system is that they inevitably impact adversely upon physical activity. Mobility is compromised, and there develops a complex physiological interplay between the consequences of reduced mobility, the ageing process, and functional ability in general (see Chapter 8). Such interplay often leads to the establishment of a cycle of decreased activity and increasing impairment, arising from some original pathology but not dependent upon it. This has the effect of intensifying or accelerating deterioration of structure and function. This issue is explored in more depth, below, and also in the final section of this chapter.

Considerations in practice

Box 7.2 presents the case of Mrs Robinson, which illustrates the interplay of pathology with restricted physical activity, and the impact upon multiple body systems, leading into a potential cycle of deterioration of health and function.

By considering Mrs Robinson's story, it becomes apparent that occupational assessment must be comprehensive whenever mobility and movement functions are compromised. It could be argued that every body structure and function affects, and is affected by, movement. It is known that physical exercise beneficially affects mood due to the stimulatory effect upon endorphin release in the brain. Assessment of functions at impairment level, such as mood, cognition, sensory function, motor function, joint range of movement, muscle function, is relevant. Activity and occupational assessment are also vital to determine habits, patterns, routines, task demands and the individual's capacity and performance abilities.

One occupational goal that should always be included in any intervention with any person who has restricted mobility and movement difficulties, is to seek ways to maintain, if not improve upon, levels of physical activity within daily routines. Movements that occur within occupational contexts are more likely to be performed and repeated because they serve meaningful and valued ends, and the skill of the therapist is to incorporate beneficial movement and posture within occupational performance. This should include attention to joint range of movement, quality and quantity of muscle work, application of forces

---

Box 7.2   Mrs Robinson with osteoarthritis of the knees.

Mrs Robinson, aged 77, has **osteoarthritis** of both knees. She has the following impairments:
Reduced movement of knee joints, especially into flexion, due to joint surface damage, osteophyte formation, thickening and stiffening of joint capsule, and pain on movement.

Acitivity limitations:
Limited amount of walking, and frequency of standing up and sitting down, during a day because of pain.
Sits in an armchair with legs raised on a stool to limit flexion.
When climbing steps and stairs she leads with the less affected leg to avoid flexing the other knee.
She experiences difficulty with getting in and out of the bath, car, and with sitting and standing when using the toilet.
When walking, Mrs Robinson does not adequately flex her knees, so brushes the floor with her feet and is at risk of catching her toe and stumbling.

Functional and systemic consequences:
Habitual avoidance of fullest possible range of movement at the knees encourages joint capsule stiffening and shortening of the fibres on the extensor aspect of the knee.
Limited joint movement reduces the circulation of synovial fluid which reduces nourishment of the cartilages.
Both flexor and extensor muscles of the knee are used less, leading to muscle atrophy and loss of sarcomeres (fibre shortening).
Blood supply to the muscles is reduced due to the reduced contraction activity. General reduction in activity (mobility) and exercise contributes to reduced respiratory capacity, and cardiac deconditioning.
Venous return will be less efficient.
Lack of mechanical stress upon bones will increase calcium resorbtion and the risk of osteo-porotic change.
Reduced muscle activity will impair heat production.
A decline in cardiorespiratory fitness makes her more vulnerable to chest infections.
Pain and fear of falling limit her social activities and restrict community access, leading to increased stress response activation, anxiety and risk of depression.
Reduced activity leads to loss of appetite, and difficulties with mobilising discourage cooking, leading to risk of nutritional deficiency.
Lack of movement and dietary change contribute to risk of constipation.

---

through the skeleton, and variations in posture and positioning throughout the day. Not to do so, as has been illustrated in Box 7.2, leaves the way open to further, possibly avoidable, deterioration in multiple body systems.

The digestive system

The ICF considers the structure and functions of the digestive system to involve ingestion and digestion of food and elimination of waste (WHO 2001). Nutrition and diet are important throughout the lifespan to maintain health and this is especially true in older age (see Chapter 8). However, many older people are often at nutritional risk because of restricted access to food, or to a variety of foods (under- and malnutrition), or due to impaired ingestion, digestion, absorption and utilisation of nutrients because of chronic disease and drug-nutrient interactions.

Ingestion and digestion

As discussed in Chapter 6, sensation of smell and taste decline as part of the normal ageing process (Morley, 2001) and are also affected by medication and some diseases. Flavour is an important component in the experience of eating, and the reduction in ability to detect and discriminate flavours has implications not just for pleasure and enjoyment, but also for the ability to detect excess/absence of food constituents (salt, sugar) and freshness or contamination. The ability to chew food is important and many older people with poor dentition may reduce the range of foods they eat. For many older people with few of their own teeth, well-fitting dentures are crucial to chew and masticate food suffi- ciently, to maintain an appropriate calorie intake. Older people with stroke or Bulbar Palsy might find it difficult to have well-fitting dentures. For many older people, loss of teeth is caused by periodontal disease because of poor oral hygiene, and therefore regular, efficient cleaning and brushing of teeth and gums is important to optimise nutritional intake. A reduced production of saliva and a dry mouth are often associated with ageing; these also affect chewing and consequent swallowing of food. However, these are often induced by medication or as a result of interventions such as radiotherapy (Phillips 2003).

Atrophy of the stomach mucosa occurs in a third of older people over 60 (Horwarth 2002), causing a reduction in the secretion of gastric acid, pepsin and intrinsic factor. These cause a reduction in the absorption of vitamin B12, folate, calcium and iron – with deficiencies in vitamin B12 and folate being associated with reduced cognitive function and immunity, calcium with bone density and iron with iron deficiency anaemia (Phillips 2003). Malabsorption of calcium is also associated with a deficiency of vitamin D. Ageing is also associated with a slowing of gastric emptying which prolongs the sensa- tion of meal-induced fullness, and may lead to anorexia and weight loss. Alterations to levels of leptin and cholecystokinin which are gastrointestinal hormones also cause the sensation of satiety in response to fat in older people, causing the 'anorexia of ageing' (Morley 2003).

The pancreas is affected by ageing with a reduction in the pancreatic enzyme impairing the digestion of fats. Its endocrine functions also change, with reduced insulin efficiency therefore increasing the incidence of glucose intolerance and non-insulin-dependant diabetes mellitus (NIDDM).

The liver is said to have a progressive decline of volume and blood flow with increasing age. Whereas this may not have much impact on normal liver function it could cause slower elimination of some medications from the body. However, more age-related changes occur in the gallbladder, which concentrates and secretes bile acids that make fats present in the intestine soluble and more easily digested. A reduction in the secretion of these acids probably leads to the higher incidence of gallstones in older people, which may lead to the need for surgical removal in cases of severe upper abdominal pain, pancreatitis and jaundice (Bateson 1999).

Elimination

Changes in the small and large intestine do not seem to occur with ageing, so that the motility of food and waste through these organs is not affected. However, many older people do complain of changes to bowel habits with increasing age, such as constipation or, more distressingly, faecal incontinence. Constipation can be difficult to determine as this has different connotations for different people. Whereas current older people were given laxatives as children to 'keep them regular' the emphasis on daily defaecation is no longer in vogue.

Pathologies of the system

There is conflicting evidence for swallowing difficulties in normal ageing (known as presbyphagia) (Leslie et al. 2003, Robbins et al. 2006); however, this is often compromised by central nervous system disturbances following a stroke, Parkinson's disease, or Bulbar Palsy (known as dysphagia), because of impairment to the swallowing reflex. Such swallowing difficulties are identified in 60% of clients with stroke and are consequently linked to the incidence of chest infection in this client group. Swallowing is a complex action involving the appropriate cessation of respiration and closure of the airways. Any problems therefore need thorough and rapid investigation to ensure appropriate nutritional intake, homeostasis and prevention of aspiration of food into the lungs.

Faecal incontinence is more distressing and occurs in 7% of over 65-year-olds. It is the second most common reason for admission to residential care, with a third of older residents in care homes faecally incontinent (Kamm 1998).

Faecal incontinence can either be seen as 'an inevitable consequence of old age or as a failure of medical and nursing management' (Allen 1998, p. 62). It causes embarrassment, humiliation and fear in an older person – proof of regression into a second childhood and many who suffer from it curtail both physical and social activity. For many carers it is the 'last straw' in their ability to cope with an older relative. Causes of faecal incontinence are:

- Constipation with overflow
- Faecal impaction
- Colorectal disease (Irritable Bowel Syndrome)
- Diarrhoea
- Drug induced
- Impaired absorption of food and constituents by stomach, small or large intestine.
- Gastro-intestinal infection
- Neurogenic incontinence (reduced cortical inhibition – common in dementia)
- Environmental (poor mobility, inability to get to toilet, cope with clothing, etc).

Considerations for practice

For occupational therapists, an awareness of impairment of digestive function in older age is important. Occupational therapists can advise older people about nutritional intake and supplementation, as well as ensuring that they can eat adequately and safely. This can be achieved through the simple provision of modified cutlery or a non-slip mat and/or by improving positioning. With a client with swallowing difficulties it is useful to work jointly with a speech and language therapist. Reinforcement and facilitation through the use of assistive products of good oral hygiene is also important. An awareness of the interaction of medications with the digestive system and possible causes of constipation and faecal incontinence is crucial, especially where environmental factors may be a barrier.

Occupational therapists have an important role collaborating with dieticians and health promotion experts to advise on food budgeting and planning low-cost, nutritious meals, including enjoyable food preparation 'for one'. To provide an opportunity to eat with and to cook for others, e.g. at luncheon clubs, restaurants, 'pop-in' cafés and to encourage older people to use the internet for food shopping and recipe selection can also be part of the occupational therapist's role.

Metabolism

Metabolism is defined as 'the regulation of essential components of the body such as carbohydrates, proteins and fats, the conversion of one to another and their breakdown into energy' (WHO 2001, p. 85). Metabolism is fuelled by the nutrients and fluid we take in and regulated by the endocrine system, hence it is dealt with in this section of the chapter.

Basal (or resting) metabolic rate (BMR) is the rate of energy expenditure required to keep the body functioning at rest. This is said to decline with age with the BMR of a 70-year-old being 9–12% lower than of a 30-year-old. The reduction in BMR is mainly caused by reduction in lean body mass due to muscle loss (Phillips 2003). Such a decline in BMR impacts on calorie intake and weight regulation. Metabolism of minerals is also affected as part of normal ageing, with some loss of bone density due to removal of minerals and collagen matrix; more accelerated loss is associated with osteoporosis, as already discussed.

Water and electrolyte balance are controlled by thirst, hunger and renal functions, which all change with normal ageing. These changes do not impact upon the body's homeostasis in normal events but puts an older person on a 'knife-edge' of control so that an infection, changes in weather, or use of medications can cause an imbalance of water and electrolytes within the body (Allen 1998). Older people have a delayed and less intense response to thirst, which inhibits water intake. Dehydration is the most common cause of water and electrolyte imbalance in older people (Brownie, 2006) and in mild cases can cause dry skin, cognitive changes, lethargy or syncope but may, in extreme situations, contribute to stroke, heart attack or renal failure. It is therefore necessary for older people to be encouraged to drink not only plenty of water but also to replenish sodium levels at times of illness or hot weather to prevent serious consequences of dehydration.

The endocrine system

Hormone production is essential for maintenance of circadian rhythms, energy metabolism and also for dealing with intrinsic and extrinsic stressors (Morley 2003). Ageing of the endocrine system creates a 'change in the smooth oscillatory release of hormones to a more chaotic pattern of release' (Morley 2003, p. 333). A decline in the efficiency of hormonal receptors and effector mechanisms in older people also causes the endocrine system to become sluggish and respond less effectively to stress (Bennett and Ebrahim 1995).

Some key hormone changes that occur with ageing are described in Table 7.1. They are characterised by dysregulation in the production of many hormones, which disrupts functions in multiple body systems. For example, decreasing insulin production disrupts glucose metabolism, and reduction in thyroid hormones slows cell metabolism. Reduction in production of testosterone and oestrogen can contribute to poorer cognitive function, loss of strength, muscle mass and bone mineral density as well as loss of fertility (Drake et al. 2000, Morley 2003). Conversely, cortisol levels rise in old age, and this is part of a complex series of interconnected changes to the immune and endocrine systems that lead to an increase in inflammatory processes. In turn, these are implicated in the genesis of a range of decremental changes to body systems, and of chronic disease conditions (Hunt et al. 2010a, b).

Hormone replacement therapy has been considered and most successfully carried out with oestrogen replacement. Benefits include better cognitive functioning and the reduction in bone loss and cardiovascular risk. Disadvantages includeg the risk of breast and endometrial cancer. Testosterone replacement therapy in men has been shown to increase muscle strength and mass as well as libido, bone density and cognition; however, supplementation can increase the risk of stroke with long-term risks not known. Vitamin D supplements are also given, but more successful for the housebound and those in residential care is a 30-minutes a day exposure to sunlight (outdoors) to restore levels (Reid et al. 1986).

Effects of changes in other body systems

Many endocrine processes are regulated by the autonomic nervous system (ANS) through a combination of neural and hormonal signalling. Hypothalamic function (the hypothalamus being the control centre of the ANS) and feedback mechanisms are key to the regulation of many physiological processes – sexual maturity and reproduction, growth, hunger and satiety, stress responses and immune functions to name but a few. Changes to other body systems therefore influence the release of hormones either by direct influence upon endocrine organs or through their effect upon the hypothalamus. Some examples are discussed below.

Reduced absorption and manufacture of vitamin D leads to poorer absorption of calcium from the diet. Falling blood concentrations of calcium in turn stimulate a rise in production of parathyroid hormone (PTH), and an increase in resorption of calcium from bone, contributing to loss of bone mass.

Atherosclerosis can affect the renal arteries and reduce blood flow to the kidneys. This initiates the renin-angiotensin-aldosterone (RAA) pathway response which, through a series of steps, leads to stimulation of the adrenal glands to produce aldosterone. Aldosterone acts upon the kidneys to prevent water loss, and is a powerful vasoconstrictor. The outcome of these actions is an increase blood volume and pressure which, in situations of dehydration or blood loss, would restore blood flow to the kidneys

(Tortora and Derrickson 2009). However, when resulting from a disease process such as atherosclerosis, the result is to increase already high blood pressure and increase strain upon the cardiovascular system, aggravating the atherosclerotic process further. ACE (angiotensin converting enzyme) inhibitors are a group of drugs designed to break this cycle and help to control blood pressure.

The hypothalamus activates the stress response as a result of stimulatory inputs, including proprioceptive feedback from moving joints and muscles, and changes in blood gas composition as we start to exercise. Such stress responses are important to enable cardiovascular and musculoskeletal responsiveness for exercise. If an older person becomes less physically active and more sedentary, the reduction in release of hormones such as adrenaline, through lack of physiological stimulation, plays a part in deconditioning, loss of response variability and accelerated muscle tissue loss.

Pathologies of the system

Conversely, psychological distress can lead to prolonged activation of the stress response (Lovallo 2005). This gives rise to a complex series of changes affecting the neuro-, endocrine and immune systems, with adverse consequences for cardiovascular and mental health, immune and digestive functions, sleep, appetite, and affective state. Though not primarily arising from pathology of the endocrine system, chronic stress and its associated health risks represent a maladaptation of neuroendocrine homeostatic mechanisms in the face of situations the human body is not evolutionarily adapted to. Older people face many sources of psychological stress, including bereavement, being a carer of an ill or disabled spouse, financial worries, personal disability, chronic ill-health, and hospitalisation.

Hypo- and hyperthyroidism are conditions that can occur at any age, but hypothyroidism is the most common thyroid disorder of old age. It is an autoimmune disorder that most commonly occurs from middle age onwards, affecting approximately 2% of older women but only 0.2% of men. Common early symptoms include weight gain, feeling tired and lethargic, constipation, dry skin and hair, brittle nails, and increased sensitivity to cold. It may be insidious in onset, due to a gradual failure of the thyroid gland, its symptoms therefore dismissed as a part of a general feeling of being run down, or attributed to the menopause. Consequently, it is likely to be underdiagnosed, and is often only found in blood test results that may have been taken for other reasons. Hormone replacement medication is highly effective.

Another primary and increasingly common endocrine disorder is Type 2 diabetes. This manifests as an insulin insensitivity and a failure of the pancreas to secrete insulin in compensation, resulting in rising blood glucose levels (National Collaborating Centre for Chronic Conditions (NCCCC) 2008). Although it has been hypothesised that insulin secretion and sensitivity are impaired as part of the ageing process, this is still debated (Barbieri et al. 2001, Ning et al. 2010). However, environmental factors, including obesity, inactivity, social deprivation and diets with a high saturated fat content appear to be factors in the development of Type 2 diabetes, because its incidence is rapidly increasing. Other factors known to be associated with a higher risk for developing Type 2 diabetes are a family history of diabetes and Asian or African-Caribbean genes (NCCCC 2008).

Table 7.5   Occupational interventions to support endocrine system functioning.

Occupational intervention	Endocrine system benefit
Relaxation training/stress management	Reduction in frequency or amount of stress hormone release, reducing adverse effects of chronic stress response activation
Engagement in community activities (physical and social, such as luncheon clubs, activity groups, keep-fit, swimming)	Counters social isolation, and provides sources of support, helping to reduce experiences of stress (as above). Increases physical activity with healthy activation of endocrine stress responses to exercise (maintaining cardiovascular and musculoskeletal health)
Environmental adaptation for access, and mobility equipment	Easier mobility, facilitates increased physical activity; healthy stimulation of endocrine mediated responses as above.
Self-care: feeding	Improved nutrition and hydration, supporting calcium homeostasis and bone density. Maintains energy levels for activity Management of blood glucose levels
Domestic ADL: cooking skills	As above

Considerations in practice

Even though endocrine function may seem far removed from the sphere of occupational therapy, it is obvious from the foregoing discussion that it plays an essential part in the functioning of most body structures, and is essential to physiological and mental health. Health professionals must have an understanding of the commoner endocrine disorders that affect older people, such that occupational interventions can be designed to support endocrine function, and the therapist is able to recognise signs and symptoms of possible pathology that may be developing, yet unrecognized, in the affected individual (such as hypothyroidism or early diabetes) (see Table 7.5).

Taking a simple supplementation of vitamin D, for example, is one that an occupational therapist can encourage in older clients to help prevent osteoporosis.

Structures and functions of the genito-urinary systems

Urinary system

Ageing processes within the kidneys impact not only on renal function in the excretion of urine, but also on the cardiovascular system in the control of blood pressure. The kidney is said to shrink from approximately 300 g at age 20 to 200 g by the age of 80, with a 40% loss in the number of functioning glomeruli by the age of 80 (Tortora and Derrickson 2009). The filtration rate of the glomeruli steadily declines from the age of 40 and is associated with a rise in blood pressure. There is also a declining ability for the loop of Henlé to reabsorb sodium, causing a reduced ability to concentrate urine during periods of water depletion. This has serious consequences for older people, potentially leading to more rapid dehydration in hot weather, and the need to for nighttime micturition (Bennett and Ebrahim 1995). A slowing glomerular filtration rate also slows the clearance of many medications through the kidney, causing drug toxicity if they accumulate (Mangoni and Jackson 2003).

Involuntary loss of urine from the body (incontinence) causes misery for many older men and women, being seen as a social and hygiene problem. More than 20% of older people have urinary incontinence and this figure rises above 50% for those older people living in long-term residential care. More women than men suffer from incontinence of urine (Thakar and Stanton 2000).

Continence of urine (or voluntary control) requires a well-functioning lower urinary tract, with central nervous system inhibition and facilitation by the basal ganglia, frontal cortex and cerebellum, as well as good cognitive functioning, motivation, mobility and manual dexterity. Incontinence should not be accepted as a normal part of growing older but is associated with disease processes and problems that commonly occur with ageing such as stroke and dementia.

Incontinence can either be transient or established, with transient incontinence being more common in older people. Causes of transient incontinence are:

- Delirium
- Urinary tract infection
- Urethritis and vaginitis
- Alcohol and drug use
- Mental health problems such as depression
- Excessive output due to high fluid intake
- Use of diuretics (including caffeine)
- Restricted mobility
- Impacted stools (Lui 2007).

There are three main types of established incontinence – detrusor overactivity, stress incontinence and outlet obstruction – which are caused by structural and functional problems within the bladder and urethra, or due to CNS control. In older people, the capacity and contractility of the bladder decrease with age, as does the ability to postpone voiding. Bladder contractions are increasingly uninhibited by CNS control and residual volumes within the bladder after voiding increase. Both the urethral length and sphincter strength decline with age in women and the prostate enlarges in men (Abrams 1995, Thakar and Stanton 2000).

Considerations in practice

Management of established incontinence varies – with detrusor overactivity responding to bladder retraining, by emptying the bladder on a regular 2–3 hourly basis. This is especially useful for those older people after stroke and also with dementia. Weight loss (where appropriate) and treatment of the precipitating cause of outlet incompetence (e.g. cough) can be sufficient, but otherwise the use of pelvic floor exercises is said to be successful in all age groups. Medication to alleviate the symptoms of outlet obstruction may be sufficient but otherwise resection of the prostate is carried out (Abrams 1995, Thakar and Stanton 2000).

Occupational therapists are involved in more behavioural approaches to the management of urinary incontinence. A reminder for regular use of the toilet can be necessary and, more importantly, an assessment of dressing ability to establish whether the client can easily manage clothing when going to the toilet. Access to the toilet might be difficult because of poor mobility and a risk assessment may be necessary to eliminate or reduce any environmental hazards for both day and night time usage. Ensuring that clients can manage pads if supplied with clothing may also be necessary as part of a dressing assessment.

Sexual functions

There has been an assumption both within the literature and by most professionals that older people do not have intimate sexual relationships and this is explored in more detail in Chapter 8. For many older people the physical changes to sexual functions make coitus more difficult and few seek advice about these impairments, perhaps perceiving them as an inevitable part of ageing.

Effects of changes in other body systems

Reduction in hormones, as already discussed, as well as cardiovascular insufficiencies, diabetes and some medications, impact on sexual functioning,. The presence of disease processes such as arthritis or respiratory conditions could cause pain, reduced physical capacity and an increase in discomfort. Such problems may also reduce desire as a result. Women experience less sexual dreaming as they get older and this is associated with a reduction in testosterone levels, which also causes loss of libido in men (Miracle and Miracle 2001). A reduction in oestrogen levels in women with the menopause causes physical changes such as atrophy of the uterus, contraction and shortening of the vagina with loss of elasticity, thinning of the epithelium and reduction of vaginal lubrication. All of these cause discomfort during penetration and reduce desire (Bennett and Ebrahim 1995).

Older men have a more gradual decline in sexual functioning and structures, maintaining fertility almost throughout their lives. However, secretion of testosterone declines by approximately 30% by the age of 80, with decreased production of sperm, seminal fluid and greater need for stimulation to achieve an erection and a shorter time for ejaculation to occur. Erectile dysfunction occurs in 50% of men aged 40 to 70 years and this increases with age. However, ageing does not cause erectile dysfunction, which is more likely to be caused by vascular, neurological, endocrine or iatrogenic factors. Vascular disorders are the most common cause of erectile dysfunction in older men; especially arterial disease, with this being an early symptom of atherosclerosis. Many other factors influence sexual functioning:

- Post-event anxiety (after a cardiovascular event or stroke) – however, intercourse should not be hazardous if blood pressure is controlled
- Stroke – can reduce erectile function, vaginal lubrication and sensation
- Arthritis – inflammation of joints, fatigue, weakness, pain, restricted range of moment (especially hips)
- Alcohol – long-term cumulative effect can inhibit libido
- Surgery – long-term effects are rare, even after hysterectomy or prostatectomy
- Medications – corticosteroids reduce libido, tranquillisers, antidepressants, beta blockers cause impotence
- Diabetes – causes erectile dysfunction

- Incontinence of urine and catheterisation
- Sexually transmitted diseases – AIDsAQ has increased by 22% in older people in the last 10 years, as older people equate the use of condoms with fertility rather than 'safe sex'.

(Read 1999, Miracle and Miracle 2001)

Considerations in practice

Occupational therapists should not avoid advising older people about their sexual activity and may have to deal with their own beliefs and attitudes and be explicit about the boundaries of the therapeutic relationship. The need for advice on alternative positioning or energy conservation may be necessary as well as a health promotion role of 'safe sex' education. Miracle and Miracle (2001) describe the PLISSIT intervention model – Permission, Limited Information, Specific Suggestions, Intensive Therapy. For the majority of occupational therapists, the first two aspects of permission and limited information could be within their scope, with referral for more specific help or therapy by a more experienced colleague. However, like any other aspect of daily life, it is crucial that the occupational therapist acknowledges the need for help by the most appropriate professional and the older person is dealt with sensitively and professionally at all times.

Key threats in the relationship between physiology, homeostatic disruption and occupation

In this final section of this chapter, we consider some key issues affecting health and wellbeing in older people. These highlight the interactions between changes in physiology, functional activity levels and pathology, and how these compound or accelerate functional decline and ill-health. Such interactions must be understood by occupational therapists if they wish to work effectively to enhance the health and wellbeing of older people.

Physical inactivity

Physical activity is an important modulator of risk factors for ill-health, particularly obesity, heart and other cardiovascular diseases. Reduction in physical activity is a common feature of ageing, and may occur for a number of reasons that are longstanding or new – retirement from an active job, obesity, chronic disease and pain, or a period of illness. Sedentary behaviour is recognised as a risk factor for chronic ill-health, morbidity and mortality in older populations (DiPietro 2001). Physical exercise, and the promotion of physical activity, has emerged as an important feature of health maintainance and ill-health prevention regimes in the older population. Physical activity promotes beneficial changes in the musculoskeletal system, impacting also upon cardiovascular, respiratory, metabolic and endocrine functions, and evidence for its relationship to improved health in older adults has been established through research (for example, Purath et al. 2009, Spirduso and Cronin 2001, Blair and Wei 2000).

Absence of, or greatly reduced, physical activity can initiate a spiral of functional and health decline. Refer back to the case of Mrs Robinson (Box 7.2) and the earlier discussion of the neuromusculoskeletal system for a reminder of the effects of reduced mobility on this system. Atrophy of muscle fibres, reduced muscle metabolism, and reduced joint movements impact upon joint stability and muscle force generation. Venous return becomes less efficient as the skeletal muscle pump is not active, with the risk of venous thrombosis. Peripheral tissues may become oedematous. As muscles atrophy, so their capillary beds shrink, reducing their blood supply. Cardiac output decreases in the absence of demand from the muscles. Even a short period of immobility (a few weeks in bed due to illness, a period of hospitalisation) will quickly lead to changes. Over time, cardiac deconditioning may occur, reducing the system's ability to respond to changing demands, and with the identified musculoskeletal changes, the person's ability to resume normal levels of activity could be seriously impaired.

Additionally, if nutritional intake is compromised such that calcium intake and Vitamin D become deficient (illness and lack of activity may contribute to lack of appetite; remaining indoors), and without the stimulus of physical forces acting on bone, there is a shift in endocrine activity with an increase in PTH production and decrease in calcitonin. This shifts the balance further towards the demineralisation of bone, as calcium is reabsorbed into the bloodstream and excreted. Loss of mobility frequently leads to a reduction in social interactions and difficulty engaging in meaningful occupations. This impacts upon mood, and could add to feelings of fatigue and lethargy, reducing motivation for engagement in activity, further compounded by loss of appetite and a reduction of food intake, thereby reducing energy levels. In consequence, a person who seeks to resume an activity after a period of much reduced physical movement may find that the same activity requires more physical and mental effort than before, leading to a perception of that activity as difficult, and a reduction in willingness to engage in it. Hence a reduction in physical activity could initiate a sequence of physiological changes that lead to further reduced capacity and tolerance for activity, and further decline in physiological systems. The end result could be a decline into a state of frailty.

Frailty

Frailty has been defined as a state or syndrome characterised by loss of homeostatic regulation with increased vulnerability to stressors due to age-related decline in multiple body systems. This leads to a loss of resilience and physiological reserves necessary to recover to full health following an episode of illness or incapacity (Lang et al. 2009, Kuh et al. 2007). (The reader is also signposted to Chapter 2, where frailty has been discussed in terms of occupational transitions and successful ageing).

Lang et al. (2009) described it as a progressive process that features two stages: firstly, a pre-frail stage that is clinically silent, with apparent recovery from external stressors. This is followed eventually by a frail stage in which there is incomplete recovery from illness, with clinically measurable deterioration to a 'complication state' associated with negative health outcomes.

Essentially, all people eventually become frail in old age, but it occurs later in 'healthy' individuals. The period of frailty might be short, immediately preceding death, or extended, depending upon underlying health and other factors in the person's life (e.g. co-morbidities). The foregoing discussion of physical inactivity clearly illustrates how this state could develop, and also thereby indicates that frailty is a syndrome that should be modifiable by some form of intervention, both in the extent to which it develops, and over what time course. It further suggests that susceptibility to it, and those at greater risk of developing it, should be identifiable through assessment of risk factors in their lives.

Frailty has been described as a separate condition to, and not synonymous with, disability. A person may have a disability but be healthy, whilst a person may be generally frail but have no specific disability. Although not conclusive, frailty could be diagnosed in the presence of two or more of the following: undernutrition, dependence, prolonged bed rest, pressure ulcers, gait disorder, general weakness, extreme old age, weight loss, anorexia, fear of falling, hip fracture, confusion, going outdoors infrequently, polypharmacy (survey of American geriatricians cited in Kuh et al. 2007).

Kuh et al. (2007) proposed a 'Life Course' approach to frailty: that factors across the life course and in early life determine/influence ageing and frailty onset. These comprise of:

• Modifiable factors – nutrition, activity, chance events
• Non-modifiable factors – genetic inheritance, gender.

Therefore it can be argued that risk of frailty is influenced by biological capital acquired during early years, even pre-natally. Further, optimum physiological attainment in adulthood and rate of decline (when and how much) vary and early social, environmental and developmental characteristics (e.g. growth, cognitive ability) influence capabilities and performance in later life. Both of these views support the argument that interventions for health and wellbeing in old age need to start from the beginning of life and should take a life-course approach.

Undernutrition, malnutrition and obesity

Undernourishment in older people is an important but under-reported and under-recognised issue. An alarming 40% of the patients admitted to hospital and 10% of patients in the community are undernourished (Royal College of Physicians 2002). Groups of older people that appear to be most at risk are older people in care homes (Ministry of Agriculture, Food and Fisheries and the Department of Health 1998) and those with long-standing illness (Margetts et al. 2003). Other risk factors include dysphagia, slow eating, low protein intake, poor appetite, presence of a feeding tube and age (Keller 1993). Poor nutritional intake can hinder recovery from illness and is an associated risk factor for skin ulceration and also thermoregulation. Reduced calorie intake as part of a reduction of energy needs also means that older people need to eat foods with high nutritional value to compensate for this lower intake (Phillips 2003). For many older people, eating well and poor nutritional status could also be affected by low social status and monetary income, living alone, and travel restrictions, leading to limited access to a wide variety of foods, and greater preference for easy-to-prepare foods and less fresh fruit and vegetables (Horwath 1989). Unexplained weight loss and poor nutrition are both strong indicators for and contributors to the development of frailty.

Malnutrition is not just a problem manifested as weight loss and undernourishment in old age. It is also an issue of excess and unbalanced food intake, resulting in obesity.

Whilst the typical 'picture' of the frail older person is one of low body weight, obesity is posing a greater problem in industrialised societies as an increasing percentage of people become obese and continue so into old age. In 2008, the percentage of people aged 65–74 in England who were obese (BMI of $30 kg/m^2$ or more) was reported as 33%, with the total prevalence of overweight (BMI between 25 and $30 kg/m^2$), including obesity, being 83%. In the 75+ age group, a total of 72% were overweight, with 23% being obese (National Health Service 2008).

Obesity is associated with increased risks of Type II diabetes, cardiovascular diseases and stroke, and musculoskeletal disorders (joint degeneration, back pain). Metabolic syndrome, or cardiometabolic syndrome, are terms that have been used to refer to the constellation of adverse homeostatic changes that occur in obesity, and which predispose the sufferer to these specific pathological conditions.

Directly, obesity could result in reduced activity levels and poor exercise tolerance, resulting in activity limitations and participation restrictions. Of growing concern is the interaction between obesity and its associated metabolic changes, with sarcopenia, the progressive loss of muscle mass that occurs with aging. 'Sarcopenic obesity' is the term that has been coined to describe this state, in which low muscle strength combined with excessively high body (fat) mass creates a situation of frailty (Blaum et al. 2005; Stenholm et al. 2009) and accelerated development of pathologies. In particular, bio-chemical changes that occur in old age (arising from immunosenescence, endocrine senescence and muscle tissue breakdown), and also arise as a direct consequence of excessive adipose tissue being present in the body, are increasingly believed to contrib-ute in a cumulative way to increased and abnormal levels of inflammatory activity. Dysregulated inflammation is increasingly recognized as a critical component in the gen-esis of a range of chronic pathologies including atherosclerosis, cardiovascular diseases, some cancers, osteoporosis and rheumatoid arthritis (Graham et al. 2006), as these diseases are all associated with elevated serum concentrations of inflammatory proteins (Hunt et al. 2010a).

Thermal dysregulation and hypothermia

Regulation of body heat to prevent either hypothermia or hyperthermia in older people is crucial to preventing pathological events within body functions or structures, including exacerbation of existing conditions or even death. Thermoregulation is a finely-tuned process maintaining the core temperature at the optimal level for the body's biochemical processes to take place (Worfolk 1997). Regulation of body heat is carried out by both intrinsic and extrinsic means, with intrinsic regulation through functioning of the cardio-vascular, respiratory, neuromuscular, digestive and endocrine systems and extrinsically with nutrition and medication (Knies 1996).

As discussed in previous sections, much of the body's heat is generated as a by-prod-uct of metabolism in the organs and muscles and regulated by the hypothalamus through neuroendocrine and autonomic nervous system mechanisms. Activity in most of these organs and systems declines from the age of 70 onwards. Loss of subcutaneous fat, reduced vasoconstriction and ability to shiver (due to loss of muscle mass) all impact on maintenance and response to heat changes. Response to body temperature changes is also impaired with the ageing process (more so in 80-year-olds and upwards, and the very frail) with reduction in the number of thermal, chemical and mechanical receptors, and also a reduced sensitivity, perception and processing of changes in both body and environmental temperatures.

A reduced ability to sweat in high ambient temperatures and a reduced thirst sensation can lead to heat stroke if poorly monitored. Increased cardiovascular activity to release heat through radiation from vasodilatation of skin capillaries (which may be less in number or atherosclerotic) results in increased cardiac output and is often the cause of death rather than the exposure to higher ambient temperatures (Wilmshurst 1994). Attention should be paid to the types of clothing worn (light and loose fitting) and avoidance of unnecessary exertion (Keatinge 2004). Where possible, older people at risk of heat-related problems could benefit from taking cool showers/baths or being in air-conditioned buildings (Woolfe 2003).

Hypothermia is of greater concern in the UK due to low winter temperatures and also the age of much of the housing stock lived in by many older people. The emphasis on prevention of hypothermia within falls management programmes has been strongly recommended (Simpson et al. 1998) as mortality rates are approximately 50% in all cases of hypothermia (with those over the age of 75 five times more likely to die as a result) (Danzl 2012).

Risk factors for hypothermia are:

- Cardiovascular disease
- Diabetes
- Low physical activity
- Low body mass index
- Medications
- Low ambient temperature
- Poor nutrition (a high protein meal can increase the metabolic rate by 30% as opposed to a carbohydrate meal by 4%)
- General anaesthesia and surgery.

Occupational therapists need to be aware of declining thermoregulation in older people, especially those frailer and over 75. An increase in physical activity in either high or low ambient temperatures can further compromise impaired body functions that are already struggling to maintain homeostasis. Education about clothing, rehydration, and nutrition is important as well as maintenance of environmental temperatures and dealing with inactivity such as that experienced by many of the case study individuals discussed in Chapter 5 following a fall.

The role of the occupational therapist in supporting and enhancing physiological health

This final section has considered key physiological threats to homeostasis and health that are of particular significance for older people: physical inactivity, frailty, under- and over-nutrition, obesity, and thermal dysregulation. Whilst posing a threat to any age group, it is uniquely in older age that these threats are most likely to combine, presenting a formidable challenge to health and wellbeing. In discussing each threat, and considering the foregoing discussions of age-related change to body systems, it is possible to discern some common lessons for the practice of occupational therapy that should be incorporated into our work with older people. Essentially, there is a clear argument that physiological needs and homeostatic function must be understood and considered with every client if our practice is to properly address occupational needs.

In addition to the primary occupational performance needs (activity limitations, performance restrictions) for which a client may have been referred to occupational therapy services, the underpinning body structures and functions that enable function must be supported through our interventions. Attention to these will provide a means of promoting ongoing good health and homeostatic resilience, and preserving existing capacity for performance. Occupational interventions should include consideration and/or monitoring of:

- Adequacy of diet – range and amount of nutrients, and hydration
- Bladder and bowel function
- Quality and amount of sleep
- Physical exercise and activity – incorporation into ADL
- Basic functional abilities (balance, mobility, cognition)
- Mood (affective state)
- Degree of choice and autonomy in daily life, and personal relationships
- Uptake of vaccinations
- Anticipation of stressful events (e.g. planned surgery) and coping mechanisms for existing stressors
- Effective rehabilitation after stressful events (nutrition, mobilisation and resumption of activities).

Neglect of these factors has the potential to create physiological stress for the individual, whose ability to withstand stress is reducing. The ageing process, though not pathological in itself, renders the older person increasingly vulnerable to homeostatic disruption and morbidity. This stems from the multiple sources of decrement and dysregulation of body structures and functions that develop as we age, and the greatly increased risk of impairment occurring as a result.

To illustrate the importance of the central messages in this chapter, return to the example of Mrs Robinson (Box 7.2) and consider how ageing, pathology and functional limitation would create a cycle of deterioration.

Summary

This chapter has discussed those body functions and structures involved in the integumentary, cardiovascular, respiratory and immune systems, neuromusculoskeletal system, digestive, metabolic and endocrine system and genitourinary and reproductive systems in relation to normal ageing and also those pathological processes that occur during older age. The consequences of impairments in body functions and structures have, where possible, been related to occupational performance and the role of the occupational therapist has been discussed.

The interrelationship of body functions has been explored, culminating in an examination of some key physiological threats to the health of older people.

Occupational therapists must have knowledge and understanding of the physiology of ageing if they are to be truly holistic in their practice, and able to work effectively to enable older people to improve and maintain health and wellbeing. This chapter has presented illustrations and explanations of why this is so, and what occupational therapists should consider and address.

References

Abrams, P. (1995) Fortnightly review: Managing lower urinary tract symptoms in older men. *BMJ* **310**, 1113–1117.

Allen, S.C. (1998) *Medicine in Old Age*, 4th ed. Edinburgh: Churchill Livingstone.

Barbieri, M., Rizo, M.R., Manzella, D. and Paolisso, G. (2001) Age-related insulin resistance: Is it an obligatory finding? The lesson from healthy centenarians. *Diabetes/Metabolism Research and Reviews* **17(1)**, 19–26.

Bassey, E.J. (2001) Exercise for prevention of osteoporotic fracture. *Age and Ageing* **30** (Supplement 4), 29–31.

Bateson, M.C. (1999) Gallbladder disease. *BMJ* **318**, 1745–1747.

Bennett, G. and Ebrahim, S. (1995) *The Essentials of Health Care in Old Age*, 2nd ed. London: Edward Arnold.

Blair, S. and Wei, M. (2000) Sedentary habits, health, and function in older women and men. *American Journal of Health Promotion* **15(1)**, 1–8.

Blaum, C.S., Li Xue, Q., Michelon, E., Semba, R.D. and Fried, L.P. (2005) The association between obesity and the frailty syndrome in older women: The Women's Health and Aging Studies. *Journal of the American Geriatric Society* **53**, 927–934.

Bonder, B.R. and Dal Bello-Haas, V. (2009) Functional Performance in Older Adults. third edi. Philadelphia: F.A. Davis Company,.

British Heart Foundation Heart Disease Statistics Website (2010) Accessed 14/12/2010 http://www.heartstats.org/datapage.asp?id=9075

Brownie, S. (2006) Why are elderly individuals at risk of nutritional deficiency? *International Journal of Nursing Practice* **12**, 110–118.

Crepeau, E.B., Cohn, E.S. and Boyt Schell, B.A. (2009) *Willard & Spackman's Occupational Therapy* 11th edition. Philadelphia: Lippincott Williams & Wilkins.

Danzl, D.F. (2012) Hypothermia. In: *The Merck Manual for Health Care Professionals*. Accessed 16/07/2012 at: http://www.merckmanuals.com/professional/injuries_poisoning/cold_injury/hypothermia.html?qt=hypothermia&alt=sh

DiPietro, L. (2001) Physical activity in aging: Changes in patterns and their relationship to health and function. *Journals of Gerontology: SERIES A*. Vol. **56A** (Special Issue II), 13–22. Accessed 06/01/11 at: http://biomedgerontology.oxfordjournals.org/content/56/suppl_2

Drake, E.B., Henderson, V.W., Stanczyk, F.Z., McCleary, C.A., Brown, W.S., Smith, C.A., Rizzo, A.A., Murdoch, G.A. and Buckwalter, J.G. (2000) Associations between circulating sex steroid hormones and cognition in normal elderly women. *Neurology* **54(3)**, 599–603.

Graham, J.E., Christian, L.M. and Kiecolt-Glaser, J.K. (2006) Stress, age, and immune function: Toward a lifespan approach. *Journal of Behavioural Medicine* **29(4)**, 389–400. Accessed 04/01/2011 at http://web.ebscohost.com

Herbert, R. (1991) The normal ageing process reviewed. *Nursing Standard* **5(51)**, 36–39.

Horwath, C.C. (1989) Marriage and diet in elderly Australians: Results from a large random survey. *Journal of Human Nutrition and Dietetics* **2(3)**,185–193.

Hunt, K.J., Walsh, B.M., Voegeli, D. and Roberts, H.C. (2010a) Inflammation in aging Part 1: Physiology and immunological mechanisms. *Biological Research for Nursing* **11(3)**, 245–252. Accessed 10/01/11 at http://brn.sagepub.com/content/11/3/245.full.pdf+html

Hunt, K.J., Walsh, B.M., Voegeli, D. and Roberts, H.C. (2010b) Inflammation in aging Part 2: Implications for the health of older people and recommendations for nursing practice. *Biological Research for Nursing* **11(3)**, 253–260. Accessed 10/01/11 at http://brn.sagepub.com/content/11/3/253.full.pdf+html

Kamm, M.A. (1998) Faecal incontinence. *BMJ* **316**, 528–532.

Keatinge, W.R. (2004) Death in heat waves. *BMJ* **327**, 512–313.

Keller, H.H. (1993) Malnutrition in institutionalised elderly: How and why? *American Geriatric Society* **41(11)**, 1212–1218.

Kiecolt-Glaser, J.K., Marucha, P.T., Malarkey, W.B., Mercado, A.M.and Glaser, R. (1995) Slowing of wound healing by psychological stress. *Lance.* **346**, 1194–1196.

Knies, R.C. (1996) Geriatric trauma: What you need to know. *International Journal of Trauma Nursing* **2(3)**, 85–91.

Kuh, D. and New Dynamics of Aging Preparatory Network (2007) A life course approach to healthy aging, frailty, and capability. *Journal of Gerontology* **62A**: 7, 717–721.

Lang, P., Michel, J. and Zekry, D. (2009) Frailty syndrome: A transitional state in a dynamic process. *Gerontology* **55**, 539–549. Published online, accessed 17/12/2009.

Leslie, P., Carding, P.N. and Wilson, J.A. (2003) Investigation and management of chronic dysphagia. *BMJ* **326**, 433–436.

Lovallo, W.R. (2005) *Stress and Health: Biological and psychological interactions*, 2nd ed.Thousand Oaks: Sage Publications.

Lui, P.D. (2007) Urinary incontinence. In: *The Merck Manual for Health Care Professionals.* Accessed 16.07.2012 at http://www.merckmanuals.com/professional/genitourinary_disorders/voiding_disorders/urinary_incontinence.html#v1051498

Mangoni, A.A. and Jackson, S.H.D. (2003) Age-related changes in pharmacokinetics and pharmacodynamics: Basic principles and practical applications. *British Journal of Pharmacology* **57(1)**, 6–14.

Margetts, B.M., Thompson, R.L., Elia, M. and Jackson, A.A. (2003) Prevalence of risk of undernutrition is associated with poor health status in older people in the UK. *European Journal of Clinical Nutrition* **57(1)**, 69–74.

Ministry of Agriculture, Fisheries and Food and the Department of Health (1998) *Report of the Diet and Nutrition Survey*. Volume **1**. London: HMSO.

Miracle, A.W. and Miracle, T.S. (2001) Sexuality in late adulthood. In: Bonder, B.R. and Wagner, M.B. (eds) *Functional Performance in Older Adults*, 2nd ed. Philadelphia: FA Davis Co., pp. 218–235.

Morley, J.E. (2001) Decreased food intake with aging. *Journals of Gerontology: Series A*, **Vol**. **56A** (Special Issue 11), 81–88. Accessed 06/01/11 at http://www.biomedgerontology.oxfordjournals.org

Morley, J.E. (2003) Hormones and the aging process. *Journal of the American Geriatrics Society* **51(7)**, s333–s337.

National Collaborating Centre for Chronic Conditions (2008) *Type 2 Diabetes: National clinical guideline for management in primary and secondary care (update).* London: Royal College of Physicians.

National Health Service (2008) *Health Survey for England – 2008 trend tables.* The NHS Information Centre for health and social care. Accessed on 14/01/11 at http://www.ic.nhs.uk/ pubs/hse08trends

NHS Choices: High blood pressure (hypertension). Accessed December 2011 at: http://www.nhs. uk/Conditions/Blood-pressure-(high)/Pages/Introduction.aspx

Ning, F., Tuomilehto, J., Hammar, N., Ho, S.Y., Söderberg, S., Zimmer, P.Z., Shaw, J.E., Nakagami, T., Moha,n V., Ramachandran, A., Lam, T.H., Andersson, S.W., Janus, E.D., Boyko, E.J., Fujiimoto, W.Y. and Pang, Z.C. (2010) Does abnormal insulin action or insulin secretion explain the increase in prevalence of impaired glucose metabolism with age in populations of differnet ethnicities? *Diabetes/Metabolism Research and Reviews* **26**, 245–253.

Phillips, F. (2003) Nutrition for healthy ageing. *Nutrition Bulletin.* British Nutrition Foundation **28**, 253–263.

Purath, J., Buchholz, S.W. and Kark, D.L. (2009) Physical fitness assessment of older adults in the primary care setting. *Journal of the American Academy of Nurse Practitioner* **21**, 101–107. Accessed 13/01/11 at: http://web.ebscohost.com/ehost/pdfviewer/pdfviewer?hid=17&sid=c671c40f-6264- 4c1a-b77f-e27aa6c605d7%40sessionmgr12&vid=6

Read, J. (1999) Sexual problems associated with infertility, pregnancy and ageing. *British Medical Journal* **318**, 587–589.

Reid, I.R., Gallagher, D.J.A. and Bosworth, J. (1986) Prophylaxis against vitamin D deficiency in the elderly by regular sunlight exposure. *Age and Ageing* **15(1)**, 35–40.

Robbins, J.A., Bridges, A. and Taylor, A. (2006) Oral, pharyngeal and esophageal motor function in aging. In: *Goyal and Shaker's GI Motility Online.* New York: Nature Publishing Group,. doi:10.1038/gimo 39. Accessed 16/07/2012 at:http://www.nature.com/gimo/contents/pt1/full/ gimo39.html

Royal College of Physicians (2002) *Nutrition and Patients: A doctor's responsibility.* London. Royal College of Physicians.

Scullion, J. and Holmes, S. (2011) Palliative care in patients with chronic obstructive pulmonary disease. *Nursing Older People* **23(4)**, 32–39.

Simpson, J.M., Marsh, N. and Harrington, R. (1998) Managing falls among elderly people. *British Journal of Occupational Therapy* **61(4)**, 165–168.

Spirduso, W.W. and Cronin, D.L. (2001) Exercise dose-response effects on quality of life and independent living in older adults. *Medicine & Science in Sports & Exercise* **33(6S)**, S598–S608.

Stenholm, S., Alley, D., Bandinalli, S., Griswold, M.E., Koskinen, S., Rantanen, T., Guralnik, J.M. and Ferrucci, L. (2009) The effect of obesity combined with low muscle strength on decline in mobility in older persons: Results from the In CHIANTI Study. *International Journal of Obesity* **33**, 635–644.

Swigris, J.J., Brown, K.K., Make, B.J. and Wamboldt, F.S. (2008) Pulmonary rehabilitation in idiopathic pulmonary fibrosis: A call for continued investigation. *Respiratory Medicine* **102**, 1675–1680.

Thakar, R. and Stanton, S. (2000) Management of urinary incontinence in women. *BMJ* **321**, 1326–1331.

Tortora, G.J. and Derrickson, B.H. (2009) *Principles of Anatomy and Physiology*, 12th ed. New York: John Wiley & Sons, Inc.

Tortora, S.R. and Grabowski, G.J. (2009) *Principles of Anatomy and Physiology*, 10th edition. Chichester: John Wiley & Sons Ltd.

Trombly, C.A. and Radomski, M.V. (2002). *Occupational Therapy for Physical Dysfunction*, 5th edition. Philadelphia: Lippincott. Williams and Wilkins.

Weiskopf, D., Weinberger, B. and Grubeck-Loebenstein, B. (2009) The aging of the immune system – Review. *Transplant International*, Journal compilation, European Society for Organ Transplantation, **22**, 1041–1050. Accessed at: http://web.ebscohost.com on 04/01/2001

Victor, C. (2010) *Ageing, Health and Care*. Bristol: The Policy Press.

Wilmshurst, P. (1994) Temperature and cardiovascular mortality. *BMJ* **309**, 1029–1030.

Woolfe, R.W. (2003) Beware of fans. *BMJ* **327**, 512.

World Health Organization (2001) *The International Classification of Functioning Disability and Health*. Geneva: World Health Organization.

Worfolk, J. (1997) Keep frail elders warm! *Geriatric Nursing* **18(1)**, 7–11.

Chapter 8

Occupation and successful ageing – activity and participation

Anne McIntyre (with contributions from Lesley Wilson)

The 'doing' and taking part in occupations and activities are an important part of everyday life in many cultures. What we do (and are perceived and expected to do) provides us with our personal and social identity and role within our families, work and social environment. Indeed, the importance of activity to self-esteem and identity in older people was observed by Bullington (2006). Occupation is perceived to encompass activity and participation, as described by the WHO (World Health Organization [WHO] 2001). Activity and participation are considered crucial elements of functioning and disability alongside body functions and structures, interacting with the personal and environmental context of an older person. This chapter discusses the activity and participation issues of older people, which could be considered the key elements of occupational performance.

Within the ICF, the WHO (2001) provides the following definitions:

- Activity – 'the execution of a task or action by an individual'
- Participation – 'the involvement in a life situation'

with

- Activity limitation – 'difficulties an individual may have in executing an activity'
- Participation restriction – 'problems an individual may experience being involved in a life situation'.

The WHO (2001) also differentiates between capacity and performance of activities in the ICF, with capacity being what an individual can do as opposed to performance – what they do do. Differentiation between these two concepts is important in practice, along with self-report of activity performance, as it is debated whether older people's actual performance (especially the oldest-old) matches their self-report (Boostma-van der Wiel et al. 2001, Bravell et al. 2011).

Chapters 6 and 7 discussed the ageing body, and the need for occupational therapists to consider body functions and structures. However, it is important that these are part of our activity and occupational analyses to ensure that the focus of intervention remains on the older person's occupations. The promotion of health and wellbeing through engagement in occupation has been discussed in Chapter 2. How we engage in occupation

Occupational Therapy and Older People, Second Edition. Edited by Anita Atwal and Anne McIntyre.
© 2013 Blackwell Publishing Ltd. Published 2013 by Blackwell Publishing Ltd.

is taken further in this chapter. Even though the terms 'activity' and 'occupation; are used interchangeably in practice, Creek (2003) and Harvey and Pentland (2003) consider that there is a task-activity-occupation hierarchy, with tasks and activities only being meaningful when placed in a personal and environmental context.

Whereas 'occupation' may be unfamiliar terminology outside the profession, the use of the term 'activities of daily living' (ADLs) is familiar to many. However, universal agreement of the concept and definition of ADL has been problematic – with the subdivision of ADL into basic or personal ADLs (BADL, PADL) and instrumental or extended ADLs (IADL, EADL). The inclusion and exclusion of activities within these subdivisions can vary between professions, organisations, and geographical boundaries. It could be argued that the concept of ADL ignores the contexts of individuals, and therefore such performance has no meaning, lacking client-centredness. Therefore, the consideration of the contextual factors for an individual on their activity and participation in the ICF (WHO 2001) is to be welcomed, as is the meeting of two opposing models – the medical and social model of disability into a bio-psycho-social model. However, the introduction of universally-agreed domains within the ICF does not always fit seamlessly with established occupational therapy use.

External factors such as health and social care practices, traditions and organisational policies all influence occupational therapy practice as well as professional philosophy and beliefs; including the conceptual understanding of activity and occupation. These external factors influence the way we work, the outcome measures and the interventions we carry out. It will also influence the evidence base and research methodologies we use.

Occupational therapy research has identified age-related deterioration in everyday activity in older people (Hayase et al. 2004) and more so in all older people with dementia (Oakley et al. 2003). Although these researchers concentrated on motor and processing skills in activity capacity, rather than considering actual performance, the evidence provides us with baseline information to inform practice. Also of interest is the work of Fricke and Unsworth (2001) which highlighted the different perceptions of important instrumental ADLs between older people and their occupational therapists. Whereas older participants rated activities related and contributing to leisure as most important (use of telephone, transportation (including driving), reading) occupational therapists listed more activities related to self-care (use of telephone, medication management and snack preparation). Such evidence reinforces the need for client-centred practice, the importance of meaningful occupation and use of appropriate outcome measures to enhance our evidence base.

Many outcome measures are presented in Chapter 5, with some using the traditional concepts of ADL. Increasingly more occupational therapy-specific outcome measures are being devised to address client-centred practice and engagement in occupation. The reader is directed to Unsworth (2000), Law et al. (2005), Hemphill-Pearson 2008, Laver Fawcett 2007).

Of the nine domains listed in the ICF, the first six domains could be considered the more 'traditional' activities of daily living and related to 'doing' and the remaining three are perhaps more participatory in nature. Lesley Wilson also discusses the importance of spirituality for occupational balance. The domains discussed in this chapter are summarised in Box 8.1.

Box 8.1 Domains within the Activity and Participation components of the ICF.

Learning and applying knowledge

- Purposeful and sensory experiences
- Basic learning
- Applying knowledge

General tasks and demands

- Undertaking single tasks
- Undertaking multiple tasks
- Carrying out daily routine
- Handling stress and other psychological demands

Communication

Mobility

- Changing and maintaining body position
- Carrying, moving and handling objects
- Walking
- Climbing stairs

Self care

- Washing oneself
- Caring for body parts
- Toileting
- Dressing
- Eating
- Drinking
- Looking after one's health

Domestic life

- Acquisition of necessities
- Household tasks
- Caring for household objects and assisting others

Interpersonal interactions and relationships

- Basic interpersonal interactions
- Complex interpersonal interactions
- Relating with strangers
- Formal relationships
- Informal relationships
- Family relationships
- Intimate relationships

Major life areas

- Informal education
- School education
- Higher education
- Remunerative employment
- Basic economic transactions
- Economic self-sufficiency

Community, social and civic life

- Community life
- Recreation and leisure

- Religion and spirituality
- Human rights
- Political life and citizenship

(Source: WHO 2001*)*

Learning and applying knowledge

Defining learning and applying knowledge

The first domain of the Activities and Participation component classified by the ICF is learning and applying knowledge. Without the ability to learn and the skill to apply that learning, activity is limited. The WHO (2001) considers that this domain also includes problem-solving and decision-making skills. All of these elements are crucial to occupational therapy intervention with older people to ensure that new skills are learned or modification to previously-acquired skills takes place. Assessment of potential for rehabilitation involves consideration of all of these aspects as this often informs the choice of intervention approach. It is important to acknowledge that learning and applying knowledge apply equally to the occupational therapist working with older people, at every stage of involvement. Clinical reasoning involves active consideration of each experience, problem solving, identification of learning needs, decision making and application of existing knowledge (Mattingly and Fleming 1994). It is important to have a sense of how decisions emerged, especially in the complex settings encountered when working with older people.

Purposeful sensory experiences

Sensory experiences require the body structure to receive the sensory input, and the body function to process it (as already discussed in Chapter 6), with the environment having equal significance as a provider of stimuli.

Although Mrs Walker (see Box 8.2) was unable to use her visual sense, she was able to use other senses such as smell and sense of touch with other parts of her body, such as the back of her hand and her face, as well as her hearing to establish when her kettle had boiled. Mrs Walker's loss of peripheral sense of touch and visual sensations were gradual

---

Box 8.2   Mrs Walker who smelt her clothes.

Mrs Walker lived on her own in a warden-controlled flat. Unfortunately, she had a severe visual impairment for many years as a result of poor control of her diabetes. She also had peripheral neuropathy that affected her sense of touch in her fingers. However, Mrs Walker was fiercely independent and prided herself on her problem-solving and organisational skills. Everything in her flat was kept in a specific place so that she would know where to find it. For example, cups and plates would be on one particular shelf and tea and coffee on another, so she could make herself a hot drink. She also used equipement provided by the Royal National Institute for the Blind (RNIB). She was always immaculately clothed, and as her new OT I was surprised that she had no help with dressing. She told me how she had her clothes stored by colour in her bedroom and she thoroughly smelt her clothes before she put them on, to ensure that they were clean and not stained.

and therefore she was able to compensate for this loss over a period of time. Barriers to Mrs Walker's independent functioning were often the involvement of other people, including unfamiliar home carers who did not understand why she had organised her home in a particular way in order to make best use of her remaining senses.

It is important to establish that an individual is able to receive and process sensory experiences prior to attempting to learn new skills or apply knowledge. Practical strategies such as ensuring the use of hearing aids or glasses when required can have a defining impact on the success of an intervention. However, even when these strategies are used, a person might still have difficulty recognising sensory input, and compensatory strategies might need to be developed, using the other senses to trigger an appropriate response. For example, Mrs Walker could not see when her cup was full of water, but could hear the beeping noise made by her liquid level indicator indicating when to stop pouring.

Basic learning

Whilst this category is titled 'basic learning', it actually encompasses the range of learning from imitation to mastery of complex skills. Learning takes place from the start of therapy, as names are exchanged and the purpose explained. The prescription of equipment involves a learning process: the occupational therapist demonstrates how to use equipment and ensures that this is understood by observing its use by the older person. The use of products and technology could be contraindicated if it is not possible for the person to acquire the skills required to use it.

Applying knowledge

Age holds conflicting preconceptions in relation to learning: on the one hand, experience and acquisition of knowledge increase with age (Woodruff-Pak 1997), but there is a widespread belief that it is more difficult for older people to adapt and learn new skills and this is considered in this chapter alongside undertaking tasks.

Being sensitive to beliefs and values of all concerned enables the occupational therapist to structure the experience of therapy in a way that maximises opportunity for learning and applying knowledge.

General tasks and demands

Undertaking single and multiple tasks

What is a task? Interpretations vary between dictionary definitions, which consider a task to be a piece of work or a chore, and the interpretation of the WHO and the occupational therapy literature. The ICF considers a task as a component of an activity carried out by an individual (WHO 2001). Performance of a task is dependent upon its complexity and meaning, our motivation, past experience, knowledge and capacity. Therefore, task performance is highly dependent upon the performance skills (or body functions) we have available to us, our ability to learn new skills and tasks, as well as the environment and the personal context in which the task is carried out. In occupational therapy, we use tasks in a multitude of ways – with many of our assessments involving observation – either to consider the task's component performance skills, or which element of an activity the client finds problematic. The use of tasks will depend on the frame of reference we adopt.

Analysis of tasks is useful when considering intervention, as tasks can be structured and used within a programme of rehabilitation to facilitate (re)acquisition of skills and abilities, enhancing performance by giving meaning and value to the intervention as a 'means to an end'. Tasks will also form the target of a programme in that they are the building blocks within an activity or occupation that the older person client needs/wants to be able to do and are therefore crucial elements within goals of intervention.

Tasks are also considered in terms of their complexity, but interpretations of this vary. In the ICF, the WHO (2001) considers that reading a book is a simple task, but even though this may involve relatively simple motor skills it also requires complex cognitive and perceptual functions. Reed and Sanderson (1999) suggest that the number of steps or sequences can determine the complexity of a task or patterns within it, as well as the amount of structure, flexibility, or creativity allowed.

Tasks may be 'closed' with a definite beginning and end, such as opening a door, or 'open' such as cycle riding or knitting. Multiple tasks could involve the simultaneous and sequential performance of both simple and complex tasks, for example holding and speaking into a telephone whilst searching for pen and paper to write a message.

Most of the research on task performance in older people concentrates on cognitive functioning and abilities in 'laboratory' tasks rather than performance in everyday functioning. However, increasingly, research is being undertaken that considers everyday task performance. This research highlights that success at carrying out tasks – especially complex and multiple tasks – are more reliant upon cognitive functioning rather than motor agility, especially the executive functions of problem solving, planning and decision making (Carlson et al. 1999, Cahn-Wiener et al. 2000, Burton et al. 2007). Therefore, successful task performance is reliant upon the normal ageing processes within the pre-frontal and posterior parietal cortices as already discussed in Chapter 6.

Within occupational therapy, outcome measures of task performance (and the performance components) have been developed. Much of the research on task performance has involved 'laboratory' tests such as those involving executive functions rather than 'real world' tasks. However, the Large Allen's Cognitive Level Screen (LACL) devised by Allen et al. (1992), and the Assessment of Motor and Process Skills (AMPS) devised by Fisher (1995) and described in Chapter 5, use everyday tasks and activities to assess functioning.

Even though much of the research does not involve 'real world' tasks, it does provide useful evidence on task performance and implications for occupational therapy practice:

- Providing older people with more opportunity to practise tasks than younger people improves their performance above that of their younger counterparts (Welford 1958). This is relevant not only to rehabilitation but also to work (re)training programmes employing and training older people.

- It is thought that older people need to harness greater cerebral capacity to maintain task performance (Ward and Frakowiak 2003, Grady 2008) which indicates that task performance may require more concentration and attention.
- Older people use different strategies to their younger counterparts in successful completion of more complex tasks (Crawford and Channon 2002). This indicates that therapists must be aware of individual problem solving and execution strategies in older people.
- It is thought that older people perpetuate earlier mistakes in subsequent practice, resulting in error perseveration (Hasher et al. 1991). This indicates when and how often older people are given feedback on their performance in tasks and activities, to ensure that errors in performance are reduced. It also indicates that teaching of new tasks should be structured to minimise the possibility of error.
- Carrying out multiple tasks has also been under scrutiny, with recent research considering dual task performance. Therapists are aware that older people who are able to converse whilst carrying out daily living tasks are likely to be more successful and safer in their performance (Lundin-Olsson et al. 1997, Bowen et al. 2001, Verghese et al. 2002).

A small study by Muhaidat et al. (2010) also identified that their participants had difficulty with walking and carrying items (especially on stairs) and also when walking in crowded places. Gender differences were also observed, with older women having more difficulties dual-tasking with household chores and older men with outdoor activities and sport. Although a small study, this is of interest as it considers real-world scenarios such as that described in Box 8.3. Studies have been carried out to establish which tasks are the more demanding and these have implications not only for intervention but also in assessment, as a client may marshal extra attentional capacity because they are being assessed, but is unable to sustain this during actual performance in 'real' situations. Recent evidence suggests:

- Motor and higher cognitive tasks can normally be performed simultaneously with little detrimental effect on either, but performance deteriorates when two similar tasks are attempted at the same time – i.e. talking and map reading (Haggard et al. 2000).
- Speed of motor tasks and accuracy of cognitive tasks do decline in dual tasking with older adults and after acquired brain injury – e.g. stroke (Yardley et al. 2001).
- Performance in dual tasks progressively declines with clients who have increasing cognitive impairment (Hauer et al. 2003).

Box 8.3   **Mrs Wright with Parksinson's disease.**

Mrs Wright was seen by the local therapy team after her last attendance at the neurology clinic for her Parkinson's disease. When observing Mrs Wright's mobility, both the occupational therapist and physiotherapist identified that Mrs Wright was safer at some times more than others. They identified that Mrs Wright was less stable during dual tasks (i.e. walking and talking) than when performing the tasks independently. The decision was to keep verbal feedback during tasks to a minimum during intervention and also to consider Mrs Wright's environment and negotiate with Mrs Wright's family, so that it wasn't too noisy or busy when she was carrying out her everyday activities at home.

- The complexity of the task and also the length of time a task may take are also considered to impact on dual tasking (Yardley et al. 2001, Haggard et al. 2000).
- Older people with Parkinson's disease prioritise cognitive tasks over motor tasks when dual tasking (Bloem et al. 2006).

Carrying out daily routines

The WHO defines this within the ICF as 'carrying out simple or complex actions in order to plan, manage and complete the requirements for day to day procedures or duties. (WHO 2001, p. 130). We tend to believe that routines are occupations with established sequences in our daily lives (Christiansen and Baum 1997). Routines are especially important for those people with dementia (Alzheimer's Society 2000). Control over daily routines is said to be important in maintaining quality of life for the oldest-old , but where routines are imposed by others or external influences (such as in institutional care), this can be confining and a negative experience (Häggblom-Kronlöf et al. 2007).

Handling stress and other psychological demands

Stressors identified for older people are: failing senses; illness and disability of family, friends and self; pain; limited energy; fear of dependency; death of close family and friends; loneliness and isolation; and deterioration in personal control and autonomy (Pfeiffer 2002).

More personal and financial resources entail responsibilities for management and maintenance. Many older people are informal carers for family members, with over 2 million people aged over 60 caring for spouses, siblings, parents, and one quarter of all grandparents regularly caring for their grandchildren. It is common in many cultures for grandparents to look after grandchildren; this has reached crisis point in Africa where many older people are the main carer for their grandchildren orphaned by the AIDS epidemic. Many of these children also have AIDS (United Nations 2002) and the caregiver demands and responsibilities go unrecognised.

The majority of older carers are men and tend to be spouse carers. Older male carers are reported to have the greatest care burden (Ross et al. 2008), and are less likely to receive help from others (Baker and Robertson 2008). Dahlberg et al. (2007) also identify that the older the carer, the more hours of care given, with those carers (especially men) aged 80–89 years, providing 50 or more hours of care a week. A survey in the UK by The Princess Royal Trust for Carers (2011) also identified that two-thirds of older carers have their own long-term health problems, such as musculoskeletal problems, heart disease, cancer and depression. There is also evidence that carers neglect their own health, e.g. cancelling hospital appointments and routine checks, because of the burden of care (Department of Health [DH] 2010, The Princess Royal Trust for Carers 2011). In our own research, older carers shared distrust of help from services, seemingly preferring to shoulder the physical care-burden and ignoring their own health conditions to avoid potential admission to residential care for the care-recipient (McIntyre and Reynolds 2012). Caring for others is further considered in a later section in this chapter.

Even though many older people demonstrate stoicism and self-reliance in times of stress or crisis because of past experience of war and economic depression, they react to stress in different ways than younger people (see Chapter 9). Older people are less likely to seek help at times of both collective and personal crisis, because of a lack of appropriate help being provided for, or perceived by, the older person (Howse et al. 2005, Ardalan et al. 2010).

The Samaritans (2011) have identified that the suicide rates in older people are relatively high in the UK and the Republic of Ireland (16% of all suicides). In the UK, many older people commit suicide through drug overdose, and it is thought that physical illness, bereavement and interpersonal problems are often the cause in older suicides (Harwood et al. 2000, 2006).

Stress manifests itself with physical symptoms – causing deterioration in functioning and an exacerbation of existing disease processes (Pfeiffer 2002). Therefore, health promotion strategies are necessary for older people – not only encouraging them to maintain healthy lifestyles and wellbeing to prevent stress, but also to join appropriate self-help groups and take part in stress management programmes as part of secondary and tertiary health promotion.

Communication

Occupational therapists need to ensure that communication occurs in an environment in which the older person feels confident and comfortable. Privacy and confidentiality should be maintained at all times. Communication should not be rushed and occupational therapists need to ensure that the principles of client-centred practice are maintained at all times. Participation is largely dependent on a willingness and inclination to engage with others and is usually socially motivated, as it would be for anyone. It is important to remember that, when first meeting, you are a stranger to the older person. Relating with strangers is potentially an activity that older people might have some difficulty with, as new situations and unknown contexts may cause anxiety and confusion. An older person may be vulnerable in terms of their safety, although the experience that comes with age could improve their judgement.

Life experience and personality are more prescient indicators of capacity and performance than age *per se*. Indeed, some older persons may wish to form a formal relationship with the therapist where roles are clearly defined, with more structure, clear boundaries or even a contractual agreement like those that they would have with, for example, their solicitor, bank manager or doctor. In some cultures, certain family relationships may have a formal element, with the expectation of particular behaviours within that interaction. The informality of many institutions is a relatively recent phenomenon. Hence, even in situations where the roles could be expected to be less formal, older people might find a more formal approach reassuring initially, until they become more familiar with the person. Occupational therapists would come into this relationship category and an attitude of 'mutual respect' is an important and helpful starting place to build up rapport.

Ensuring that the older person has appropriate means to enable communication to take place is fundamental. This may mean checking that their hearing aid is effective, that they have their reading glasses available, and that a translator and/or trusted friend or family member is available to assist and support communication.

Mobility

The ICF describes mobility as 'moving by changing body position or location or by transferring from one place to another, by carrying, moving or manipulating objects, by walking, running or climbing and by using various forms of transportation' (WHO 2001, p. 138).

As occupational therapists, we are concerned not only about how safely a client moves or obtains a position but also the quality of the movement. Many factors (including team consultation) will determine whether an educational, advisory, or compensatory approach is required with a client. Traditionally, physiotherapists have been involved in the re-education of walking and transfers, whereas occupational therapists are more concerned about the relationship between the client's ability to move and their environment, to successfully perform their chosen occupations. The story of Mr Clark, who we met in Chapter 5, is quite a common one. Environmental adaptation, provision of mobility equipment (including bed, toilet and chair raisers) and the use of problem solving and learning of new skills facilitated his functioning in most areas of occupational performance.

How successfully a person moves is dependent on planning and programming of movement patterns through reciprocal innervation of muscle groups, sensorimotor feedforward and feedback mechanisms, as well as adequate muscle tone, bulk and strength, balance reactions, cardiovascular and respiratory efficiency and structurally sound bones and joints (discussed in Chapters 6 and 7). In older people, it is important to ascertain why they have mobility problems and there is much debate about which are part of normal ageing and which are part of pathological processes. Mobility problems after traumatic events should entail short-term need for precautionary postoperative measures. In other situations, such as those of Mr Clark, Mrs Wright and Mrs Johnson discussed in Chapter 5, recovery of previous levels of mobility may not be possible.

What is becoming a developing part of every health professional's role is the promotion of physical activity for clients of all ages, because of the increasing evidence for the relationship between physical activity such as walking or gardening and many health conditions such as cardiovascular conditions, Type 2 diabetes, obesity, bone health and fractures, muscle strength, cancer, falls, depression and cognitive functioning in adults and older adults (Young and Dinan 2005, US Department of Health and Human Services 2008). Worryingly, a recent Health Survey for England in 2008 (NHS Information Centre 2009) has identified that less than 45% of men and women aged 16+ meet the recommended weekly targets for physical activity and this declines with age (see Box 8.4). Therefore, the projected rise in health conditions and subsequent disability is a worrying prospect and strengthens the need for active or successful ageing health and social care policies.

However, the take-up of physical activity for older people is often disappointing and it is often how such formal or organised sessions are portrayed. As already discussed in Chapter 5, the uptake of falls prevention and interventions by older people already identified as at risk of falling has been low. This lack of participation and adherence was related

---

Box 8.4   Do you meet the physical activity recommendations?

The CMOs in the UK have recommended that all adults carry out 30 minutes (or more) of moderate/high physical activity at least five times per week.

Who meets the target?

- 41% of men aged 16+
- 31% of women aged 16+
- 20% of people aged 65+
- 10% of people aged 75+

How much do you do?
More information about physical activity across the lifespan can be found in the following documents:

- Department of Health and Human Services (2008) *Physical Activity Guidelines Advisory Committee Report*. Washington, DC: US Department of Health and Human Services. http://www.health.gov/paguidelines/pdf/paguide.pdf
- Department of Health, Physical Activity, Health Improvement and Protection (2011) *Start Active, Stay Active: A report on physical activity from the four home countries' Chief Medical Officers*. http://www.dh.gov.uk/prod_consum_dh/groups/dh_digitalassets/documents/digitalasset/dh_128210.pdf

---

to threats to autonomy and identity for older people (Yardley et al. 2006) and therefore 'rebranding' of falls prevention sessions has been recommended to focus on healthy lifestyles and fitness, as well as the individual needs of older people. Hardy and Grogan (2009) explored the barriers to and facilitators for older people carrying out physical activity. They established that motivation to prevent ill-health, feelings of superiority over younger people in terms of health and fitness, enjoyment of age-appropriate and organised sessions, being motivated by others (peer influence) and opportunity for social interaction all encouraged older people to participate in physical activity. These findings are important considerations when devising interventions that encourage physical activity either for an individual or a local community.

Maintaining a position

A stable position is crucial for everyday functioning. Trying to carry out an activity from an unstable position would be like trying to eat jelly whilst sitting on a bucking bronco. The ease with which an individual can adopt a position is dependent upon the balance mechanisms, muscle strength and range of movement required to maintain it. For example, lying is a very stable position with a low centre of gravity (COG) well within a large base of support (BOS), requiring little postural control or muscle activity to maintain it. Standing is less easy to maintain, with a higher centre of gravity in a narrower base of support. As one's centre of gravity rises and the base of support decreases, our balance and neuromuscular systems become more important in our ability to maintain a position from which to carry out everyday activities.

In response to a deteriorating balance system, many older people adopt a standing or sitting position that increases their stability – often at the expense of potential mobility. Many older people increase their stability in standing by having their legs further apart to widen their base of support, slightly flexing the hips and knees to lower their centre of gravity. Carrying out an activity from this position consequently means that the individual has to lean slightly forward, flattening out their lumbar spine, creating a kyphosis of the thoracic spine and poking the chin and head forward. This stooped posture is one that many would associate with old age – especially the oldest-old (Shumway-Cook and Woollacott 2012). As this stooped posture is associated with a reduction in spinal flexibility, range of movement and muscle weakness an older person who has been physically inactive is more likely to acquire this posture at an earlier age. Such a position may be less energy-efficient to maintain, requiring more muscle activity and therefore the individual may tire more easily and be able to stand for shorter and shorter periods of time.

Changing position

In the ICF, changing position is described as 'getting out of one position and moving from one location to another...' (WHO 2001. p. 138). In much of the therapy literature and assessments, this would be termed as 'ability to transfer' and refer to those more active changes in position that an individual may carry out. Confusingly, the ICF relates transfers to 'moving from one surface to another without changing position' (WHO 2001, p. 140) such as sliding transfers.

Deterioration in muscle strength, a decline in flexibility and range of movement, as well as CNS reaction times and interruption of normal movement patterns, all impact on changing from one position to another. Muscle stiffness and pain both impact on flexibility at any age with a consequential change in movement strategy and speed when, for example, rolling over and getting out of bed (Box 8.5).

Strategies to achieve independent standing from sitting are an important part of an occupational therapy role – whether it is teaching a client new and safer strategies using appropriate positioning of the head, body and feet and use of biomechanical principles, or environmental adaptation such as a bed or armchair raise. Shumway-Cook and Woollacott (2012) identify that 8% of older people aged 65 and over living in the community have difficulty standing from sitting. It would seem that older people use different movement strategies and patterns to optimise performance, often using momentum rather than muscle effort to stand from sitting. It is also observed that older people use different strategies to stand from sitting that not only rely upon multiple physiological and psychological processes but also on extrinsic factors such as the height, depth and firmness of the seat and the presence of armrests (Lord et al. 2002).

Getting up from the floor is an important transfer in relation to falls management, with more than 47% of older people at risk of falling being unable to get up off the floor (Reece

---

Box 8.5

Many people with hemiplegia and parkinsonian problems are observed to have problems with rolling over in bed because of impairments in body functions. Whereas Mrs Wright has difficulty with initiating rolling over and sitting up in bed, Mr Clark has difficulty in coordinating and utilising his right side, to roll over and getting his right leg into bed at night.

and Simpson 1996). Individuals can spend many minutes or hours on the floor and the consequences of a 'long lie' are hypothermia, dehydration, bronchopneumonia, pressure sores as well as anxiety and depression (Wild et al. 1981). Strategies such as 'backward chaining' are useful and necessary techniques to teach an older person how to get up off the floor and are recommended as part of a falls management programme (College of Occupational Therapists 2006).

Carrying, moving and handling objects

Our ability to carry, reach and handle objects with the upper limbs is essential for all self-care activities and most occupations. The upper limbs also have a protective role as part of the body's saving reactions when overbalancing (McIlroy and Maki 1994). This parachute response, a protective mechanism against injury during a fall, is developed in babyhood, and accounts for the occurrence of one of the most common fractures in older people (especially women), the Colles fracture (Singer et al. 1998).

Other impairments impact upon upper limb function with the ageing process affecting the soft tissues around the shoulder joint causing a decline in active range of movement, especially flexion, abduction, lateral and medial rotation (Desrosiers et al. 1995). Such decline in upper limb function can be noted over a relatively short period of time; however, it is not necessarily related to chronological age but previous activity levels (Desrosiers et al. 1999).

Carrying items also reduces postural stability by raising the centre of gravity up and out of the base of support and also putting potentially weaker shoulder and upper limb muscle groups under greater demand. However, the most significant changes are noticed in manual dexterity due to reduction in muscle mass, hand–eye coordination, sensory loss and cutaneous changes (e.g. skin slipperiness) (Desrosiers et al. 1999, Ranganathen et al. 2001). Grip strength is perceived to be a good indicator of an older person's general health and possible frailty, as well as a marker of sarcopaenia (Ashfield et al. 2010) with Carmeli et al. (2003) observing that deterioration in hand function occurs secondary to age-related changes in the neurological, musculoskeletal and cardiovascular systems. It is also considered that ageing of the CNS increases the time taken to manipulate and grasp objects by 40% between the ages of 25 and 70 years (Shumway-Cook and Woollacott 2012). Deterioration in manipulation and grip strength has impact on an older person's ability to carry out many everyday tasks, such as opening jars, milk cartons, and medication bottles.

There are several standardised upper limb and hand function assessments; however, the provision of normative data and the reliability and validity of these have not been fully explored with older people, so in many instances older people's upper limb function and activity is compared with that of younger people (Shiffman 1992). Some assessments that do consider older adults are discussed in relation to Val with colles fracture in Chapter 5.

Upper limb activity is also affected by our ability to maintain a position independently. Where sitting balance is compromised, for example, many individuals find that they have to 'fix' their position by holding onto armrests of chairs and wheelchairs for support if they do not have adequate postural support provided within the chair. The use of walking products to alleviate weight bearing through the legs after a lower limb fracture or to redistribute body weight because of poor balance immediately hampers an individual from any upper limb activity such as carrying items or opening doors. Therefore, other strategies have to be considered, such as the provision of a perching stool for washing or meal preparation, and a kitchen trolley to transport meals, drinks and any other items from room to room.

Walking

The Health Survey for England (HSE) identified that more than 30% of over 65-year-olds and 50% of over 80-year-olds living in the community consider that they have mobility problems, which compares to 36% of over 70-year-olds in the US (DH 2000, Iezzoni et al. 2001). The HSE (DH 2000) identified that problem with walking is the most common disability in older people.

It is debated whether gait and walking problems are due to normal ageing processes within the body or are due to pathological changes associated with lack of physical activity (Shumway-Cook and Woollacott 2012). As already discussed, the impact of lifestyle (e.g. exercise, nutrition) cannot be discounted and the concept of 'use it or lose it' is highly pertinent with walking. However, changes in walking (or gait) in older people are observed, with a reduction of walking speed, step length and step rate. As changes in body functions and structures occur due to ageing it is not surprising that this has an impact on walking which is a highly complex task. Deterioration in walking has already been discussed as an element in dual task performance. Other factors such as use of medication, pain, anxiety, fear of falling and the environment all contribute to walking problems. Iezzoni et al. (2001) found that most older people who could identify a cause for their mobility problems said that they were due to arthritis and musculoskeletal problems, followed by heart conditions, stroke and falls.

Occupational therapists are concerned about walking as part of occupational performance – in that the client wishes to walk to perform an occupational activity such as shopping, going to the toilet, carrying washing to the clothesline. Many assessments include mobility (i.e. walking) along with self-care items in personal activity of daily living assessments; however, these do not always discriminate between different walking demands. It is therefore necessary to consider walking in the context of the activity being carried out, as this will determine how far, how quickly, where and when an individual walks. Walking indoors, for example, has different demands of body functions (such as vision, balance) than walking outdoors on uneven ground. Fear of walking outdoors is also reported by older people and this is not only associated with musculoskeletal disease and slow walking speed but also poor conditions of roads and pavements, hills and slopes and noisy traffic (Rantakokko et al. 2009). It is also observed that many older people walk at a slower pace than that required to cross roads using signal-operated pedestrian crossings (Knoblauch et al. 1996) and this speed is affected by use of mobility aids, presence of inclines, width of road and amount of traffic. Therefore, this also adds to anxiety for older people when walking outside.

Stair climbing

Falling on the stairs is the most common accident in the home, and is more likely to happen when descending rather than ascending the stairs (Verghese et al. 2008), with 10% of older people in England unable to climb stairs (Office for National Statistics 2002).

Stair climbing and descending use a similar movement pattern as walking, with a swing through and stance phase; however, stair climbing requires greater range of movement and muscle strength in the legs, either to carry the body upward on an extending knee or controlling the descent on a flexing knee. Deterioration in lower limb muscle strength observed in older people can make stair climbing difficult, impossible or hazardous. The reliance upon sensory input to determine an appropriate strategy (especially visual cues), when stair climbing must also be appreciated (Shumway-Cook and Woollacott 2012).

Box 8.6   Consider an older person you know or one of the case studies in Chapter 5.

Identify what personal and external factors facilitated their mobility.
Consider any potential barriers.
What could an occupational therapist and/or team offer to optimise their potential?
Is there any place for health promotion strategies for this individual and people in their situation?

Self care

Whereas movement suggests the physical interaction between the person and their immediate environment, the domain of self-care is very much concerned with the person and their body. Self care is classified with the ICF as washing, caring for body parts, toileting, dressing, eating and drinking and looking after one's health (WHO 2001).

A recent survey of older Americans receiving Medicare identified that 28% of those aged 65+ experienced problems with self-care activities, with 7% of older people living in the community having problems with three or more self-care activities (Federal Interagency Forum on Aging-related Statistics 2010). These difficulties can arise equally from a mental health problem as from a physical disability (such as that experienced by many of the case studies in Chapter 5). Independence in self-care (or B/PADL) is commonly assumed in all adults and, traditionally, striving to maintain independence has been a key issue for occupational therapists. However, not all older clients wish for independence, which may be due to cultural differences (Gibbs and Barnitt 1999), due to fear and anxiety (e.g. falling again), having an over-protective carer or through disengagement (see Chapter 1 for ageing theories) (Sirkka and Bränholm 2003).

Older people seem to experience a deconditioning in self-care activities and mobility whilst in the acute care setting. Two small studies from Australia have explored occupational therapy involvement to promote occupational performance (especially in self-care tasks) and prevent deconditioning on discharge, with older adults admitted to acute care settings as a result of trauma or need for surgical intervention (Eyres and Unsworth 2005, O'Brien et al. 2012). A study in the US by Landa-Gonzalez and Molnar (2012) also explored the use of occupation-based interventions (including self-care) for older people with arthritis living in the community. This study, like the others, identified an improvement in self-care activities and quality of life for the older participants. These are pertinent (albeit small) studies that emphasise the need for an occupational performance focus for intervention with older people to maintain successful ageing.

Washing oneself

How often do you wash? This question could be considered intrusive, and yet personal hygiene is critical to our social acceptance. It is important to recognise the significance of the cleansing process. Within the ICF, washing oneself also includes showering and bathing and many recipients of occupational therapy services will emphasise the spiritual, relaxing, pain-relieving and purifying effect of immersion in water (Gooch 2003). Thus the occupation of bathing has multiple meanings; however, this is not always recognised in eligibility criteria for equipment – the emphasis on personal hygiene prevails, which causes conflict between service users and occupational therapy services.

Bathing could also be considered a dangerous activity, especially for older people, with RoSPA (2002) and Gooptu and Mulley (1994) identifying the risk of burns, falling (and drowning) in the bath as well as inability to get out of the bath leading to pressure sores, hypothermia and psychological consequences. The occurrence of these distressing incidences with older people demonstrates not only the impairment of body functions but, more importantly, the barriers within their environments, through poor bath design, poor thermal regulation, lack of or poorly positioned assistive products and alarms. However, most bathing assessments are undertaken in 'dry' or simulated situations, assessing capacity, whereas the actual performance of the activity is what should be assessed in the client's own home observing a 'wet' bath (Gooch 2003).

Caring for body parts

This category separates out those body parts which require more care than washing and drying. The absence of older people in media imagery associated with skin, hair and nail care may influence the lack of attention given to these aspects of self-care in many occupational therapy and ADL assessments. It could be argued that that skin, foot care, and dental hygiene are not traditionally domains of occupational therapy; as already discussed in Chapter 7, but these all impact both directly and indirectly on occupational performance. A prime example is the contribution of poor foot care (and long toenails) to balance problems and falls in older people (Burns et al. 2002). For older people with peripheral neuropathy and/or diabetes, advice on well-fitting shoes and socks will form part of an occupational therapy assessment for both client and carer. Therefore, the occupational therapist has a responsibility to older people to ensure that these aspects of self-care are addressed.

Toileting

Toileting is a complex activity, requiring ability in mobility, transfers and dressing as well as body functions and structures to maintain continence in both urine and faeces. Some of the difficulties considered by occupational therapists in relation to toileting have already discussed in this chapter, and the issue of urinary and faecal continence in Chapter 7. For many older people, problems with toileting can restrict their participation in social and leisure activities because of environmental barriers and poor design of public toilets for those people with mobility problems. Many older people (46%) in residential care have problems with toileting (Department of Health 2000), and for the older person loss of independence in this activity is accompanied by a loss of privacy and dignity reminiscent of early childhood.

Dressing

The ICF describes dressing as the action of putting on clothes and footwear, and taking them off (WHO 2001). Dressing is a complex activity involving many subtasks and demands on body functions and structures. Choosing clothes appropriate for the climate, culture and time is important and will determine what is worn, and the complexity and number of stages. Whereas difficulties with the physical manipulation of clothes may be easier to identify, the challenge for many occupational therapists working with older people is to unravel the problems arising from cognitive, perceptual and affective disorders. Because of its complexity, dressing involves those specific cognitive functions of sustained and selective attention as well executive functions, which are, as already stated in Chapter 6, most noticeably impaired in clients with Alzheimer's disease, learning disability, stroke and Parkinson's disease (Bellelli et al. 2002). Spatial neglect following stroke also impacts on successful dressing, with failure to dress the affected side, and apraxia which causes problems with the sequencing of the order of dressing (Walker et al. 2003).

The skills of the occupational therapist will be to determine when and what type of assistance an older person may require. for example teaching energy-conserving techniques to those with cardiovascular or respiratory conditions, or to carers where physical or verbal assistance are required. The use of compensatory techniques involving the use of dressing products might overcome difficulties with reaching, gripping clothing and managing fastenings. For some older people, changing the type of clothing worn might be acceptable, as less energy and cognitive functioning may be required to put on light stretchy clothing with fewer fastenings.

Eating and drinking

Eating and drinking are separate categories in the ICF, in contrast to other classification systems (such as the Occupational Therapy Practice Framework) which incorporate drinking within the categories of eating and feeding (American Occupational Therapy Association 2008). Rather than considering eating and drinking as only bringing food or drink to the mouth, the ICF has a wider view of the whole process of consuming food and drink (WHO 2001).

For many older people in residential care, eating and drinking are problematic (Department of Health 2000). Jacobsson et al. (2000) describe the experiences of many older people after stroke:

- Fear of choking
- Discomfort in the mouth and throat
- Discomfort from food,
- Thirst from not being able to drink from a glass

- Shame from their appearance – such as dribbling and facial paralysis
- Humiliation at dependence in being fed
- Feelings of clumsiness due to poor manual dexterity.

The need for good nutrition, dentition and swallowing in later life is addressed in Chapter 7, with the recommendation of a healthy diet for successful ageing discussed in Chapter 2. Studies show that a good diet in later years helps in reducing both the risk of and managing diseases such as heart disease, cancers, diabetes, stroke, and osteoporosis, which are the leading cause of death and disability among older people. This in turn can enable older people to maintain their independence.

Recent evidence has revealed the lack of concern about the nutritional status of older people. Indeed, there is a high incidence of malnutrition in older people, including amongst those who are obese. Although there is increasing awareness of malnutrition of older people in hospitals (14% of over 65s), 15–40% of older people living in the community are also reported to be malnourished. Contributing factors for community-living older people are social isolation, poverty, limited access to shops, inability or lack of knowledge about food preparation, cooking and nutrition. For older people in hospital or in care homes, limited choice, poor presentation and inflexible mealtimes contribute to malnutrition. Other risk factors for malnutrition are insufficient time allocated to eat, lack of assistance, missing dentures or poor dentition, difficulty reaching food, opening packaging or using cutlery, specific nutritional, religious or cultural requirements not met (European Nutrition for Health Alliance 2005, Hickson 2006, Age Concern 2010).

Occupational therapists need to consider all aspects of access and management of a healthy diet for older clients, from planning and acquisition of healthy balanced meals, to preparation, storage, feeding and eating. It must also be remembered that not all difficulties with eating relate to older people with physical disability. One of the problems associated with later stages of dementia is malnutrition, either through lack of interest in food or increasing difficulty in being able to chew or swallow. Clarke (2009) reported on the use of menu picture cards, food choice and the use of cooking activities to encourage motivation, choice and participation for older people with dementia. Creating cookery groups for older people, including 'breakfast groups', are also increasingly popular.

Eating and feeding is an activity where many members of the interprofessional team could be working alongside each other. The speech and language therapist and physiotherapist are concerned with the body functions and structures involved with swallowing and positioning, such as muscle tone, reflex activity and sensation; the nurse and dietician are concerned with nutritional and digestive issues; and the occupational therapist is more concerned with activity and environmental issues such as positioning, compensatory techniques and assistive equipment. Eating and drinking provides a good example of the use of the ICF as a framework in identifying different roles of team members working on the same activity with an older person.

Looking after one's health

Looking after one's health is central to the WHO's policy on active ageing and ethos of health promotion (WHO 2002a). Health professionals are required to ensure the older person has opportunities to access information and resources that promote a healthy lifestyle, and to live in a healthy and conducive environment. Current concepts indicate a broader interpretation of what constitutes a healthy lifestyle. In the past, being independent in self-care was considered an important indicator of health, even when it involved the use of assistive products. The three main components within the ICF of this category are:

- Ensuring one's physical comfort
- Managing diet and fitness
- Maintaining one's health.

What would stop an older person being able to ensure their own physical comfort? Discomfort is usually indicated by pain or altered sensation, so impairment of sensory perception, especially the sense of touch, will impair the ability to perceive discomfort. An occupational therapist will have particular responsibility for pressure care for those who are immobile for significant periods of time: this could involve interventions such as prescribing cushions for wheelchair users and also educating the older person, their family and carers about skin and pressure care. Discomfort can also be experienced in terms of temperature and so heating and ventilation should comprise part of a home assessment (see Chapter 9).

The benefits of physical exercise and good nutrition are important throughout the lifespan, with McCarter and Kelly (1993) suggesting that not only do these facilitate prevention of disease but also prolong healthier lives with an improvement in the biological age by 10–20 years. As already discussed, age itself is not a barrier to physical exercise and current theories of ageing (discussed in Chapter 2) consider that a decline in physical activity is not necessarily a part of normal ageing. However, a decline in physical activity is associated with an increase in chronic diseases, and therefore an increase in or maintenance of physical activity throughout life and into old age maintains activity and active participation and decreases or slows the onset of disability (Penninx et al. 2001). The literature identifies that regular exercise in older adults reduces the risk of cardiovascular disease (Manson et al. 2002), osteoporosis and Type 2 diabetes (NIDDM) (Young and Dinan 1994), cognitive decline (Yaffe et al. 2001) and is said to improve depressive symptoms in older adults (Mather et al. 2002). As already discussed in this chapter, 30 minutes of moderate exercise is advocated five times each week. Even though moderate exercise includes stair climbing, housework, gardening, lifting weights and wheelchair use; the most common form of exercise undertaken is walking. This is dependant on the access to safe, conducive, and healthy environments (WHO 2002b) and many local authorities in the UK provide organised walks or dedicated ramble routes, as well as physical activity programmes, as part of their health promotion initiatives. It is therefore relevant for occupational therapists to consider the health and wellbeing of communities and not just individuals, by assessing local environments for adequate lighting, street furniture (including signage) and even surfaces to encourage outdoor mobility, social and community participation.

The implications of a good diet and regular exercise are not only to maintain health but also to prevent the onset of disease or disability. However, many older people take medication because of disability or disease, and the use of medication increases with age. The Health Survey for England (HSE) (Department of Health 2000) identified that 80% of older people regularly take prescribed medication with 35% of over 75-year-olds taking four or more different prescribed medications daily (polypharmacy). Even though these treat the symptoms of disease, many risks are associated with taking medication in older age, especially polypharmacy. Complex dosage schedules and interactions of multiple medications, adverse drug reactions, misuse and incorrect self-medication are all associated with polypharmacy with the risks of mortality, re-admission to hospital and falls (Milton et al. 2008). Issues with medication in older people are:

- A narrower margin between therapeutic and toxic dosage due to an age-related decline in renal function, meaning that the wrong dose is often prescribed
- Inappropriate prescription of contra-indicated drugs and adverse drug reactions resulting in:
  ○ hypotension as a result of hypnotic or diuretic medication increasing risk of falls
  ○ gastro-intestinal bleeding from non-steroidal anti-inflammatories (NSAIDs)
  ○ increase in postural sway and increased risk of falls from Benzodiazepines
- Under-prescribing of appropriate and evidence-based medication
- Medications are used incorrectly or over/underused by older people
- Repeat prescriptions are wasted or inappropriately used
- Difficulty accessing general practitioner's surgery or pharmacy
- Inability by older person to read or understand medication information or open packaging
- Potential for more than one prescriber because of probable multiple co-morbidities

(Department of Health 2001, Milton et al. 2008).

Maintaining the health of older people should be promoted through initiatives to encourage a healthy lifestyle, regular exercise and healthy eating, cessation of smoking and excessive alcohol consumption, home safety and prevention of accidents, social support and welfare benefit advice, uptake of immunisations (influenza vaccinations), bereavement counselling, monitoring of blood pressure and a regular review of medication (British Geriatrics Society 2002). As much of this is reliant on the older person having insight and motivation to maintain a healthy and safe lifestyle, it is important that the

---

Box 8.7　Occupational performance and medication.

As an occupational therapist it is important to appreciate what medication an individual takes, when and how often because of the impact on occupational performance. It is important to consider the following:

- Can the older person get a regular supply of their medication?
- Can the older person understand and be able to take the medication as required?
- Can they open the medicine bottle, dosette box or blister pack?
- Is the medication 'doing the job' required?
- Has the older person had their regular review of medication (every six months for 4+ medications, annually for 1–3) and by whom?

Consider Mrs Wright (from Chapter 5) and the role of medication in the 'on-off' phenomena she experiences and how it affects her occupational performance. What are the issues for Mrs Wright? How and why might the OT be involved?

occupational therapist can enable and facilitate their older clients to look after their own health (see Box 8.7). It is also important to understand what older people perceive as being in good health so that they can be supported to make healthy lifestyle choices. Miller and Iris (2002) investigated the perspectives of 45 older adults via focus groups and questionnaires. They wanted to know what the participants thought about health and well-being. The themes emerging suggested aspects of health in older age: 'functional independence, self-care management of illness, positive outlook, and personal growth and social contribution'. Health was much more than the absence of disease. Meaningful occupation was recognised as promoting health, and the authors recommended that health promotion programmes expand to consider aspects beyond exercise and diet.

Domestic life areas

Home is the setting for domestic and daily life and the base from which the wider community and social networks are experienced (as described in Chapter 3). The ICF classifies domestic life as including:

> "…acquiring a place to live, food, clothing and other necessities, household cleaning and repairing, caring for personal and other household objects, and assisting others."
> (WHO 2001)

The majority of older people wish to age in familiar surroundings, with known social connections and resources (Cook et al. 2007). Peel et al. (2007) observed that those older participants who had lived in their home for longer than five years had greater psychosocial resources to draw upon. Successive governments have long accepted the importance of older people remaining in their own home for as long as possible, known internationally as 'ageing in place' (Sixsmith and Sixsmith 2008). The home environment may have defined areas: privacy for self-care activities, refuge for rest and communal spaces for socialising.

Occupational therapy involvement in an older person's home environment is usually through the provision of assistive technology, adaptation to the physical environment or recommendation for formal carers to enable the older person to live at home safely, and these are discussed further in Chapter 9. It is worth considering that these interventions focus on the home as a house or a building. It is therefore important that we consider what the home environment means and provides for the older person if we are going to facilitate and enable them to successfully age in place. For many older people, home reinforces their sense of identity, autonomy, provides memories and links with family and friends through the objects within it and symbolises independence, freedom and security (Dahlin-Ivanoff et al. 2007, Haak et al. 2007). Therefore, home is a functional place that facilitates belief in their own capacity, everyday routines and habits, provides challenges and opportunity to take risks and the place where they can make choices and govern their daily life. Moreover, provision of assistive technology, removal of treasured objects and provision of care within the home can be viewed as a sign of reduced competence, loss of autonomy and freedom in daily routines (Dahlin-Ivanoff et al. 2007, Haak et al. 2007) and threaten the emotional attachment to home. It is therefore important that when assessing an older person's occupations for successful ageing in place, we must consider how we can enable an older person to continue to govern their daily life and maintain their autonomy in a well-designed home that is fit for purpose.

Acquisition of goods and services

Older people can be entitled to an overwhelming array of public services and benefits, and both the service and eligibility criteria can change at an alarming rate. Inadequate services can lead to exclusion, forcing dependence and therefore disability onto many older people. Many older people use their local shops to acquire their food and household shopping, services to carry out financial transactions and maintenance of their home and community centres for participation in social events. Changes to the local environment can impact on the older person's ability to age successfully by reducing feelings of self-efficacy and independence. Changes such as closure of local shops and services as well as limited public transportation are obvious factors for creating a shrinking world for older people. Less obvious changes, such as merchandise being inappropriate to the older person's needs, unfamiliar out-of-town shopping centres as well as supermarkets with large shop floors, can lead an older person to feel insecure, fatigued and ignored. Although the increasingly popular use of the internet amongst older people (see Chapter 9) has meant that older people have greater access to information and services, this discriminates against those older people who are not computer literate and also reduces opportunities for social interaction in the local community.

Household tasks

Preparation of meals

Nutritional requirements change as people age and an inadequate intake of food and fluid is associated with diverse symptoms. These issues have already been discussed and it is important for the occupational therapist to consider what is being consumed as well as how it is consumed. A home-based assessment is a good opportunity to explore what routines for eating and drinking are established. Many routines and habits associated with meal preparation are culturally determined or reflect a particular problem-solving strategy (Gibbs and Barnitt 1999).

In meal preparation, there are many ways of grading the complexity, which should always reflect what might realistically be expected or achieved on a long-term basis. The longer a meal takes to prepare, the more complex the preparation will be and the more demands it places on the person preparing it.

Both Creek (1996) and Fair and Barnitt (1999) have studied the activity of making a cup of tea in more detail, establishing the complexity, cultural, regional and generational differences that need to be considered in an assessment that occupational therapists carry out on a regular basis. Creek (1996) suggests that occupational therapists should concentrate on the process of tea-making rather than the outcome, and this principle can be applied to many everyday activities, such as dressing, where the task is complex and requires interplay between body functions and structures with personal and environmental contexts for successful completion. By considering the process of carrying out the activity, problem areas can be observed and analysed so that problems with successful completion can be identified, or possible future problems prevented.

Caring for household objects

Occupational therapy assessment will rarely involve direct observation of all these elements of housework, and a client-centred approach will highlight what is a priority. Impairment of body function could impact on the housework required: for example, incontinence and/or feeding difficulties could result in extra laundry and the need to change bedding daily. Movement disorders might create difficulties in cleaning and using household appliances: for example, manoeuvring a vacuum cleaner or operating controls on cookers and disposing of rubbish (Sirkka and Bränholm 2003), changing lightbulbs or tending to a prized garden.

Caring and assisting others

This section considers the role of older people in caring for others. As already discussed in other sections of this chapter, many older people are involved in assisting others, usually their spouse. This section particularly considers the positives and negatives of caring for family or friends. It is not fully known how many people are informal carers for others. Many people see the care they give as an extension of their role of spouse, partner, parent, sibling or friend, and would therefore not consider themselves as a carer. Other people do not explicitly acknowledge themselves as a carer because of the perceived stigma of the health condition of, or relationship with, the care-recipient (Department of Health 2010, Knochel et al. 2011).

There are many definitions and concepts of caring. Even recent surveys organised by the UK government have different definitions (see Box 8.8).

Examination of the UK Census (2001) data identified that 10% of the UK population are carers (5.9 million) (Dahlberg et al. 2007). It had also been identified from the English Longitudinal Survey of Ageing (ELSA) in 2002, that 10% of the population over age 52 are carers, 39% of whom care for their spouse and 34% care for their parents/in-laws (Ross et al. 2008, Vlachantoni 2010).

As previously stated, carer burden is experienced by older carers and this can be considered in terms of subjective burden (carer feelings, attitudes and emotional reactions) or objective burden (concrete events, physical care) (Morgan and Laing 1991). It is said that

---

Box 8.8   Definitions of caring.

- Providing active support to another in the preceding week of the survey (Hyde and Janevic 2004)
- Provide unpaid care for family members, neighbours, or others who are sick, disabled or elderly (Office of National Statistics 2006)

80% of spouse-carers of older people with dementia experience carer burden (Etters et al. 2007). From the ELSA, Ross et al. (2008) identified that care-recipients' health, independence in personal activities of daily living and experience of pain did not seem to impact on the spouse-carer's quality of life, but there were significant correlations between the care-recipients' reduced independence in instrumental activities of daily living (mainly community living and integration) and memory function, on the spouse-carers' quality of life. Often care burden is not associated with the care-recipient but with the availability of social support (Zarit et al. 1980). The research literature indicates differing experiences of caring between the genders and also for spouses and children of older care-recipients. However, many older people have positive experiences, with research by Graham and Bassett (2006) revealing the empowering and enabling nature of caring for the carer. Many older spouse-carers perceive caring as an extension of their marital role and relationship: husband carers of older people with dementia try to maintain their past lives as couples, with wife-carers trying to protect their husband with dementia from recognising their deterioration (Perry and O'Connor 2002).

There are many international policies and guidelines that relate to carers and the principles within these documents relate to respect for the carer's human rights, dignity, security, health and wellbeing. Box 8.9 provides details of the UK and Australian carer strategies.

Box 8.9   Carer strategies from Australia and the UK.

Australian Government (2011) *National Carer Strategy*. Commonwealth of Australia, Productivity Commission. Accessed 20/07/2012 at http://www.fahcsia.gov.au/sites/default/files/documents/06_2012/national_carer_strategy.pdf

Department of Health (2010) *Recognised, Valued and Supported: Next steps for the Carers' Strategy*. London: Department of Health. Accessed 20/07/012 at: http://www.dh.gov.uk/prod_consum_dh/groups/dh_digitalassets/@dh/@en/documents/digitalasset/dh_122393.pdf

---

Interpersonal relationships

The WHO (2001) considers interpersonal relationships to involve basic and complex interactions with family, friends, lovers and strangers in a socially and contextually appropriate way. In this section, relationships with partners are discussed, with formal relationships discussed earlier as part of communication, and relationships with friends discussed in Chapter 3.

The WHO (2002a) suggests that there are several ageist myths about older people: one is that older people are asexual and another is that they are heterosexual. Intimate relationships are not always addressed or considered in occupational therapy practice, particularly sexual relationships between older people. Although there are changes in sexual functions with ageing, these do not exclude older people from being sexually active or from having intimate relationships. Amongst health care professionals, sexuality is assumed not to be a priority for older people, and consequently this does not get discussed. In care home settings particularly, health care staff face the dilemma of ensuring a person's human rights are not breached, but also that vulnerable individuals are protected. Environmental issues of shared and public places and limited privacy in care homes create difficulties for those residents who wish to have intimate relationships with others (Royal College of Nursing 2011).

It is also important not to assume that lesbian, gay, bisexual or transgender (LGBT) older people have the same needs and requirements as heterosexual older people (Knochel et al. 2010). Although there are some similar challenges for older people in LGBT relationships as for heterosexual couples, there are also differences. Lack of legal recognition of the relationship means that access to benefits, pensions or services can be restricted (Age UK 2010). Fear of discrimination and stigmatisation also means that older LGBT carers are less likely to seek help either from their family of origin, from the community or residential care services (Age Concern 2010, Hughes et al. 2011, Knochel et al. 2011). Surveys by Hughes et al. (2011) and Knochel et al. (2011) in the USA identified that local services were often not meeting the needs of LGBT older people or acknowledging that they needed to be addressed. There is also some evidence of ageist attitudes within the LGBT community itself, which leads to a lack of support for older people seeking help (Heaphy 2007, Hughes et al. 2011).

Acknowledgement and understanding of the sexual relationship and orientation of older people are crucial for successful ageing. Many organisations provide good practice guidelines for professionals to ensure that these important aspects and relationships in older peoples lives are not ignored (see Box 8.10). For a practising occupational therapist these provide useful resources that can ensure occupational justice prevails.

The emotional relationship between couples and family members is an important factor to consider when working with older people, especially those who are more frail and dependent in everyday activities. The desire to work within a client-centred framework can inadvertently lead to the needs of the referred individual being considered in isolation rather than in the context of their relationships with partners and families. However, there are many expectations of spouses/partners and families to care, monitor and supervise an older person when their everyday functioning and independence decline. There is an increasing awareness that the needs of the couple need to be considered in intervention and service provision because of their interdependence, especially when the carer is older and has their own health problems (McIntyre and Reynolds 2012). Indeed, the Australian national carer strategy explicitly highlights that caring occurs as an interrelationship between the carer and the care-recipient. This strategy suggests that, even though needs

---

Box 8.10   Guidance for professionals on intimate relationships of older people.

Age Concern (2002) Good practice guidance: Opening doors: working with older lesbians and gay men. Accessed 18/07/2012 at: http://www.ageuk.org.uk/documents/en-gb/for-professionals/equality-and-human-rights/gpg115_opening_doors_working_with_older_lesbians_and_gay_men_2001_pro.pdf?dtrk=true

Royal College of Nursing 2007 Older people in care homes: sex, sexuality and intimate relationships. A RCN discussion and guidance document for the nursing workforce. Accessed 18/07/2012 http://www.rcn.org.uk/__data/assets/pdf_file/0011/399323/004136.pdf

of individuals should be addressed, it is important to understand that the needs of either member of the relationship can change because of their interdependence on each other and changing life circumstances (Australian Government 2011). Understanding of 'couplehood' (as described by Kaplan 2001, and Hellström et al. 2005) enables the therapist to understand the mutual support and needs of older couples.

Education, work and employment

The concepts of education, work and employment fit with the occupational performance term 'productivity'. Although the older population may be perceived to have retired from employment and completed their education, a demographic shift towards an older population, anti-discriminative legislation and current financial constraints mean that older people are working for longer. There is also an increasing recognition and emphasis on lifelong learning. The social capital of older people is increasingly realised. Older workers are seen to be more collaborative, motivated and have valued accrued knowledge and experience. For the older worker themselves there is evidence of improved cognitive functions (Biggs et al. 2012). However, the working environment appears more hostile for older manual workers, as they are perceived to be slower, have lower physical fitness and lack of experience in new techniques (Gibb 2008).

Lifelong learning takes many forms and it has to be considered that many older people who remain in the workplace require training in new skills and techniques. In many instances there is an assumption that older people are unable to learn new skills (Biggs et al. 2012); however, as can be seen in earlier chapters and the section on tasks and demands, an older person is able to learn new skills and information, but may require different strategies for successful learning to take place.

A study by Withnall and Thompson (2003) established that older people are interested in a wide range of learning opportunities for self-satisfaction, intellectual stimulation and enjoyment. Whereas some older people choose more formal routes such as university or further education classes, others participate in the University of the Third Age (U3A). The U3A started in France in 1973 specifically to meet the needs of older learners, and this concept has been adopted worldwide. In most of Europe, U3A groups are associated with universities, althoughin the UK, the U3A groups are organised by members. More recently, an online U3A has been developed to enable those more isolated older people to study, network and access resources.

Many older people remain in productive roles after their retirement through volunteering, with approximately 40% of people aged 75 and under having a regular commitment as a volunteer. Volunteering is perceived to be more beneficial than other forms of social engagement as it increases role enhancement, self-esteem, self-efficacy and social networks. However, it is unclear whether volunteering contributes to successful ageing by increasing self-perception of health and functioning through better coping strategies and psychosocial resources or through actual reduction in mortality and morbidity (Lum and Lightfoot 2005, Wahrendorf et al. 2006). These studies also identify that commitment to volunteering declines in older people aged 75+, with McMunn et al. (2009) indicating that associated factors for ceasing voluntary work were ill-health and financial circumstances.

A study by Tang et al. (2010) found that, in the USA, remaining as a volunteer was determined by the level of support and training given by the organisation, the length and regularity of the commitment by the individual, and their income and health (especially mental health). It would seem that better training and support would not only enable the older person to continue as a volunteer and maintain self-esteem, quality of life and social networks, but also provide the organisation with a valuable resource. The opportunity to take up other voluntary roles rather than drop this activity as the person becomes older is also of relevance, as older people do not necessarily have to drop activities but perhaps swap them for similar ones such as advocated by Atchley's continuity theory (1971). The implications for such changes can, however, be that older people reduce their social networks so that they are at more risk of poorer quality of life, health and wellbeing (Silverstein and Parker 2002).

Community, social and civic life

The WHO (2001) considers community participation to be involvement in organised social events outside of the family. This concept overlaps with volunteering in local organisations and charities already discussed in the previous section. Other aspects of community life are considered here, namely recreation and leisure, religion and spirituality, political life and citizenship.

Recreation and leisure

Older people's participation in recreation and leisure activities has received increasing attention in research, because of the strengthening association with successful ageing (and therefore primary health promotion) through better cognitive and physical health and quality of life. One could argue that an older person who pursues their own meaningful leisure and recreational activities has no need of occupational therapy; however, the well elderly studies by Clark et al. (1997, 2001, 2011) discussed in Chapter 2 demonstrate the power of occupation-focused programmes in primary heath promotion for well older people. In the UK this has informed the NICE guidance for occupational therapy to improve the mental wellbeing of older people (NICE 2008).

The role of leisure activities in contributing to successful ageing has also been explored, with a study by Glass et al. (1999) identifying that social activities such as visits to the cinema or playing cards, bingo, board games and productive activity (shopping, preparing meals, and gardening) conferred equal survival advantages as physical activity. These researchers hypothesised that it is not only physical activities that influence mortality but also those activities with little or no physical exertion as they may have psychosocial and physiological benefits (i.e. reduction of stress and impact on immune response). Activities such as crossword puzzles, reading, board games, playing musical instruments and dancing were also associated with a lower risk in cognitive impairment and dementia. Frequency of these activities was also significant; those carrying out these leisure activities four times per week were 47% less at risk of dementia than those carrying out their activities once a week (Verghese et al. 2003).

Other aspects of activities have been considered for their contribution to successful ageing, with Fisher and Specht (1999), Menec (2003), Maier and Klumb (2005) and Litwin and Shiovitz-Ezra (2006) concluding that, whereas social and productive activities infer benefits such as longevity and independence in functioning, solitary and creative activities have psychological benefits such as problem solving, self-efficacy and a sense of engagement and satisfaction in life. Participants in the studies by Reynolds (2009) and Tzanidaki and Reynolds (2011) also expressed a sense of continuity through taking up their arts and crafts in older life.

The relevance of social engagement in older age has been explored in Chapter 3, and has been considered the link between activity and successful ageing. Evidence from several studies suggest that engagement in social activity such as volunteering, dancing or bingo indicates the presence of social networks for an individual that can provide support, reciprocal connection with the community and others, as well as providing a sense of purpose and self-esteem (Bassuk et al. 1999, Mendes de Leon 2005, Litwin and Shiovitz-Ezra 2006). It is suggested that such self esteem is also associated with active engagement in better health care practices such as smoking cessation and uptake of immunisation and therefore social engagement is a crucial part of public health care policy for older people.

It is also pertinent to consider potential gender differences in the role of leisure activities in successful ageing. Agahi and Parker (2008) suggest that, although men and women benefit from participating in leisure activities such as reading, cultural visits, gardening, dancing, singing and other hobbies, women benefit more, with significantly lower mortality rates. It was also found that older women benefit from leisure activities that involve social engagement, whereas men benefit more from solitary hobbies or gardening. It could be said that solitary and social leisure activities have differing performance demands and involve different body functions and structures. Whereas the use of group activity is widely accepted (and perhaps currently more prevalent), the importance of solitary activity for successful ageing should not be overlooked.

Civic and political life

The involvement of older people in community and civic life fits within the WHO Active Ageing policy (WHO 2002a). In the UK, there has been a push for public services to be fit for purpose and therefore meet the needs of their service users. As older people are the largest group to use health and social care services they have often been involved in service development, commissioning and evaluation. However, their involvement has been patchy and with mixed success. Scourfield and Burch (2010) suggest that the involvement of older people has ranged from tokenism to consultation. However few service consultation and commissioning processes have been older people-led or involved them in decision-making, which Arnstein (1969) advocated as true participation in civic life. Scourfield and Burch (2010) and Wistow et al. (2011) suggest that current involvement of older people in service development and commission is a well-intentioned attempt at civic participation but is potentially ill-informed, unprepared and therefore possibly more harmful to older people's autonomy and sense of engagement.

In the UK and the USA, where voting is optional, more older people vote in political elections than other age groups. However, it could be argued whether the political parties and process meet their needs or address their issues (Binstock 2010). In the UK, although older people are more likely to vote, their participation in political activity is declining. Postle et al. (2006) suggest that there are implicit barriers to political activity, such as the timing, cost and venue of meetings, especially for those with transportation difficulties and caring roles. In other instances, it is observed that there has been a lack of representation of older people on local committees and working parties where decisions are made. Other barriers to political activity seem to be attitudinal, in that older people felt that political parties were disengaged and undemocratic. It would seem that older people felt more able to have more involvement at a local level through local forums and through member organisations such as Age UK or AARP in the USA (Postle et al. 2006).

It would seem that to involve older people in civic and political life to uphold social justice requires political parties and public services to consider how best to facilitate older people's participation by removing environmental and attitudinal barriers as well as considering issues such as levels of fatigue, attention, co-morbidities and other responsibilities and demands. Such consideration would enable older people to contribute greater social capital and enable their own successful ageing.

Religion and spirituality by Lesley Wilson

The terms 'religion' and 'spirituality' are often bracketed together, as indeed they are by the ICF. However, they are by no means synonymous. Religion is concerned with a recognised set of beliefs, values and behaviours within a formal framework, usually in connection with devotion to a God. Spirituality is experienced as being less formal and more concerned with personal interpretations of life and the inner experience. This inner experience can of course also encompass religion, and although the two terms are not always interchangeable, they can be inclusive of each other. There is some evidence that older people in particular are quite comfortable with combining these concepts (Ortiz and Langer 2002).

The definition of terms continues to be a challenge, both in practice and in the wider literature (Wilson, 2010) and this is reflected in the ongoing uncertainty amongst occupational therapists about how to address spiritual matters with their clients (Udell and Chandler 2000, Belcham 2004).

Occupational therapists value the spiritual dimension of occupation and also acknowledge the importance of spirituality as part of their holistic, client-centred approach. However, much of the literature on this topic is nearly 20 years old and has come from North America (e.g. Egan and Delaat 1994, 1997, Christiansen 1997, Enquist et al. 1997). More recent studies in the UK have highlighted spirituality in relation to particular client groups (e.g. Feeney and Toth-Cohen 2008), including older people (Bursell and Mayers 2010) but on the whole these studies are still small in scale and numbers.

The ICF (WHO 2001) focuses on the activities associated with religious and spiritual practice, such as going to places of worship or praying and chanting. Studies have shown that those older people with strong religious convictions have higher levels of life satisfaction, and are more likely to be at ease with their personal past and the prospect of death (Ayele et al. 1999, Coleman et al. 2002). In particular, spiritual care comes to the fore at the end of life and in the hospice setting but is still less conspicuous in the everyday care of older people despite recent government initiatives to bring spiritual care into its end of life care strategy (Department of Health 2008).

In the health domain, spirituality and religion have traditionally been seen to be the responsibility of the hospital chaplain, although the medical profession and occupational therapists, amongst others, have also acknowledged the value of a belief system and the ability to draw on inner resources as part of the healing process.

From a practical perspective, occupational therapists can assist older people in carrying out the occupations associated with their spiritual needs in many ways. Some examples include ensuring access to places of worship, including transport and ramped wheelchair entrances, by recommending or designing comfortable seats and even suggesting larger and clearer print for songsheets or religious texts. Many churches are now fitted with loop systems to enhance hearing, which community occupational therapists can recommend if appropriate.

Spiritual leaders are also willing to visit people in their own homes or in a residential setting and it may fall to the occupational therapist to arrange this if the need is not identified by others in the care team. Additionally, occupational therapists may become involved in running groups to meet the spiritual needs of older people as part of a team approach as described in Box 8.11.

Box 8.11

An example of the occupational therapist and chaplain working together is described by Bryant and Law (1990). A teamwork project was set up to meet the spiritual needs of elderly mentally ill people in hospital. Weekly services were conducted in the hospital chapel and themes were identified and presented to reflect the liturgical and seasonal patterns of the year. In this way, the spiritual side of the patients' lives, which is often ignored in institutional settings, was acknowledged and nourished. Interestingly, the team also looked after its own spiritual needs by having a day away once a year. This aspect of looking after oneself in order to care for others is often overlooked in healthcare practice.

Summary

This chapter has considered the nine domains within activity and participation, as conceptualised by the WHO (2001). It focuses on older peoples' 'doing' and 'being', discussing how both the ageing body and contextual factors can either facilitate or hamper occupational justice and successful ageing. Although this chapter has not instructed the reader in particular interventions, it is hoped that further tools and information are provided to support and enable clinical reasoning. It is also hoped that the chapter reveals different dimensions of an older person's experience so that their potential can be fulfilled in intervention.

References

Agahi, N. and Parker, M.G. (2008) Leisure activities and mortality: Does gender matter? *Journal of Ageing and Health* **20**, 855–871.

Age Concern (2002) Good practice guidance: Opening doors: Working with older lesbians and gay men. Accessed 20/06/2012 http://www.ageuk.org.uk/documents/en-gb/for-professionals/equality-and-human-rights/gpg115_opening_doors_working_with_older_lesbians_and_gay_men_2001_pro.pdf?dtrk=true

Age Concern (2010) *Hungry to be Heard: The scandal of malnourished older people in hospital.* London: Age Concern.

Allen, C.K., Earhart, C.A. and Blue, T. (1992) *Occupational Therapy Treatment Goals for the Physically and Cognitively Disabled.* Bethesda, MD: The American Occupational Therapy Association Inc.

Alzheimer's Society (2000) *Maintaining Skills: An advice sheet for carers.* London: Alzheimer's Society.

American Occupational Therapy Association (2002) Occupational therapy practice framework: Domain and process. *American Journal of Occupational Therapy* **56(6)**, 609–639.

American Occupational Therapy Association (2008) Occupational Therapy Practice Framework: Domain and process, 2nd edition *American Journal of Occupational Therapy* **62(6)**, 25–683.

Ardalan, A., Mazaheri, M., Naieni, K.H., Rezaie, M., Teimoori, F. and Pourmalek, F. (2010) Older peoples' needs following major disasters: A qualitative study of Iranian elders' experiences of the Bam earthquake. *Ageing and Society* **30(1)**, 11–24.

Arnstein, S.R .(1969) A ladder of citizen participation. *Journal of the American Institute of Planners* **35(4)**, 216–224.

Ashfield, T.A., Syddall, H.E., Martin, H.J., Dennison, E.M., Cooper, C. and Aihie Sayer, A. (2010) Grip strength and cardiovascular drug use in older people: Findings from the Hertfordshire Cohort study. *Age and Ageing* **39**, 185–191.

Atchley, R.C. (1971) Retirement and leisure participation: Continuity or crisis? *The Gerontologist* **11**, 13–17.

Australian Government (2011) *National Carer Strategy.* Commonwealth of Australia, Productivity Commission.

Ayele, H., Mulligan, T., Gheorghiu, S. and Reyes-Ortiz, C. (1999) Religious activity improves life satisfaction for some physicians and older patients. *Journal of the American Geriatric Society* **47(4)**, 453–455.

Baker, K.L. and Robertson, N. (2008) Coping with caring for someone with dementia: Reviewing the literature about men. *Aging & Mental Health* **12(4)**, 413–422.

Bassuk, S.S., Glass, T.A. and Berkman, L.F. (1999) Social disengagement and incident cognitive decline in community dwelling elderly persons. *Annals of Internal Medicine* **131(3)**, 165–173.

Belcham, C. (2004) Spirituality in occupational therapy: Theory in practice? *British Journal of Occupational Therapy* **67(1)**, 39–46.

Bellelli, G., Lucchi, E. and Cipriani, G. (2002) Executive dysfunction and depressive symptoms in cerebrovascular disease (letter). *Journal of Neurology, Neurosurgery and Psychiatry* **73(4)**, 460–464.

Biggs, S., Carstensen, L. and Hogan, P. (2012) Social capital, lifelong learning and social innovation. In: Beard, J., Biggs, S., Bloom, D., Fried, L., Hogan, P., Kalache, A. and Olshanky, J. (eds) (on behalf of the World Economic Forum) *Global Population Ageing: Peril or promise?* Geneva: World Economic Forum Global Agenda Council on Ageing Society, pp. 39–41.

Binstock, R.H. (2010) From compassionate ageism to intergenerational conflict? *The Gerontologist* **50(5)**, 574–585.

Bloem, B.R., Grimbergen, Y.A.M, van Dijk, J.G. and Munneke, M. (2006) The "posture second" strategy: A review of wrong priorities in Parkinson's disease. *Journal of the Neurological Sciences* **248**, 196–204.

Bootsma-van der Wiel, A., Gussekloo, J., de Craen, A.J.M., van Exel, E., Knook, D.L., Lagaay, A.M. and Westendorp, R.G.J. (2001) Disability in the oldest-old: Can do or "do do"? *Journal of the American Geriatrics Society* **49(7)**, 909–914.

Bowen, A., Wenman, R., Mickelborough, J., Foster, J., Hill, E. and Tallis, R. (2001) Dual task effects of talking while walking on velocity and balance following a stroke. *Age and Ageing* **30(4)**, 319–323.

Bravell, M.E., Zarit, S.H. and Johansson, B. (2011) Self-reported activities of daily living and performance-based functional ability: A study of congruence amongst the oldest-old. *European Journal of Ageing* **8**, 199–209.

British Geriatrics Society (2002) *Standards of Care for Specialist Services for Older People.* London: British Geriatrics Society.

Bryant, W. and Law, M. (1990) A spiritual lift from a world of confusion. *Therapy Weekly* February 1.

Bullington, J. (2006) Body and self: A phenomenological study on the ageing body and identity. *Journal of Medical Ethics* **32**, 25–31.

Burns, S.L., Leese, G.P. and McMurdo, M.E.T. (2002) Older people and ill fitting shoes. *Postgraduate Medicine Journal* **78(3)**, 344–346.

Bursell, J. and Mayers, C.A. (2010) Spirituality within dementia care: Perceptions of health professionals. *British Journal of Occupational Therapy* **73(4)**, 144–151.

Burton, C.L., Strauss, E., Hulstch, D.F. and Hunter, M.A. (2007) Cognitive functioning and everyday problem solving in older adults. *The Clinical Neuropsychologist* **20(3)**, 432–452.

Cahn-Wiener, D.A., Malloy, P.F., Boyle, P.A., Marran, M. and Salloway, S. (2000) Prediction of functional status from neuropsychological tests in community-dwelling elderly individuals. *The Clinical Neuropsychologist* **14(2)**, 187–195.

Carlson, M.C., Fried, L.P., Xue, Q.-L., Bandeen-Roche, K., Zeger, S.L. and Brandt, J. (1999) Association between executive attention and physical functional performance in community-dwelling older women. *Journal of Gerontology: Social Sciences* **54B(5)**, S262–S270.

Carmeli, E., Patish, H. and Coleman, R. (2003) The aging hand. *Journal of Gerontology: Medical Sciences* **58A(2)**, 146–152.

Christiansen, C. (1997) Acknowledging a spiritual dimension in occupational therapy practice. *American Journal of Occupational Therapy* **51(3)**, 169–180.

Christiansen, C.H. and Baum, C. (1997) Understanding occupation: Definition and concepts. In: Christiansen, C.H. and Baum, C. (eds) *Enabling Function and Well-Being*, 2nd ed. New Jersey: Slack Inc.

Clark, F., Azen, S.P., Zemke, R., Jackson, J., Carlson, M., Mandel, D., Hay, J., Josephson, K., Cherry, B., Hessel, C., Palmer, J., and Lipson, L. (1997) Occupational therapy for independent-living older adults: A randomised controlled trial. *Journal of the American Medical Association* **278(16)**, 1321–1326.

Clark, F., Azen, S.P., Carlson, M., Mandel, D., LaBree, L., Hay, J., Zemke, R., Jackson, J. and Lipson, L. (2001) Embedding health-promoting changes into the daily lives of independent-living older adults: Long-term follow-up of occupational therapy intervention. *Journals of Gerontology Series B Psychological and Social Sciences* **56(1)**, P60–63

Clark, F., Jackson, J., Carlson, M., Chou, C.P., Cherry, B.J., Jordan-Marsh, M., Knight, B.G., Mandel, D., Blanchard, J., Grander, D.A., Wilcox, R.R., Lai, M.Y., White, B., Hay, J., Lam, C., Marterella, A. and Azen S.P. (2011) Effectiveness of a lifestyle intervention in promoting the well-being of independently living older people: Results of the Well Elderly 2 Randomised Controlled Trial. *Journal of Epidemiology Community Health*, doi: 10.1136/jech.2009.099754

Clarke, L. (2009) Improving nutrition in dementia through menu picture cards and cooking activities. Nursing Times.net

Coleman, P., McKieran, F., Mills, M. and Speck, P. (2002) Spiritual belief and quality of life: The experience of older bereaved spouses. *Quality and Ageing – Policy, Practice and Research* **3(1)**, 20–26.

College of Occupational Therapists (2006) *Falls Management*. London: College of Occupational Therapists.

Cook, C.C., Martin, P., Yeams, M. and Damhorst, M.L. (2007) Attachment to "place" and coping with losses in changed communities: A paradox for ageing adults. *Family and Consumer Sciences Research Journal* **35(3)**, 201–214.

Crawford, S. and Channon, S. (2002) Dissociation between performance of abstract tests of executive functioning and problem solving in real-life-type situations in normal aging. *Aging and Mental Health* **6(1)**, 12–21.

Creek, J. (1996) Making a cup of tea as an honours degree subject. *British Journal of Occupational Therapy* **59(3)**, 128–130.

Creek, J. (2003) *Occupational Therapy Defined as a Complex Intervention*. London: College of Occupational Therapists.

Dahlberg, L., Demack, S. and Bambra, C. (2007) Age and gender of informal carers: A population-based study in the UK. *Health and Social Care in the Community* **5**, 439–445.

Dahlin-Ivanoff, S., Haak, M., Fänge, A. and Iwarsson, S. (2007) The multiple meaning of home experienced by very old Swedish people. *Scandinavian Journal of Occupational Therapy* **14**, 25–32.

Department of Health (2000) *The Health Survey for England (HSE)*. London: HMSO.

Department of Health (2001) *National Service Framework for Older People*. London: Department of Health.

Department of Health (2008) *End of Life Care Strategy*. London: HMSO.

Department of Health (2010) *Recognised, Valued and Supported: Next steps for the Carers Strategy*. London: Department of Health.

Department of Health and Human Services (2008) *Physical Activity Guidelines Advisory Committee Report*. Washington, DC: US Department of Health and Human Services http://www.health.gov/paguidelines/pdf/paguide.pdf

Department of Health, Physical Activity, Health Improvement and Protection (2011) *Start Active, Stay Active: A report on physical activity from the four home countries' Chief Medical Officers*. http://www.dh.gov.uk/prod_consum_dh/groups/dh_digitalassets/documents/digitalasset/dh_128210.pdf

Desrosiers, J., Hebert, R., Bravo, G. and Dutil, E. (1995) Shoulder range motion of healthy elderly people: A normative study. *Physical and Occupational Therapy in Geriatrics* **13(1/2)**, 101–128.

Desrosiers, J., Hebert, R., Bravo, G. and Rochette, A. (1999) Age-related changes in upper extremity performance of elderly people: A longitudinal study. *Experimental Gerontology* **34(3)**, 393–405.

Egan, M. and Delaat, D. (1994) Considering spirituality in occupational therapy practice. *Canadian Journal of Occupational Therapy* **61(2)**, 95–101.

Egan, M. and Delaat, D. (1997) The implicit spirituality of occupational therapy practice. *Canadian Journal of Occupational Therapy* **64(1)**, 115–121.

Enquist, D., Short-DeGraff, M., Gliner, J. and Oltjenbruns, K. (1997) Occupational therapists' beliefs and practices with regard to spirituality and therapy. *American Journal of Occupational Therapy* **51(3)**, 173–180.

Etters, L., Goodall, D. and Harrison, B. (2007) Caregiver burden among dementia patient caregivers: A review of the literature. *Journal of the American Academy of Nurse Practitioners* **20** 423–428.

European Nutrition for Health Alliance (2005) *Malnutrition within an Ageing Population: A call to action*. London: European Nutrition for Health Alliance,

Eyres, L. and Unsworth, C. (2005) Occupational therapy in acute hospitals: The effectiveness of a pilot program to maintain occupational performance in older clients. *Australian Occupational Therapy Journal* **52**, 218–224.

Fair, A. and Barnitt, R. (1999) Making a cup of tea as part of a culturally sensitive service. *British Journal of Occupational Therapy* **62(5)**, 199–205.

Federal Interagency Forum on Aging-related Statistics (2010) *Older Americans 2010: Key indicators of well-being*. Washington DC: Federal Interagency Forum on Aging-related Statistics.

Feeney, L. and Toth-Cohen, S. (2008) Addressing spirituality for clients with physical disabilities. *OT Practice* **13(4)**, 16–18, 20.

Fisher, A.G. (1995) *The Assessment of Motor and Process Skills*. Colorado: Three Star Press.

Fisher, B.J. and Specht, D.K. (1999) Successful aging and creativity in later life. *Journal of Aging Studies* **13(4)**, 457–472.

Fricke, J. and Unsworth, C. (2001) Time use and importance of instrumental activities of daily living. *Australian Journal of Occupational Therapy* **48(3)**, 118–131.

Gibb, A. (2008) *Understanding the older worker in construction*. Report to Ageing Research Going Places. Strategic Promotion of Aging Research Capacity.

Gibbs, K.E. and Barnitt, R. (1999) Occupational therapy and the self-care needs of Hindu elders. *British Journal of Occupational Therapy* **62(3)**, 100–106.

Glass, T.A., de Leon, C.M., Marottoli, R.A. and Berkman, L.F. (1999) Population based study of social and productive activities as predictors of survival among elderly Americans. *BMJ* **319**, 478–483.

Gooch, H. (2003) Assessment of bathing in occupational therapy. *British Journal of Occupational Therapy* **66(9)**, 402–408.

Gooptu, C. and Mulley, G.P. (1994) Survey of elderly people who get stuck in the bath. *BMJ* **308**, 762.

Grady, C.L. (2008) Cognitive neuroscience of aging. *Annals of New York Academy of Science* **1124**, 127–144.

Graham, J.E. and Bassett, R. (2006) Reciprocal relations: The recognition and co-construction of caring with Alzheimer's disease. *Journal of Aging Studies* **20**, 335–349.

Haak, M., Fänge, A., Iwarsson, S. and Dahlin-Ivanoff, S. (2007) Home as a signification of independence and autonomy: Experiences among very old Swedish people. *Scandinavian Journal of Occupational Therapy* **14**, 16–24.

Haggard, P., Cockburn, J., Cock, J., Fordham, C. and Wade, D. (2000) Interference between gait and cognitive tasks in a rehabilitating neurological population. *Journal of Neurology, Neurosurgery and Psychiatry* **69(4)**, 479–486.

Häggblom-Kronlöf, G., Hultberg, J., Eriksson, B.G. and Sonn, U. (2007) Experiences of daily occupations at 99 years of age. *Scandinavian Journal of Occupational Therapy* **14(3)**, 192–200.

Hardy, S. and Grogan, S. (2009) Preventing disability through exercise: Investigating older adults' influences and motivations to engage in physical activity. *Journal of Health Psychology* **14(7)**, 1036–1046.

Harvey, A.S. and Pentland, W. (2003) What do people do? In: Christiansen, C.H. and Townsend, E.A. (eds) *Introduction to Occupation: The Art and Science of Living*. New Jersey: Prentice Hall.

Harwood, D.M.J., Hawton, K., Hope, T. and Jacoby, R. (2000) Suicide in older people: Mode of death, demographic factors, and medical contact before death. *International Journal of Geriatric Psychiatry* **15**, 736–743.

Harwood, D.M.J., Hawton, K., Hope, T., Harriss, L. and Jacoby, R. (2006) Life problems and physical illness as risk factors for suicide in older people: A descriptive and case-control study. *Psychological Medicine* **36**, 1265–1274.

Hasher, L., Stoltzfus, E.R. Zacks, R.T. and Rypma, B. (1991) Age and inhibition. *Journal of Experimental Psychology: Learning, Memory and Cognition* **17(1)**, 163–169.

Hayase, D., Mosenteen, D., Thimmaiah, D., Zemke, S., Atler, K. and Fisher, A.G. (2004) Age-related changes in activities of daily living ability. *Australian Occupational Therapy Journal* **51**, 192–198.

Hauer, K., Pfisterer, M., Weber, C., Wezler, N., Kliegel, M. and Oster, P. (2003) Cognitive impairment decreases postural control during dual tasks in geriatric patients with a history of severe falls. *Journal of the American Geriatric Society* **5(11)**, 1638–1644.

Heaphy, B. (2007) Sexualities, gender and ageing: Resources and social change. *Current Sociology* **55(2)**, 193–210.

Hellström, I., Nolan, M. and Lundh, U. (2005) "We do things together": A case study of "couple-hood" in dementia. *Dementia* **4(7)**, 7–22.

Hemphill-Pearson, B.J. (2008) *Assessments in Occupational Therapy Mental Health: An integrative approach*. Thorofare: Slack Inc.

Hickson, M. (2006) Malnutrition and ageing. *Postgraduate Medical Journal* **82**, 2–8.

Howse, K., Ebrahim, S. and Gooberman-Hill, R. (2005) Help-avoidance: Why older people do not always seek help. *Reviews in Clinical Gerontology* **14**, 63–70.

Hughes, A.K., Harold, R.D. and Boyer, J.M. (2011) Awareness of LGBT ageing issues among aging service network providers. *Journal of Gerontological Social Work* **54**, 659–677.

Hyde, M. and Janevic, M. (2004) Social activity. In: Marmot, M., Banks, J., Blundell, R., Lessof, C. and Nazroo, J. (eds) *English Longitudinal Study of Ageing: Health, wealth and lifestyles of the older population in England: The 2002 English Longitudinal Study of Ageing*. London: Institute for Fiscal Studies, pp. 167–179.

Iezzoni, L.I., McCarthy, E.P., Davis, R.B. and Siebens, H. (2001) Mobility difficulties are not only a problem of old age. *Journal of General Internal Medicine* **16(4)**, 235–243.

Jacobsson, C., Axelsson, K., Österlind, P.O. and Norberg, A. (2000) How people with stroke and healthy older people experience the eating process. *Journal of Clinical Nursing* **9**, 255–264.

Kaplan, L. (2001) A couplehood typology for spouses of institutionalised persons with Alzheimer's disease: Perceptions of "We" – "I". *Family Relations* **50(1)**, 87–98.

Knoblauch, R.L., Pietrucha, M.T. and Nitzburg, M. (1996) Field studies of pedestrian walking speed and start-up time. *Transportation Research Record* 1538. U.S. Department of Transportation.

Knochel, K.A., Quam, J.K. and Croghan, C.F. (2011) Are old lesbian and gay people well served? Understanding the perceptions, preparartion and experiences of aging services providers. *Journal of Applied Gerontology* **30(3)**, 370–389.

Landa-Gonzalez, B. and Molnar, M. (2012) Occupational therapy intervention: Effects on self-care, performance, satisfaction, self-esteem/self-efficacy, and role functioning of older Hispanic females with arthritis. *Occupational Therapy in Health Care* **26(2–3)**, 109–119.

Laver Fawcett, A. (2007) *Principles of Assessment and Outcome Measurement for Occupational Therapists and Physiotherapists: Theory, skills and application*. Chichester: John Wiley & Sons.

Law, M., Baum, C. and Dunn, W. (2005) (eds) *Measuring Occupational Performance: Supporting best practice in occupational therapy*. 2nd edition..Thorofare, NJ: Slack.

Litwin, H. and Shiovitz-Ezra, S. (2006) The association between activity and wellbeing in later life: What really matters? *Ageing and Society* **26**, 225–242.

Lord, S.R., Murray, S.M., Chapman, K., Munro, B. and Tiedemann, A. (2002) Sit-to-stand performance depends on sensation, speed, balance and psychological status in addition to strength in older people. *The Journal of Geronontology: Series A* **57(8)**, M539–M543.

Lum, T.Y. and Lightfoot, E. (2005) The effects of volunteering on the physical and mental health of older people. *Research on Aging* **27**, 31–55.

Lundin-Olsson, L., Nyberg, L. and Gustafson, Y. (1997) "Stops walking when talking" as a predictor of falls in elderly people. *Lancet* **349**, 617.

Maier, H. and Klumb, P.L. (2005) Social participation and survival at older ages: Is the effect driven by activity content or context? *European Journal of Ageing* **2**, 31–39.

Manson, J.E., Greenland, P., LaCroix, A.Z., Stefanick, M.L., Mouton, C.P., Oberman, A., Perri, M.G., Sheps, D.S., Pettinger, M.B. and Siscovick, D.S. (2002) Walking compared with vigorous exercise for the prevention of cardiovascular events in women. *New England Journal of Medicine* **347(10)**, 716–725.

Mather, A.S., Rodriguez, C., Guthrie, M.F., McHarg, A.M., Reid, I.C. and McMurdo, M.E.T. (2002) Effects of exercise on depressive symptoms in older adults with poorly responsive depressive disorder. *British Journal of Psychiatry* **180**, 411–415.

Mattingley, C. and Fleming, M.H. (1994) *Clinical Reasoning*. Thorofare: Slack.

McCarter, R.J. and Kelly, N.G. (1993) Cellular basis of ageing in skeletal muscle. In: Coe, R.M. and Perry, H.M. (eds) *Ageing, Musculoskeletal Disorders and Care of the Frail Elderly*. New York: Springer.

McIlroy, W.E. and Maki, B.E. (1994) Compensatory arm movements evoked by transient perturbations of upright stance. In: Taguchi, K., Igarashi, M. and Mori, S. (eds) *Vestibular and Neural Front*. New York: Elsevier Science.

McIntyre, A. and Reynolds, F. (2012) There's no apprenticeship for Alzheimer's: The caring relationship when an older person experiencing dementia falls. *Ageing and Society* **32(5)**, 873–896.

McMunn, A., Nazroo, J., Wahrendorf, M., Breeze, E. and Zaninotto, P. (2009) Participation in socially-productive activities, reciprocity and wellbeing in later life: Baseline results in England. *Ageing and Society* **29(5)**, 765–782.

Mendes de Leon, C.F. (2005) Social engagement and successful aging. *European Journal of Ageing* **2**, 64–66.

Menec, V.H. (2003) The relationship between everyday activities and successful ageing: A 6-year longitudinal study. *Journal of Gerontology, Series B, Psychological Sciences and Social Sciences*, **58**, 74–82.

Miller, A.M. and Iris, M. (2002) Health promotion attitudes and strategies in older adults. *Health Education and Behaviour* **29(2)**, 249–267.

Milton, J.C., Hill-Smith, I. and Jackson, S.H.D. (2008) Prescribing for older people. *BMJ* **336**, 606–09.

Morgan, D.G. and Laing, G.P. (1991) The diagnosis of Alzheimer's disease: Spouses' perspectives. *Qualitative Health Research* **1(3)**, 370–377.

Muhaidat, M., Skelton, D., Kerr, A., Evans, J. and Ballinger, C. (2010) Older adults' experiences and perceptions of dual tasking. *British Journal of Occupational Therapy* **73(9)**, 405–412.

NHS Information Centre (2009) *Health Survey for England 2008 Physical Activity and Fitness: Summary of key findings*. London: NHS Information Centre.

NICE (2008) NICE public health guidance 16: Occupational therapy interventions and physical activity interventions to promote the mental wellbeing of older people in primary care and residential care. London: NICE.

Oakley, F., Dura,n L., Fisher, A. and Merritt, B. (2003) Differences in activities of daily living motor skills of persons with and without Alzheimer's disease. *Australian Occupational Therapy Journal* **50(2)**, 72–78.

O'Brien, L., Bynon, S., Morarty, J. and Presnell, S. (2012) Improving older trauma patients' outcomes through targeted occupational therapy and functional conditioning. *American Journal of Occupational Therapy* **66**, 431–437.

Office for National Statistics (2002) *Living in Britain: Results from the 2001 general household survey*. London: Office for National Statistics.

Ortiz, L.P.A. and Langer, N. (2002) Assessment of spirituality and religion in later life: Acknowledging clients' needs and personal resources. *Journal of Gerontological Social Work* **37(2)**, 5–21.

Peel, N.M., McClure, R.J. and Hendrikz, J.K. (2007) Psychosocial factors associated with fall-related hip fracture. *Age and Ageing* **36**, 145–151.

Penninx, B.W., Messier, S.P., Rejeski, W.J., Williamson, J.D., DiBari, M., Cavazzini, C., Applegate, W.B. and Pahor, M. (2001) Physical exercise and the prevention of disability in activity of daily living in older persons with osteoarthritis. *Archives of Internal Medicine* **161(19)**, 2309–2316.

Perry, J. and O'Connor, D. (2002) Preserving personhood: (Re)Membering the spouse with dementia. *Family Relation* **51(1)**, 55–62.

Pfeiffer, B. (2002) Understanding Older People's Stress. Accessed16/03/2012 at: http://www.outreach.missouri.edu/cmregion/thriving/archives2002/2002%20November/Understanding%20Older%20People's%20Stress.html

Postle, K., Wright, P. and Beresford, P. (2006) Older people's participation in political activity – making their voices heard: A potential support role for welfare professionals in countering ageism and social exclusion. *Practice: Social Work in Action* **17(3)**, 173–189.

Princess Royal Trust for Carers (2011) *Always On Call, Always Concerned: A survey of the experiences of older carers*. Woodford Green: The Princess Royal Trust for Carers.

Ranganathen, V.K., Siemionow, V., Sahgal, V.and Yue, G.H. (2001) Effects of ageing on hand function. *Journal of the American Geriatrics Society* **49 (11)**,1478–1484.

Rantakokko, M., Mänty, M., Iwarsson, S., Törmäkangas, T., Leinonen, R., Heikkinen, E. and Rantanen, T. (2009) Fear of moving outdoors and development of outdoor walking difficulty in older people. *Journal of American Geriatric Society* **57**, 634–640.

Reece, A.C. and Simpson, J.M. (1996) Preparing older people to cope after a fall. *Physiotherapy* **82(4)**, 227–235.

Reed, K.L. and Sanderso, S.N. (1999) *Concepts of Occupational Therapy*, 4th edition. Philadelphia: Lippincott. Williams and Wilkins.

Reynolds, F. (2009) Taking up arts and crafts in later life: A qualitative study of the experiential factors that encourage participation in creative activities. *British Journal of Occupational Therapy* **72(9)**, 393–400.

RoSPA (2002) *Can the Home Ever Be Safe?* Birmingham: Royal Society for the Prevention of Accidents.

Ross, A., Lloyd, J., Weinhardt, M. and Cheshire, H. (2008) *Living and Caring? An investigation of the experiences of older carers*. London: National Centre for Social Research.

Royal College of Nursing (2007) Older people in care homes: Sex, sexuality and intimate relationships. A RCN discussion and guidance document for the nursing workforce. Accessed 18/07/2012 at: http://www.rcn.org.uk/__data/assets/pdf_file/0011/399323/004136.pdf

Samaritans (2011) *Suicide Statistics Report*. London: Samaritans. Accessed 20.05.2012 at: http://www.samaritans.org/pdf/Samaritans%20Suicide%20Statistics%20Report%202011.pdf

Scourfield, P. and Burch, S. (2010) Ethical considerations when involving older people in public service participation processes. *Ethics and Social Welfare* **4(3)**, 236–253.

Sirkka, M. and Bränholm, I.-B. (2003) Consequences of a hip fracture in activity performance and life satisfaction in an elderly Swedish clientele. *Scandinavian Journal of Occupational Therapy* **10**, 34–39.

Shiffman, L.M. (1992) Effects of ageing on adult hand function. *American Journal of Occupational Therapy* **46(9)**, 785–792.

Shumway-Cook, A. and Woollacott, M.H. (2012) *Motor Control: Theory and applications*, 4th edition. Baltimore: Lippincott Williams and Wilkins.

Silverstein, M. and Parker, M.G. (2002) Leisure activities and quality of life among the oldest old in Sweden. *Research on Aging* **24(5)**, 528–547.

Singer, B.R., McLauchlan, G.J., Robinson, C.M. and Christie, J. (1998) Epidemiology of fractures in 15,000 adults: The influence of age and gender. *Journal of Bone and Joint Surgery* **80(2)**, 243–248.

Sixsmith, A. and Sixsmith, J. (2008) Ageing in place in the United Kingdom. *Ageing International* **32**, 219–235.

Tang, F., Morrow-Howell, N. and Choi, E. (2010) Why do older adults stop volunteering? *Ageing and Society* **30(5)**, 859–878.

Tzanidaki, D. and Reynolds, F. (2011) Exploring the meanings of making traditional arts and crafts among older women in Crete using interpretative phenomenological analysis. *British Journal of Occupational Therapy* **74(8)**, 375–382.

Udell, L. and Chandler, C. (2000) The role of the occupational therapist in addressing the spiritual needs of clients. *British Journal of Occupational Therapy* **63(10)**, 489–495.

United Nations (2002) *Building a Society for All Ages: HIV/AIDs and older people.* Accessed 16/03/2004 at:. http://www.un.org/ageing/prkit/hivaids.htm

Unsworth, C. (2000) Measuring the outcome of occupational therapy: Tools and resources. *Australian Journal of Occupational Therapy* **47(4)**, 147–158.

Verghese, J., Buschke, H., Viola, L.. Katz, M., Hall, C., Kuslansky, G. and Lipto,n R. (2002) Validity of divided attention tasks in predicting falls in older individuals: A preliminary study. *Journal of the American Geriatric Society* **50(9)**, 1572–1576.

Verghese, J., Lipton, R.B., Katz, M.J., Hall, C.B., Derby, C.A., Kuslansky, G., Ambrose, A.F., Sliwinski, M. and Buschke, H. (2003) Leisure activities and the risk of dementia in the elderly. *New England Journal of Medicine* **348(25)**, 2508–2516.

Verghese, J., Wang, C., Xue, X. and Holtzer, R. (2008) Self-reported difficulty in climbing up or down stairs in nondisabled elderly. *Archives of Physical Medicine and Rehabilitation* **89(1)**, 100–104.

Vlachantoni, A. (2010) *The Demographic Characteristics and Economic Activity Patterns of Carers over 50: Evidence from the English Longitudinal Study of Ageing. Population Trends (141).* London: Office for National Statistics.

Walker, C.M., Walker M.F. and Sunderland, A. (2003) Dressing after stroke: A survey of current occupational therapy practice. *British Journal of Ovccupational Therapy* **66(6)**, 263–268.

Ward, N.S. and Frackowiak, S.J. (2003) Age-related changes in the neural correlates of motor performance. *Brain* **126(4)**, 873–888.

Wahrendorf, M., von dem Knesebeck, O. and Siegrist, J. (2006) Social productivity and well-being of older people: Baseline results from the SHARE study. *European Journal of Ageing* **3(2)**, 67–73.

Welford, A.T. (1958) *Ageing and Human Skill.* Oxford: Oxford University Press.

Wild, D., Nayak, U.S. and Isaac, B. (1981) How dangerous are falls to older people at home? *BMJ* **282**, 266–268.

Wilson, L. (2010) Spirituality,occupation and occupational therapy revisited: Ongoing consideration of the issues for occupational therapists. *British Journal of Occupational Therapy* **73(9)**, 437–440.

Wistow, G., Waddington, E. and Davey, V. (2011) *Involving Older People in Commissioning: More power to their elbow?* London:, Joseph Rowntree Foundation.

Withnall, A. and Thompson, V. (2003) *Older People and Lifelong Learning: Choices and experiences.* Sheffield: ESRC Growing Older Programme.

Woodruff-Pak, D.S. (1997) *The Neuropsychology of Aging.* Malden, USA: Blackwell Publishing.

World Health Organization (2001) *The International Classification of Functioning Disability and Health.* Geneva: World Health Organisation.

World Health Organization (2002a) *Active Ageing. A Policy Framework.* Geneva: World Health Organization.

World Health Organization (2002b) *Physical Activity Through Transport as Part of Daily Activities.* Geneva: World Health Organization Regional Office for Europe.

Yaffe, K., Barnes, D., Nevitt, M., Lui, L. and Covinsky, K. (2001) A prospective study of physical activity and cognitive decline in elderly women. *Archives of Internal Medicine* **161(14)**, 1703–1708.

Yardley, L., Gardner, M., Bronstein, A., Davies, R., Buckwell, D. and Luxon, L. (2001) Interference between postural control and mental task performance in patients with vestibular disorder and healthy controls. *Journal of Neurology, Neurosurgery and Psychiatry* **71(1)**, 48–52.

Yardley, L., Donovan-Hall, M., Francis, K and Todd, C. (2006) Older people's views of advice about falls prevention: A qualitative study. *Health Education Research* **21(4)**, 508–517.

Young, A. and Dinan, S. (1994) ABC of Sports Medicine: Fitness for older people. *BMJ* **309**, 331–334.

Young, A. and Dinan, S. (2005) Activity in later life. *BMJ* **330**, 189.

Zarit, S.H., Reever, K.E. and Bach-Peterson, J. (1980) Relatives of the impaired elderly: Correlates of feelings of burden. *The Gerontologist* **20(6)**, 649–655.

Chapter 9

Environmental impacts, products and technology

Anita Atwal, Sarah Buchanan, Marcus Sivell-Muller, Anthony Slater and Sue Vernon

The ICF (WHO 2001, p. 171) makes a significant step in emphasising that loss of independence is not only related to bodily functions but also environmental factors. The term 'environmental factor' is used to describe factors that 'make up the physical, social and attitudinal environment, in which people live and conduct their lives'. Environmental factors can interact with a health condition to either create a disability and/or restore functioning, depending on whether the environmental factor can be regarded as a facilitator or a barrier. Consequently, disability can no longer be regarded as a feature of the individual, but rather as the outcome of an interaction of the person with a health condition and the environmental factors. This in turn has meant that the recognition of the central role played by environmental factors has changed the locus of the problem and, hence, focuses of intervention, from the individual to the environment in which the individual lives (Schneidert et al. 2003). In many of the case studies in Chapter 5, environmental barriers prevent participation in valued activities. For example, Mrs Smith with coronary heart disease is unable to play bridge as she can no longer climb the stairs.

Factors such as the social and attitudinal environment have been considered in Chapters 3 and 4. In this chapter other, more physical, environmental factors are discussed. These are:

- Transport and driving
- Assistive technology and home modification
- Natural events and those caused by humans.

Environmental factors place large and important restrictions on the amount to which older adults can fully participate in society. Occupational therapists need to focus on educating members of the public, architects and builders on ways to overcome barriers that prevent older people participating in their chosen activities. Outdoor environments can be particularly challenging. A study by White et al. (2010) considered the features of the neighbourhood environment and their association with disability in older adults. These researchers found that parks and walking areas, disabled parking, and accessible public transport were all important features of the local environment for older adults with existing functional limitations, not only for general physical activity but for recreational and social activity as well. Some narratives outlining how the environment impacts upon

Occupational Therapy and Older People, Second Edition. Edited by Anita Atwal and Anne McIntyre.
© 2013 Blackwell Publishing Ltd. Published 2013 by Blackwell Publishing Ltd.

Box 9.1   Narratives outlining importance of environment on social occupations for persons with polio and post-polio syndrome.

'I think I've stopped socialising in the villages much. I'm only in a little village and I can't get into my head using the scooter in the village and the little village hall is just too far to walk there and to walk back.'

   'Mobility and access meant unable to attend child's schools, concerts, parents' night, etc; unable to carry the job I trained for, due parking restrictions with loss of access to clients, suppliers, trade fairs. Denied access to jury service due to parking limitations, and court refused to reserve disabled parking space or cover taxi fare. Very limited social life.'

   'The difficulties of getting around, especially into friends/family homes, is making me feel isolated and depressed.'

---

a person's occupations and wellbeing are outlined in Box 9.1. These narratives are from people with polio and post-polio syndrome

Transport and Driving – Sue Vernon

Being able to mobilise within the community is important for maintaining social relationships and independence. In Chapter 3, Mrs Jameson is unable to get out of her house and therefore has difficulty seeing other people. A literature review published by the UK Department of Transport (Dunbar et al. 2004) found that older people aged 70+ make more journeys on foot even in rural areas. Mobilising on foot, however, can result in injuries for older adults, for example due to uneven paving stones which might result in falls. It is a dangerous way to travel, resulting in the high number of accidents and deaths in older adults (Dunbar et al. 2004).

   Older adults do utilise public transport; however, there are many barriers to using public transport which are outlined in Box 9.2. Access to transport is important for maintaining social relationships and independence (Gilhooly et al. 2003). Therefore, occupational therapists have an important role in enabling older people to use transport and to instigate wellbeing opportunities such as security and safety, and environmental issues. This might include giving advice on methods of transport both for well older people and those older people who have experienced a change in their functional ability.

   The National Travel Survey (1996–1998) found that the single factor most affecting travel by older people is access to a car (both as a driver and as a passenger). Driving is an occupation that contributes to engagement in other areas of occupation such as social and leisure occupations (Stav et al. 2011). The ability to drive also fosters a sense of control over one's life because of the convenience, flexibility, and spontaneity associated with driving (Gardezi et al. 2006). It is not possible to use licence-holding statistics to determine exactly how many drivers are over a certain age, because having a driving licence does not mean one is still driving. Many people stop driving but keep their licence updated for identification purposes. Nevertheless, population demographics and longer life expectancy are increasing the number of older drivers on our roads. By 2035, the number of people aged 85 and over is projected to be almost 2.5 times larger than in 2010, reaching 3.5 million and accounting for 5% of the total population (Office for National Statistics 2011).

Box 9.2   Barriers to using public transport.

- Personal security – especially at night
- Risk of falls on moving transport
- Carrying heavy loads (e.g. shopping)
- Unreliable services
- Isolated stops with a long distance between them
- Poor lighting in waiting areas
- Cost of travel
- Difficulty boarding and alighting from vehicles
- Confusion over use and access to information

For the older driver, using the car continues to be very enabling as personal mobility declines and confidence to try new things, such as using public transport, lessens. Unfortunately, at the same time it becomes more likely that health reasons will make it to necessary to retire from driving. Such a change of lifestyle at this time can be difficult to accept and adjust to. Even when personal mobility remains good, it is not easy to accommodate to being without a car. During a brief spontaneous interview with a fit and mobile ex-driver in her 80s, her initial thoughts about the negative aspects included:

- Inconvenience – 'You have to plan journeys. It was easier when the car was sat outside waiting for you to use at any time'
- Difficulty getting to local parks, certain shopping areas, visiting friends and family and attending concerts
- Some places are not accessible by bus.

She listed some positive aspects of not having a car:

- Not having the worry or the responsibility of looking after a car
- Driving conditions are stressful these days because other drivers are impatient
- More economical using public transport and or a taxi.

However, retiring from driving brings its inevitable losses, grieving and adjustment as described since it is an unwelcome reminder of deteriorating abilities and increasing age (Whitehead et al. 2006). Occupational therapists therefore may want to provide information such provision of information resources, practical journey planning and community mobility projects, which would help in the adjustment for those retiring from driving.

Fitness to drive

In some countries, specific guidance and regulations about fitness to drive are available. However, there is often uncertainty about which professionals should give give advice on fitness to drive. Encouragingly, in the UK, just over 90% of occupational therapists agreed or strongly agreed it was very important to discuss fitness to drive with their patients, and just over 80% felt it fell within their role to do so (Hawley 2010). Occupational therapists should not be misled into thinking an ordinary driving instructor or road safety expert can test their patients' driving ability. There is a need for specialist driver assessment and rehabilitation services, as ordinary driving instructors have limited knowledge of the functional implications of injuries and diseases (Unsworth 2007). In order to evaluate the on-road findings correctly, a pre-drive investigation of physical, cognitive, visual and reaction time aspects should be carried out using evidence-based tests and methods. This should be followed by an on-road evaluation designed to test for the effects of any identified clinical deficits. Each element must inform the other in order to come to a correct analysis and conclusion. These assessments are usually carried out in accredited assessment centres, which can be expensive. There is therefore a case for all occupational therapists to offer their patients knowledgeable advice and to use a degree of clinical screening so that only relevant referrals are made.

Driving and occupational therapy

Driving is an important domain for occupational therapy (Korner-Bitensky et al. 2010). Occupational therapists' knowledge of physical and cognitive assessment and rehabilitation skills form an ideal basis on which to build specific expertise for focusing on this important everyday activity. As well as assessing and advising when referral for expert driving assessment might be prudent, an occupational therapist's holistic and enabling approach means they can also facilitate planning for and activation of the decision to retire from driving. Occupational therapists face difficult ethical situations if they notify relevant organisations that an older adult needs an assessment without their consent. For example, in the UK, the College of Occupational Therapists recommends that occupational therapists do not directly report their concerns but should ask a medical practitioner to do so (College of Occupational Therapists 2012).

However, occupational therapists can:

- Provide advice to a driver
  - By ensuring all patients know the requirements of each country's driving agency
  - By providing a resource of general information on driving relevant to medical conditions, and details of driving assessments available at mobility centres
  - For the latter stages of a driving career, while driving skills remain intact, general advice as listed can help maintain mobility for as long as possible
- Maintain safe driving for the relatively fit, active older driver:
  - Assisting older people in making the correct vehicle choice, including high seat, low doorsill with minimal rubber seal to catch one's feet against
  - Other suggestions might include changing to automatic transmission to make the driving task easier before managing changes becomes a problem
  - The therapist should select as many safety-assist options as is economically viable, such as reversing sensors
  - The therapist should recommend that the older adult seeks advice on simple assistive adaptations such as panoramic rear view mirror for a driver with an arthritic neck who is unable to make direct 360 degree observations since normal mirrors alone do not cover blind spots.

Clinical screening

Screening should cover all skills required for driving, not just cognition. In listing cognitive tests the results of which correlate with driving ability. Table 9.1 outlines tests which

Table 9.1 Tests which could be used to assist clinical screening in driving.

Aspect to screen	Elements	Example tool	Evaluation
Physical	Range, power, coordination, sensation, proprioception, pain	Any approved clinical method. OT-DORA	Expert evaluation of function in relation to use of controls and adaptation options is required if deficits are found
Visual	Acuity, fields, phoria, depth, low light vision, contrast sensitivity, susceptibility to glare	Keystone driver vision screener Optec OT-DORA (Information about all three screening tools is available on their websites)	Pass/fail scores on test sheets or check visual standards. In-car evaluation and expert tuition can overcome effects of some deficits that fulfil rules but do affect driving
Cognitive	Visual perception, spatial skills, attention, divided attention, praxis, executive function, comprehension	Rookwood Driving Battery (Mckenna and Bell 2007) OT-DORA	Cutoff scores can identify those who should cease driving and those who should be referred for further expert on-road assessment
Reaction time	Speed of information processing Physical response time	RT-2S brake reaction tester (Information about screening tool is available on website)	Measure against norms for the equipment used. Consistency and speed further complement cognitive and physical findings
Medication	Drowsiness, perceptual/ attitudinal changes	Interview Observation Reaction time test OT-DORA	Check medication packet for warnings of side effects likely to affect driving Record functional concerns likely to relate to medication Obtain referring doctor's opinion

could be used to assist clinical screening. Further information about screening tools can be found on the screening tools websites.

Assessing driver fitness should include the physical, cognitive and visual-perceptual components necessary for safe operation of a motor vehicle (Vrkljan et al. 2011). There are many clinical tests which inform what physical, visual or cognitive deficits an older person might have, but unless the test has been specifically researched for use as a driver screening tool, it is not possible to say how the result correlates with actual on-road performance.

Even though the best test batteries have improving correlations, results should only be used as indicators for when referral for an expert in-car evaluation is prudent. An example set of tests often used in pre-drive screening is listed below, but included also is a new battery, the recently-released OT-DORA (Occupational Therapy Driver Off-Road Assessment). Further information can be found on this website: http://www.drivingotser-vices.com/off-road-assessment.html. However, only an expert in-car evaluation can tell whether the older adult could have compensated for their deficits when actually in the car.

Vision and driving

Older adults should have regular check-ups with an optician. In the UK, the visual acuity standard requires the driver to read a new-style numberplate at 20 metres in good daylight. Regular eye tests every two years (minimum) are important, as eyesight can deteriorate steadily in the older driver without the individual being aware of any deterioration. Spectacles and vehicle windows should be kept clean.

Drivers with developing cataracts should test their ability to read a numberplate much more frequently because, as they develop towards the point that surgery can be considered, acuity often reduces to less than the legal limit and a short time off driving is required. Driving at night is a situation best avoided due to oncoming vehicle headlight glare and glare from low winter sun in the day. If visual deficits of any kind have been found with a driver vision-screening tool the occupational therapist should make a referral for more a expert review by an optical specialist. It may also be helpful to seek advice from a driving centre concerning a practical driving assessment to check compensatory ability for visual deficits such as squints and monocular vision, which fulfil the rules but can still affect driving.

Cognition

It is not yet possible to clinically screen with sufficiently high accuracy to predict safe driving because of all the factors involved in the task and the speed and complexity of processing required in the real driving situation. The need for a practical on-road evaluation is necessary in all but the most obviously impaired cases because pre-drive screening does not show whether a driver can compensate for the cognitive deficit found. It might appear controversial to suggest that even top scoring subjects indicating lack of cognitive impairment should also have a practical in-car review, but this is because, compared to clinical table top tests, there is far greater cognitive loading in the real driving environment. Physical control of the vehicle plus the visual world moving at speed and attention on stimuli being presented in the 360 degree environment all have to be processed. The results of cognitive tests should only be used as a guide and used in conjunction with clinical reasoning and information from all available sources. Moreover, an appreciation of the prognosis (especially in a deteriorating condition), of the patient's level of insight, ability to self-monitor, risk awareness and sense of public responsibility which places other road users' safety on the same level of importance as his own personal goals should also inform screening.

Reaction time

Reaction time can be measured against norms for the equipment being used, but should also be evaluated alongside other clinical findings because it can be affected by speed of information processing and/or physical function. Psychological and attitudinal factors also sometimes contribute.

Products and assistive technology – Anita Atwal

The provision of the right and timely assistive technology (AT) is in the centre of enabling and maintaining independence and quality of life. There is evidence that the use of devices increases with age and that women use more equipment than men (Giltin et al. 2006). Occupational therapists are in the unique position that they are the only professionals with expertise in occupation but also in the environment, assistive technology and older people. The Canadian Association of Occupational Therapists (2006) strongly advocates that occupational therapists need to enable clients to select, educate and use assistive technology to support their occupational performance. The ICF defines assistive products and technology as 'product, instrument, equipment or technology adapted or specially designed for improving the functioning of a disabled person' (WHO 2001). This definition therefore incorporates a broad and diverse range of products from simple devices such as grab rails to sophisticated video surveillance products.

The scope for assistive devices is vast and complex. Successful use of AT has been found to reduce mortality rates (Gitlin et al. 2006), functional decline (Mann et al. 1999, Wilson et al. 2009) and increase self-efficacy (Sanford et al. 2006). In addition, there is evidence that the right prescription of assistive devices could have cost-saving implications for health and social care providers (Goodacre et al. 2008). Nevertheless, despite the reported benefits, there are barriers to ensuring that AT is successfully adopted and used. One barrier relates to access to AT, since not all groups have access to professionals such as occupational therapists who can advise on assistive devices. In the UK, a primary reason for limited access is the small number of occupational therapists working within social services departments who traditionally assess, prescribe and advise on AT (Mountain 2000). In England, occupational therapists make up 2% of the social services workforce but they have to deal with approximately 35% of all referrals (Riley et al. 2008), resulting in long waiting lists. These delays can impact negatively upon a person's health and wellbeing and in dissatisfaction and concern from users (Audit Commission 2004). Waiting times could be reduced if the occupational therapists' skills were used more effectively and others were able to assess for provision of minor equipment, particularly since delays in AT provision are associated with minor equipment such as grab rails. Therefore, in England, as part of the personalisation agenda, older adults will have the opportunity to self-assess for assistive technology. In addition, other professionals who are trusted assessors will also have access to minor assistive technology (Winchcombe and Ballinger 2005).

The second barrier relates to equipment abandonment, since approximately one-third of all provided assistive devices are abandoned (Scherer and Galvin 1996). Equipment abandonment is associated with a number of factors, including knowledge about the device, involvement in the process of selecting the device, attitude towards the technology and lack of fit of the assistive devise between service users and their environment (Phillips and Zhao 1993, Gitlin 1995, Wielandt and Strong 2000, Martin et al. 2012). Occupational therapists need to encompass assessing people's 'readiness' to use equipment as well as other environmental assessments they conduct. Assistive technology might also be associated with identity threats, or the dehumanisation and anonymity of care, since it could be argued that assistive technology focuses primarily on physical rather than psychosocial needs. A study by Petersson et al. (2012) also highlights that older people's own perceptions of the safety of AT and home modifications are important factors in their acceptance, as well as the perceived abilty of these to enable autonomy and independence. Threats to identity and autonomy also emerged from an earlier study of older people who had fallen, who perceived home safety checks as intrusive and patronising, resenting modifications and AT provision made without their own agreement or consultation (Simpson et al. 2003). Consequently, before occupational therapists make any type of changes to an older person's environment, they need to consider carefully why modifications are being made, and the needs and perceptions of the older person. A person-environment fit is therefore essential. Table 9.2 outlines issues which an occupational therapist should consider when considering assistive technology such as telecare, for an older adult.

Table 9.2   Points to consider when prescribing assistive technology (Adapted from Care Services Improvement Partnership, Health and Social Care Change Agent Team, 2005).

Does the person understand what the telecare is supposed to do?
Have they been given a full explanation of the options?
Have they agreed that they would like to try telecare?
Have their closest family and friends been involved in these discussions?
Have you considered how you will balance any tension or conflict between the rights and risks of all parties involved?
Have you a suitable assessment tool to identify need?
Have you planned how to introduce telecare to the person?
Have you planned how the telecare will be installed?
How will you review its usefulness?
Have you a decommissioning plan?
Have you a protocol for the use of telecare?

Categories of assistive technology

Assistive technology can be categorised into three groups. These are supportive technology, detection and reaction, and prediction and intervention (Doughty 2004).

Supportive technology

More traditional products and assistive technology, such as those for mobility, are assessed and provided to older people on a daily basis. Mobility problems in older people can be very restrictive in their performance of everyday occupations. These are evidenced within the case studies in Chapter 5. Mobility performance is dependent upon the context in which these occupations are carried out and how supportive the environment is to successful accomplishment. The use of walking products has been scrutinised by many researchers, because of reported non-use of equipment when issued to older people (Edwards and Jones 1998). It is therefore important to not only consider the impairment the client has, or may have in the future, but also their attitude and safety awareness and the environmental context, as well as the advantages and disadvantages of the various types of equipment. Provision of walking products has traditionally been considered the domain of physiotherapy colleagues; however, consideration of any walking product within an environmental context is a very relevant part of an occupational therapist's role. An awareness of the appropriateness of the product issued within the client's context is important and an understanding of the correct and safest method of usage is crucial.

The use of mobility products such as walking sticks and wheelchairs can compensate for impairment or lack of confidence, promoting independence in occupational performance through activity and participation. Over 28% of older adults use a mobility aid, with the usage increasing with age (Office of National Statistics 2002). Walking sticks are used most often (25% of all older people), with walking frames being used by 4–9% of older individuals and another 4–14% using wheelchairs (Edwards and Jones 1998, Iezzoni et al. 2001, Office of National Statistics 2002). Walking products such as sticks and frames provide useful support for those with balance problems or to redistribute weight through the upper limbs for those with lower limb muscle weakness or pain, and are most commonly used by those with musculoskeletal problems (Iezzoni et al. 2001). The use of a walking stick, crutch, quadrapod, rollator or walking frame increases stability in standing and walking, maintaining an individual's centre of gravity within an enlarged base of support. However, successful use is dependent on adequate upper limb strength and control as well as dynamic standing balance (see Chapter 6).

Occupational therapists are often involved in the assessment and provision of wheelchairs. In Chapter 5, Mr Clark requires a wheelchair to mobilise for long distances outdoors. Wheelchair design, construction and provision have been greatly influenced over the past few years by the new technologies, lighter weight materials, improvements in medical science, socio-political changes, demands and expectations of users and an increasingly ageing population. Whereas the largest group of older users have arthritis and musculoskeletal problems, the largest group of younger adults are those with neurological problems (Ham et al. 1998). In the UK, both manual and electrically-powered indoor/outdoor chairs (EPIOCs) are issued to those individuals with mobility problems. However, eligibility criteria for provision will vary from area to area. The setting of national minimum standards for wheelchair provision ensures that there should be no discrimination against clients on basis of age (National Wheelchair Managers Forum 2010). Older wheelchair users can be considered as belonging to three groups – the permanent, fulltime user who needs alternative means of mobility at all times, the part-time user (for example, outdoor use only) and the temporary user (post-operative) – and their needs and level of provision will differ. Exploration of the older person's perception and expectation of a wheelchair as part of the assessment and prescription process is essential, as wheelchairs are often perceived by many older people prior to provision as an easy means of independent outdoor transport. However, a self-propelling manual wheelchair requires 9% more energy expenditure than walking (Ham et al. 1998) and therefore those with energy-restrictive problems may find propelling a wheelchair both fatiguing and disappointing. Good upper limb strength and range of movement are also necessary for independent mobility in a manual wheelchair.

As many users will sit for long periods in their wheelchair, adequate postural support and pressure relief are crucial elements of the assessment process. Other factors for consideration are the client's method of transfer, the environment for use, access, transportation and storage, as well as when and how often the chair will be used. Many carers of older people are partners, family or friends, and might themselves be older, with their own limitations and health problems. It is therefore crucial that carers' needs also are taken into account when considering the ease of opening and folding, the weight of the wheelchair and the occupant for pushing and also lifting into a car for transportation. Maintenance and safety issues of the wheelchair, its accessories and pressure-relieving cushions, are highly important and the ability of the client or carer to take responsibility for these also needs to be assessed. The needs of the carer are also important.

Box 9.3   Using assistive technology with older adults.

Consider an older person you know and consider how assistive technology could facilitate participation in activities of daily living.

Read through the case studies in Chapter 5: would assistive technology enhance functional intendance and quality of life? What additional factors would need to be considered?

Electrically-powered chairs tend to be provided to those individuals with relatively severe physical disability. As with uses of manual wheelchairs, cognitive and perceptual problems need to be addressed to ensure safe and accurate maneuvering of the more powerful and heavier wheelchair. Regular maintenance and storage of these powered chairs is even more of an issue, so that the battery is recharged adequately in the appropriate surroundings. For many people, electrically-powered outdoor chairs enable independent participation in social and routine activities (such as shopping), thus maintaining quality of life (Brandt et al. 2004). Risk assessment is very important for both the safety of the individual and other members of the public, and maintenance, and storage issues should also be considered before purchase. Other forms of supportive technology are discussed in Box 9.4.

Box 9.4   Memory supportive technology.

Electronic calendars and/or speaking clocks are examples of simple assistive technology that can help with managing short-term memory loss. Other useful items developed by the Bath Institute of Medical Engineering (www.bath.ac.uk/bime/projects.htm) are locators for lost objects. Another useful devise is a remote day planner. A carer or a relative can write the day's appointments/events via the internet (www.ihagen.no/english.htm). An automated medicine reminder is a device that is programmed to give a bleep when it is time to take the medicine (http://www.pharmacell.se/englishk.html).

Detection and reaction technologies

Detection and reaction technologies are particularly useful devices for people with short-term memory difficulties such as Maureen and Darragh (see Chapter 5). These include devices such as gas detectors, flood detectors, smoke alarms and shut-off valves, and pressure-activated systems that enable a bath or sink to be filled only to a specific level. From our own clinical experience, one of the most challenging features is the risk that an older person might leave their gas cooker on. The current options available to occupational therapists are to remove the gas cooker, recommend the use of a hot meal delivery service (known as 'meals on wheels' in the UK), educate the client how to use a microwave, or recommend that the client moves into a residential home. However, assistive technology enables the therapist to install a cooker usage monitor, which will shut off the gas to the cooker if, for example, the saucepan is overheating. This can enable the client to maintain their independence and carry on performing occupations that have meaning and purpose. Other useful devises include lights that come on automatically when a person leaves the room, and sensors to detect intruders.

Prediction and intervention

The use of telecare in the home can facilitate independent living and occupational therapists must be familiar with the increasing amount of technology that is available to users. Telecare can only be used where there are sufficient carers or care support available to respond quickly when an alarm is raised. There continues to be a debate about the ethical issues regarding the use of telecare devices for persons within the home. However, it is essential that in all instances the consent of the person is obtained and ethical guidance is outlined (see Box 9.5; adapted from Mackenzie 2007, Wey 2007, Department of Health 2007b). Many of the case studies within Chapter 5 have discussed falling as part of their story.

Box 9.5   Ethical considerations when prescribing telecare.

Non-maleficence: Is there a risk that a piece of equipment could lead to more confusion or distress? There is a need for shared understanding of any risks and that these risks are documented (Department of Health 2007b).

Beneficence: How does the assistive technology promote health, wellbeing and quality of life of the person and their carer? Therapists may focus on managing risks resulting in physical harm but less in those relating to emotional harm, e.g. boredom, isolation (Mackenzie 2007).

Autonomy refers to respecting the person's rights to things like self determination, privacy, freedom, and choice. Thus occupational therapists need to ensure that the person is placed at the centre of the assessment process and that their needs, choices and preferences are met by the use of the technology and that these risks are documented. Consideration should also be given to civil liberties and human rights (Mackenzie 2007).

Justice means treating everyone fairly. Thus occupational therapists need to ensure that older adults have equal access to technology and that therapists acknowledge cultural and social differences. In addition, the usual legal considerations of confidentiality and data protection need to be adhered to. Carers' needs should be fully assessed and addressed (Mackenzie 2007).

> **Box 9.6 Telecare to help manage falls for people with dementia.**
>
> Pressure mats placed at the side of a bed or chair can let carers know when someone is up, and they in turn can check to see if the person is using walking aids or requires their assistance.
> Weight sensors or bed monitors can alert a carer that someone is about to rise and they in turn can respond quickly and offer support.
> Infra-red beams can be placed at key points within the bedroom, and will alert a carer when there is movement in the room.

Maureen, who has a learning difficulty and a fractureed neck of femur, could benefit from telecare (Box 9.6) to enable her to live within her own home.

Other supportive ATs include the use of memory devices. Darragh is experiencing short-term memory loss and some of the technology could be useful to help him structure his day and/or to act as a reminder so that a carer might not be needed. Such AT could take the form of wallcharts or alarms, post-it notes, diaries or electronic organisers (Caprani et al. 2006).

Technology and the internet

There are many communication devices which can be of use to older people, for example cordless telephones, memory telephone with a photo or a symbol instead of a number for family and friends, or textphones. Electronic communication devices vary and can be used to convey simple or complex messages. They display or speak words produced by the older person touching a keyboard, screen symbol or picture. There are many devices to help older people to continue to watch television; for example, a home loop system which enables hearing-aid users to hear a sound system without other extraneous sounds, subtitling and captions, personal inductive listening devices, or personal speech amplifiers.

Computers can be modified and/or adapted to interact with and be used by older people. Modification can include alternate keyboards, switches activated by pressure, touch screens, special software, and voice-to-text software. Occupational therapists need to be more aware the role the internet can play in promoting occupation. The internet offers older people an opportunity to access and gain information about a wide range of services including health and social care and access to a wide range of consumer goods, through internet shopping. Computers can be adapted to ensure that all older persons can use them effectively, for example, big keys/high contrast keyboards and screen magnifiers for older people who read large print. Keyboards can also be adapted for use on wheelchairs, or for single-handed use. Voice recognition and word prediction are useful devices for older persons with communication problemsThere is evidence that older adults are using the Internet to keep in touch with family and friends. A survey (ONC 2010) found that a total of 90 per cent of all internet users aged 16–74 who had gone online in the past three months did so to send and receive email. The fact that older adults do not feel socially isolated could lessen feeling of social exclusion. Increasingly, the Internet is being made available by Age UK in day centres, nursing homes, residential care homes and sheltered housing units in England. However it has been suggested that older adults still prefer to visit or phone for information rather than use local authority websites to find out information about services (Hislop 2010). When considering who may want to use the internet, some research has indicated that this may be influenced by the typology of the individual. The first type identified was the non-line outsider who is not generally averse to using the internet, but is hampered by fear and uncertainty. The second type is the "tech skeptic", who is critical of technology and resentful of pressure to become connected. The third type is the cautious toe-dipper, who has tentatively embraced the Internet for basic tasks but it not very adventurous. The fourth type is the digital trail-blazer, who is adventurous (Hannon and Bradwell 2007). The research found that the over 75s were more likely to be non-line outsiders, while 55–65s were more likely to be tech skeptics. Thus occupational therapists should take it account this typology when considering internet use with older adults.

Use of virtual technology within occupational therapy practice

It has been predicted that virtual reality will have an immense impact on the rehabilitation of older people. Virtual reality (VR) is an advanced technology that enables humans to simulate, visualise, interact with and manipulate existing places in the real world or optionally in imaginary worlds. VR has a variety of potential benefits in therapeutic research and process and has shown encouraging results in healthcare and therapeutic processes (Chodos et al. 2010) to train people with disabilities who are using wheelchairs (Schultheis and Rizzo 2001) and in education (Caudell et al. 2003; Stansfield et al. 2005, Weiderhold 2006).

In occupational therapy, VR is already used specifically to facilitate rehabilitation with patients in different settings. For example, Weiss et al. (2004) used VR to train stroke patients to cross the road safely although they encountered various stages of difficulty resembling the real time. Zhang et al. (2003) used VR with people recovering from brain injury to prepare a meal although, like the study by Weiss et al. (2004), it was found that it could not replicate the real-life experience. See Box 9.7 for how VR technology could be used to enhance the home visit process.

Box 9.7   How VR technology could be used to enhance the home visit process.

The 3D interior design software (3DIDS) is one application of VR technology which primarily allows individuals to design or redesign their homes virtually prior to going ahead with these changes in the real world. This technology enables occupational therapists to rapidly create the 3D representation of the patient's home and provides an interactive simulation of the home area which can be easily navigated through in real time. This would enable the client to 'walk' through their home, via a PC or laptop, and could help therapists consider barriers to everyday performance and enhance the client's insight and motivation to participate in tailored interventions. This in turn could enhance performance on a pre-discharge home visit and, possibly, in some cases, eliminate the need for a home visit (Money et al. 2011).

Visual impairment, design and assistive technology – Anthony Slater and Sarah Buchanan

About two million people in the UK have reduced vision that affects their everyday life. Around one in eight people aged over 75, and one in three people aged over 90, have serious sight loss. Less serious sight loss can have a significant effect on daily living. Most people begin to have reduced vision in later life because of normal ageing of the eye or the onset of age-related eye conditions, and the incidence of sight loss increases steeply with age.

An eye test at least once every two years should be part of everyone's health routine. Many causes of sight loss can be prevented or reduced if they are caught early by visiting an optician. The nature and degree of a person's sight loss is related to their eye condition. Few people with sight loss are totally blind. Most have some residual vision and appropriate design can help to maximise their functional vision. While there is not a single solution or response to sight loss, general approaches have been shown to be useful.

Because sight loss is common it is essential that design, management and maintenance of people's homes should address sight loss and take action to make the most of sight. Improvements do not have to involve rebuilding or major refurbishment. There is no need for a lot of money to be spent or for expenditure to be made all at the same time. Small changes, using everyday non-specialist equipment and resources as part of routine maintenance and upgrading, can benefit everyone. Good practice for sight loss will make homes safer, more secure and easier to live in and will support independence. It will help the majority of people, whether or not they have sight loss, and will also help people with other sensory loss. People usually know what they would like to be improved in their home but they may not know how to achieve it or about changes that could make a big difference to their lives. People appreciate information, advice and discussion of alterations that might help them enjoy their home more and make the most of their sight.

Bigger, brighter and bolder

Most people will find things easier to see if they are bigger, brighter and bolder. So, increasing the size of details, improving lighting while avoiding glare, and using colour and contrast to make things stand out from their background can all help. Other sensory cues can be provided, such as tactile or audible information. Clutter should be avoided so that items can be found more easily and spaces navigated more safely. Outdoors, pathways should not be overhung by plants or trees or obstructed by garden or street furniture.

Increasing the size of details makes them more visible. Thus, large-print text is generally easier to read than small print. Using a thicker pen to write notes will increase the size of the lines. Public bodies and utilities will generally supply correspondence in large print if requested. When choosing everyday articles for the home it is worth considering the

---

Box 9.8   An older person's opinions of the importance of light.

'It's a major importance to me that I can live independently and being able to see what I am taking out of cupboards is vital to me – the light makes a big difference.'

size of details. A clock with large numbers will be easier to see. A telephone with bigger buttons is probably easier to use. The larger buttons and larger size electrical switches might also be easier for people with reduced manual dexterity to use. An object can be made to appear larger by bringing it closer or using optical aids such as magnifiers. There are many different types of magnifiers and a specialist low vision practitioner can help to determine the most appropriate one for the particular person and the specific task. General lighting provides background lighting to the room. It enables people to see the size and shape of the room and the main objects within it, helping them to move around safely. General lighting should give a reasonably even illumination within a space, avoiding shadows and dark areas. Lighting levels should be similar in adjacent rooms to avoid adaptation difficulties when moving from bright areas into significantly darker ones or vice versa. General lighting can be provided by electric lighting, usually from ceiling or wall lights, or natural daylight. It is important to consider the light needed for both day and nighttime and to balance electric lighting and natural light.

For all but the smallest rooms, one light source is unlikely to be sufficient and two or more sources at different points in the space will be needed to produce an even spread of general lighting across the whole space. While the ceiling light, usually in the centre of the room, can be augmented by additional fittings located at other points on the ceiling, it may be more practical to add a free standing uplight which will bounce light off the ceiling to light a dark corner. This can be plugged into an existing electrical wall socket and avoids the need for additional wiring. With a small kitchen, it can be difficult to cook as there is limited work surface space and accidents are more likely when the surface space becomes cluttered. Glare creates dazzle which might make it hard to see and light shades will prevent a direct view of the bright electric lamp minimise glare from lights. Vertical blinds prevent glare from windows, by blocking a direct view of the sun while continuing to admit daylight.

Task lighting directs light where it is needed for detailed activities. Even with the best general lighting fitted in your home, the amount of light available could still be inadequate to enable someone to see close-up detailed tasks such as reading, writing, preparing food and continuing with hobbies such as knitting or sewing. Reading in poor or dim lighting will be more difficult and tiring. Increasing the amount of light on the task will make it easier to see and less tiring to do. Task lighting is often provided at short distances, for example one metre or less from the task. A task light 0.5 m from a book will provide 25 times more light than the same light 2.5 m away, e.g. mounted on the ceiling. Task lighting may be provided by a portable task light but fixed lighting can be used too (Box 9.9)

Box 9.9   User perception of improved lighting.

Improvements to lighting over a bathroom mirror meant 'I can now have a wet shave in the bathroom – previously I shaved by the window in the bedroom'.

Improvements to the lighting in one home meant 'it's easier to see a pot on the stove and I can see the handle – so as not to knock it over. I can also now see a cup and fill it from the kettle. I can make a sandwich without cutting my fingers'.

For instance, when preparing food on a kitchen work surface, a person mght obscure direct light from the ceiling light, casting a shadow over the task. The task can be lit by miniature fluorescent lighting mounted under kitchen wall cupboards, behind an opaque pelmet to prevent a direct view of the bright lamp causing glare. This can be powered using an existing electrical socket outlet avoiding the need for changes to fixed wiring. If all the existing sockets are in use, a simple conversion kit can change a single socket outlet to a double outlet or change a double outlet to a triple to provide the extra socket needed.

Fixed-task lighting can also be used in dark cupboards to make it easier to find items. Lighting is particularly helpful in wardrobes, placed over hanging clothes. Miniature fluorescent lamps mounted under a shelf, behind an opaque pelmet, can be controlled by a simple time lapse switch so that it is not left lit inadvertently after use. This can also be powered using an existing electrical socket outlet, avoiding the need for changes to fixed wiring.

It is harder to see an object which is similar in brightness and colour to its background. An object can be made to appear bolder by increasing the contrast between the object and its surroundings. This can be achieved by increasing the difference in brightness between the object and its background or by using different colours for object and background.

Colour contrast is achieved better with contrasting shades of one colour than with different colours in the same shade. Using different colours that are equally dark will not be effective. Contrast can be achieved by using different colours in paint or furnishings and by adding contrast colour strips. Increasing contrast between different room surfaces, such as floor and walls, can make orientation easier. Contrast between a surface and fixtures on that surface, such as sockets, handles or grab rails can make them easier to locate. For example, in a kitchen, good tonal contrast between surfaces, contrast between floor and cupboards can help orientation, contrast between the worktop and the wall behind it helps when placing objects on the worktop, contrast between the wall and the electrical switches and sockets can make them easier to locate, contrasting handles on cupboards, drawers and appliances are also helpful. Coloured stick-on markers can provide both contrast and tactile cues.

Adaptations to improve contrasts around the home can be simple and relatively cheap. Electrical switches are more visible if they contrast with the surrounding wall, perhaps by having a border painted or taped around them. Painting doors or door frames to contrast with adjacent walls will make doorways easier to find and help orientation. A contrasting strip on the front edge of stairs and steps, and between a step and adjacent walls, can reduce trip hazards. This approach can be applied to many everyday activities around the home. Preparing vegetables using a dark chopping board for cutting potatoes but a white one for cutting green vegetables or tomatoes can make the task easier and safer. Shiny objects and materials with a high gloss finish such as glossy wall tiles, worktops or floor coverings can create confusing reflections and glare, and reduce contrast. Matt surfaces, especially in bathrooms and kitchens, aid both orientation and tasks.

Tactile and audible cues

People with reduced vision can benefit from tactile and audible cues. Simple tactile cues can be provided by adding small stick-on markers (known as bump-ons) to indicate particular points, for example the point at which to set a thermostat. They can be applied to handrails to warn of a change of direction or to indicate the floor level in a multistorey building. Labels of different shapes or textures can be used to differentiate between objects. Appliances on which controls give a click at each setting as they are turned enable the user to select the desired setting by counting the appropriate number of clicks. Other useful devices, such as talking clocks and talking microwave cookers, are available. Changes in flooring materials can provide cues to help older adults find their way but must not be potential trip hazards. A change from carpet to hard flooring can be used to indicate a transition from one space into the next, or mark the approach to a potential hazard such as steps.

Home and home visits

Occupational therapists in partnership with other professionals need to ensure that older peoples' housing needs are considered in relationship to positive lifestyle choice. Occupational therapists play an important role in advising and enabling older people to apply for grants to carry out adaptations to their homes. The associations and relationships people have with their homes are varied and complex. It is essential that occupational therapists understand the meaning of home to an individual. This should be discussed prior to commencing any environmental adaption and/or any intervention that is associated with the home. Indeed, therapists need to understand that the home is often inextricably linked with relationships, memories and personal identity. Indeed, our own research into home visits found that some older adults were critical of occupational therapists for not allowing them to say 'hello' to their home, i.e. some people wanted to relax in their own homes before beginning the home visit assessment but time constraints did not allow them to do this (Atwal et al. 2008a). It is suggested, however, that if society adopts a primary health promotion approach to housing (namely the concept of lifetime homes), then home modifications will no longer be needed. Lifestyle homes are designed to meet the flexible and changing needs occurring throughout one's family life and to meet the varying needs of numerous changes of occupier in the same house (Department for Work and Pensions 2008). In the UK, all new housing will be built to these standards by 2013 (Department for Work and Pensions 2008). Investing in lifestyle homes is cost effective as it reduces the need for assistive technology within the home. Lifestyle homes can also incorporate the principles of smart housing. This term is often used to describe the electronic and computer-controlled integration of assistive technology and products in the home during its construction and can also be built into older homes.

Home visits are frequently performed by occupational therapists prior to discharge from hospital. This enables the therapist to ascertain whether the patient's home environment could be modified to promote independence and/or whether assistive technology is needed to promote independence and/or additional support may be needed. When conducting a home visit or an assessment of a person's home environment, we suggest occupational therapists read, reflect upon, and follow our guidelines in Table 9.3. These guidelines have been formulated utilising findings from our own research (Atwal et al. 2008a, b, Atwal et al. 2012). Occupational therapists also need to carefully reason why and when a home visit would occur without an older adult being present.

Table 9.3 Points to consider when conducting a home visit.

All older adults are given information both verbally and non-verbally, explaining in a clear and concise manner why the home visit is needed.
  Older adults and their carers are given time to reflect upon the home visit, and write joint goals with the occupational therapists regarding the aims and purpose of the visit.
  The older adult must be give time to discuss and talk through the home visit process.
  Home visits should not be viewed as a test. Therefore, it is essential that the occupational therapist has clinically reasoned the aims and purpose of the visit.
  The older adult makes a decision with the occupational therapist regarding whom they would like present on the home visit, and also must have suitable outdoor clothing and footwear.
  The home visit should not be time bound but its length must be determined by the goals that have been set by the older adult and the occupational therapists.
  On the home visit, the occupational therapist must allow the person to become familiar with their home environment and allow the person time to relax and feel comfortable in their home environment before the assessment commences.
  After the goals of the home visit have been achieved, the occupational therapist must discuss with the older adult the outcome of the visit.
  The older adult must understand and give their preference and consent to all decisions that are made.
  Occupational therapists need to be aware that some decisions can only be made when the person is at home.
  Occupational therapists need to ensure that at all times the person's views and rights are respected and that they are an integral part of the decision-making process, even if they are deemed not to have capacity.
  Occupational therapists must reflect upon and discuss with senior therapists and other members of the team issues that warrant and need further discussion. It is essential that older adults are not viewed as the problem or the focus of negative perceptions by health care professionals.
  Occupational therapists must take risks in order to facilitate person-centred care.
  Occupational therapists must not be 'risk averse' but risk takers in their practice with older adults.
  Occupational therapists need to balance important issues such as safety and autonomy. Frameworks have been published in the UK (Department of Health 2007b, 2010) to guide clinicians to manage risk in practice.

Occupational therapists need to reflect carefully how information is communicated to older adults and their carers (Table 9.4). A Cochrane Review (Johnson et al. 2003) recommended the use of both verbal and written health information when communicating with patients. A study by Martin et al. (2012) used a web-based questionnaire to see if consumer information and participation in the decision-making process would lead to improved satisfaction and use of AT. This study found a significant relationship between feeling informed and being satisfied with an AT device. Thus, when consumers feel informed, they are more likely to be satisfied. Likewise, a study by Chiu and Man (2004) evaluated whether an additional home training programme for bathing devices would increase the rate of use and satisfaction of AT for older adults who were recovering from a stroke. Prescription and training of bathing devices was conducted with both the control and treatment group in hospital; however' the treatment group received additional home-based training post-discharge. The findings show that the additional training at home led to significantly increased functioning. In addition, it seems that equipment was much more likely to be used if family members were present during training. The inclusion of

Table 9.4   Prompts that might facilitate occupational therapists to reflect upon and manage risks (Source: Atwal et al. 2011b).

What was your role in assessing risks? Was this a difficult process? Did you feel that the risks were managed appropriately? How did you weigh up the risks? Do you feel that the risks were acceptable? If not, why not? Were you given enough support? How did you justify taking the risks? What were you good at? What were you not so good at – why? What did you learn from the experience? How did you feel at the end? Happy, sad? Why? Was the outcome satisfactory for both you as the therapist and the client? What will you do differently next week as a result of your reflections this week? What are your perceptions about the older person's quality of life?

the carer is an integral part of occupational therapy practice but little research has been conducted regarding the involvement of the caregiver (Chen et al. 2000).

We suggest that written as well as verbal information should be given. However, the therapist needs to be mindful of the special needs of older adults when designing information leaflets (see Table 9.5 for further guidance).

Table 9.5   Guidance when preparing information leaflets (See Griffin et al. 2003, Hoffman and Worrall 2004, Marshall and Williams 2006, National Health Service 2007).

• Aim for 5/6 reading level and keep content clear, simple and concise • Involve experts and use good evidence • Provide balanced information and all relevant details • Ensure the information needs of the target audience • Use clients' questions to frame information • Ensure currency by including publication date and regularly reviewing and updating • Use at least 12 point font and restrict upper leading headings to headings and sentence beginnings • Use short paragraphs and discuss important point first • Use dark print on a light background and use adequate spacing between lines • Use bold print to highlight headings • Use short sentences • Use illustrations that are recognisable, clearly labelled, informative and complementary to the text • Involve users in the development and evaluation of the text • Avoid jargon and use non-patronising language • Include a summary section, where bullet points may be helpful • Incorporate features that will actively engage the reader • Use prose, not figures • Experts should be used to endorse the message • Emphasise the positive results of prevention behaviour • Emphasise short-term risks

In summary, assistive technology and products, if prescribed and utilised correctly, can enhance the lives of older adults. Occupational therapists must be aware of and be familiar with technology so that persons with complex needs can be supported at home.

Occupational therapists need to ensure that the assistive technology fits the person, their lifestyle and their home environment. Occupational therapists must ensure that each client is treated as an individual and that the client's concerns are always addressed, respected and acknowledged. Occupational therapists must collaborate with older people, carers, rehabilitation engineers, scientists, housing experts and other health and social care professionals to conduct interprofessional research regarding assistive technology and older people.

Natural and human-caused events – *Marcus Sivell-Muller*

In industrialised societies, it is more common for occupational therapists to consider the natural and human-made environment in terms of the physical environment of the home or public buildings used by our clients and that of the surrounding areas. As already discussed in this chapter, we have considered how the home environment can act as a barrier or facilitator to older people's activity and participation. However, it is also pertinent to consider how the physical environment and the older person's functioning within it might be affected by natural and human-made events.

Pestilence, famine, plague and war: scholars of the Bible will recognise these events as the Four Horsemen of the Apocalypse. To fit a more contemporary frame of reference, the International Classification of Functioning (ICF) has developed a refined definition that promulgates two categories – natural and human-caused events. Natural events are those extremes of nature that can cause dramatic change to the physical environment. Natural events can occur regularly or irregularly, such as earthquakes and severe or violent weather conditions such as tornadoes, hurricanes, typhoons, floods, forest fires and ice storms. Human-caused events are those that owe nothing to nature but are the creation of humankind and also bring disruption, displacement and destruction. The result of conflict or environmental disaster; these events affect not just land and homes but also the social infrastructure. Both the ICF categories affect the individual's or the community's wellbeing, in some cases right to the point of denying life and even extinction.

Occupational therapists are nurtured in the understanding of the person and their interrelation with the environment. Added to this, therapists are knowledgeable and sensitive to the context of any activity, occupation or event and its immediate significance to the individual.

Human beings have sought environments in which to live in and develop and that support their existence. Without water or a regular food source, we would simply fail to thrive. Nonetheless, humans are found living in some of the harshest climatic regions of the globe. Of course, those living in Siberia have long adapted to the harshness of the winter and the need to prepare and employ strategies with which to manage not mere survival, but to maintain an ability to continue with work and other productive activities. Since the beginning of time, human beings have demonstrated the desire to engage in leisure, or to seek opportunities from which pleasure and enjoyment are gained. Whether it is in the cold of Siberia or the heat of the Ethiopian desert, games and socialising leisure activities form the basis of social life. In such communities, cultural modes have established practices that compensate and support those older members of the community who find increasing barriers to not only social interaction, but to mere survival. The restrictions on activity are recognised and long-established strategies, and customs loaded with relevant cultural meaning are applied to ensure the impairment or restriction is limited.

For the peoples of these extreme climatic environments there is an habituation in the way the individual and the group undertake their occupational performance. In common with this learned collective understanding and an acceptance of these events, those peoples who live in regions affected by earthquakes and tsunamis, typhoons and hurricanes, demonstrate habitualised modes by which they prepare for and individually address the trauma and wreckage wrought after the crises have passed. By so doing, both the individual and community, old and young, are able to form strategies through which a lifestyle as near normal is maintained. For peoples accustomed to living for several months in freezing temperatures or searing heat; extreme elements that in temperate regions are often perceived as barriers to participating in an activity exist. However, therapists might fail to take on the significance of extreme fluctuations in temperature participation.

However, it is worth considering that although emergency plans and response programmes are devised and initiated, many older people may not be able to make use of these, because of sensory impairments such as visual or hearing loss, or because of limited mobility. Reliance upon others is a necessity and not a choice for many frail and older people. It is also suggested that emergency food provision could be inappropriate for older people, in terms of how the food is distributed and also the nutritional content (Help Age International 2012).

War, on the other hand. is the most obvious manifestation of a human- caused event, leading to disruption and dislocation of people from their everyday lives; the destruction of material, the pollution of land, water and air, and the subsequent effects on established social infrastructure are part and parcel of conflict in its many guises. Health conditions are directly and indirectly exacerbated. Affected individuals' functioning is decreased and disability is commonplace; in fact, some commentators suggest that this is a major objective of war and conflict. Depending on the nature of the conflict, it is very possible that normal day-to-day participation in activity, whether employment or leisure, is restricted, whether by direct events or the overall environmental context.

Through modern media, high intensity wars, characterised by the pooling of huge resources into vast combined coalitions (like those of the world wars and, more recently, Afghanistan and Iraq) are easy to envisage and the impact upon the individual is consequently easy to recognise. Those marked out by intermittent guerrilla tactics, as in the case of Palestine and East Timor, bring not just possible death and injury, but the effect on normal day-to-day activities for both the individual and wider group is inescapable. Major industrial accidents, like those at the Union Carbide plant in Bhopal in 1984 and the meltdown in April 1986 of Chernobyl in the Ukraine, are human-caused events. These human-caused events have had an immense impact upon the wellbeing of many people who have been, and in innumerable cases still are, affected by such an incident.

Whilst noting the success of individual and community coping strategies in dealing with catastrophic events, these have been shown to be dependent upon earlier experiences

---

Box 9.10   Guidance on working with older adults in conflict situations.

Help Age International has issued guidance on working with older adults in conflict situations. It is available at http://www.helpage.org/resources/publications/

- Ageing and development
- Crisis-affected older people in Kenya and Somalia
- Right to life without violence in old age
- Protecting older people in emergencies: Good practice guide

---

and previous exposure to crisis, in particular events of the same or similar nature. For those peoples who inhabit regions of the world where extremes of climate are the norm, we know a habituation is formed to cope with demands of existence amongst the elements. Equally, it is possible to recognise the role of previous experience in developing strategies to cope with human-made events. Humanitarian interventions have been criticised for neglecting older people, failing to address gender, social and cultural issues, using systems to discriminate against them and even undermining their ability to support themselves (Help Age International 2012, Box 9.10).

A suitable illustration of how the use of a meaningful occupation amongst this client group proved to have much broader and greater-reaching therapeutic consequences than first thought is that of a knitting group established among a group of older Bosnian women refugees in 1993. Notwithstanding other factors, there was no disguising the fact that, for many individuals in this community, this was the third time in their living memory that conflict had touched them directly. Their apparent fatalism and preparedness, demonstrated by the possessions they still maintained and their attempt to adapt to this perceived temporary dislocation, were commented on by many observers and relief workers. This differentiated older people not as a prescribed 'vulnerable group' but in fact as individuals who coped better with the changing realities. The narrative in Box 9.11 is comprised of excerpts from a diary, which one of the authors maintained working as a relief worker in the former Yugoslavia. The excerpts demonstrate the value of context, the older person experience and overcoming the trauma of community and individual brutalisation and loss.

It appeared that, with the introduction of an activity the focus of which was primarily to offer some meaningful and realistic occupation for the older women, younger women found a therapeutic environment in which to discuss and bring up what had been done to them in their eviction and forced migration. At the same time, the older women, often seen by external observers as a vulnerable group, were able to reflect upon their own experiences and offer not mere empathy and solace but also strategies and a living model of coping with events.

In this chapter, different environmental factors have been considered in relation to older people. Although not a complete discussion, the topics covered in this chapter reflect the current concerns of the authors and how older peoples' activity and participation are impacted upon by their environment. Such facilitators and barriers are evident contributors to older peoples' ability to age successfully in an occupationally just environment.

Box 9.11   Occupation and conflict: A narrative by Marcus Sivell-Muller.

Whilst working as a relief worker with a UNHCR implementing partner, I spent time at numerous collective centres throughout this region. In September 1993, I was working with 180 to 200 Bosnian refugees at a town called Posusje on the Bosnian/Croatian border. The displaced persons, as they were labelled, were accommodated in a derelict secondary school. They had split themselves into extended family groups and occupied the classrooms and offices as their accommodation. As is often the norm amongst refugee communities across the globe, the majority of this group were women and children. A further breakdown of the population revealed some 29 older men and just three men over the age of 16 but younger than 70. The rest were either children or women. At first sight, the families appeared large. Traditionally, relief work is built on a number of tenets. As a rule, these principles follow a Maslow hierarchy in addressing displaced persons' needs. Furthermore, there is an acknowledgement that 'vulnerable groups' have particular issues and these require seeking out and addressing. Finally, where at all possible, empower and encourage both user and host population to discuss, work together and come to mutually beneficial decisions and outcomes. Besides the obvious grouping of young children and pregnant women, the older people and those with health conditions and disability were focused upon. At this stage it is important to note that two months before the creation of this collective centre, European newspapers had carried stories of widespread atrocities, concentration camps and the brutalisation of the civilian population by armed militias. Of particular note were the rumours of systematic rape of the female population, including young girls.

In between creating activities for the displaced youth of the centre and ensuring continual dialogue between the local town council and the refugees on the various issues that could cause problems, I would spend time taking a short walk along the main track with several of the older women. At that time my local language was limited, but it did not stop these rural mountain people attempting to communicate with me and give me advice. They were very much interested in London, and in particular the knitted wool jumper that my grandmother had sent me to keep out the Balkan winter. After a number of weeks, it became apparent that the older women sought some wool and needles in order to undertake a similar project. The necessary equipment was found through a charitable organisation and passed on to the women. I visited the main assembly area where I found several older women sitting comfortably, knitting away and drinking coffee. I was sufficiently smug to think that through providing them with the materials to engage in a meaningful occupation, I had enabled what were often considered as 'forgotten vulnerable victims' and thus contributed to an improvement in their well being.

Over the next few weeks, the relief team noticed that after the collective domestic activities of daily living were complete the majority of the women appeared to head for the assembly hall and remain there for much of the day. On one occasion, I noticed a young woman leaving the assembly hall tearfully. I asked of another what the problem was and she explained that I should come along and see how useful the knitting group had become. Of course, in my ignorance, I thought I was going to see all the women knitting useful jumpers as it had become cold. I was astounded to sit amongst the 70 or so women and watch as some knitted and drank coffee whilst one woman spoke animatedly. It became apparent that one older woman was talking about the effects the war had had upon her and her family. But not the current conflict, a war some 50 years before. Another older woman offered similar experiences and as I tried to discern words I still had yet to master a younger woman in her late 20s began to cry and talk emotively. It was explained to me that she was describing what had had been done to her by armed men who had come to her home. More women spoke and there was a considerable outpouring of grief. I was not the only man in the room; there was a very old man who sat playing with his moustache throughout. Before I left the room, I noticed an older woman, without tears, give matter-of-fact advice.

References

Atwal, A., Murphy, S., McIntyre, A., Hunt, J. and Craik, C. (2008a) Older adults and carer perceptions' of pre-discharge occupational therapy home visits in acute care: A qualitative study. *Age and Ageing* **37(1)**, 72–76.

Atwal, A., McIntyre, A., Craik, C. and Hunt, J. (2008b) Occupational therapists' perceptions of pre-discharge home assessments with older adults in acute care. *British Journal of Occupational Therapy* **71(2)**, 52–58.

Atwal, A., McIntyre, A. and Wiggett, C. (2011a) Risks with older adults in acute care settings: UK occupational therapists' and physiotherapists' perceptions of risks associated with discharge and professional practice. *Scandinavian Journal of Caring Science* **26(2)**, 381–393, doi: 10.1111/j.1471-6712.2011.00946.x

Atwal, A., Wiggett, C., McIntyre, A. (2011b) Risks with older adults in acute care settings: occupational therapists' and physiotherapists' perceptions. *British Journal of Occupational Therapy*, **74(9)**, 412–418.

Atwal, A., Spiliotopoulou, G., Plastow, N., McIntyre, A. and McKay, E.A. (2012) Older adults' experiences of occupational therapy pre-discharge home visits: A systematic thematic synthesis of qualitative research. *British Journal of Occupational Therapy* **75(3)**, 118–127.

Audit Commission (2004) Independence and Wellbeing. Available at: http://www.audit-commission.gov.uk/SiteCollectionDocuments/AuditCommissionReports/NationalStudies/OlderPeople_overarch.pdf

Brandt, A., Iwarsson, S. and Stahle, A. (2004) Older people's use of powered wheelchairs for activity and participation. *Journal of Rehabilitation Medicine* **36(2)**, 70–72.

Canadian Association of Occupational Therapists (2006) CAOT position statement: Assistive technology and occupational therapy. Available at: http://www.caot.ca/default.asp?pageid=598

Caprani, N., Greaney, J. and Porter, N. (2006) A review of memory aid devices for an ageing population. *PsychNology* **4(3)**, 205–243.

Care Services Improvement Partnership, Health and Social Care Change Agent Team (2005) Factsheet: Telecare and Ethics. London: Department of Health.

Caudell, T.P., Summers, K.L., Holten, I.V.J., Hakamata, T., Mowafi, M., Jacobs, J., Lozanoff, B.K., Lozanoff, S., Wilks, D. and Keep, M.F. (2003) Virtual patient simulator for distributed collaborative medical education. *Anatomical Record Part B: The New Anatomist* **270(1)**, 23–29.

Chen, L.P., Mann, W.C., Tomita, M.R. and Burford, T.E. (1998) An evaluation of reachers for use by older persons with disabilities. *Assistive Technology* **10(2)**, 113–125.

Chiu, C.W.Y. and Man, D.W.K. (2004) The effect of training older adults with stroke to use home-based assistive devices. *Occupational Therapy Journal of Research* **24(3)** 113–120.

Chodos, D., Stroulia, E., Boechler, P., King, S., Kuras, P., Carbonaro, M. and de Jong, E. (2010) Healthcare education with virtual-world simulations. In: Proceedings of the 2nd Workshop on Software Engineering in Health Care, SEHC Washington DC, USA: The IEEE Computer Society.

College of Occuaptional Therapists (2012) Briefing 26 – Confidentiality and a Service User's Fitness to Drive. London: College of Occuaptional Therapists.

Department for Transport (DfT) (2000) Understanding People's Needs. Older people: Their transport needs and requirements – Summary report, London: DfT.

Department of Health (2007a) *Putting People First: A shared vision and commitment to the transformation of adult social care.* London: Department of Health.

Department of Health (2007b) *Independence, Choice and Risk: A guide to best practice in supported decision making.* London: Department of Health.

Department for Work and Pensions (2008) *Lifetime Homes, Lifetime Neighbourhoods. A National Strategy for Housing in an Ageing Society*. London: Department for Work and Pensions. London.

Doughty, K. (2004) Supporting independence: The emerging role of technology. *Housing, Care & Support* **7(1)**, 11–17.

Dunbar, G., Holland, C.A. and Maylor, E.A. (2004) *Road Safety Research Report No. 37 Older Pedestrians: A critical review of the literature*. Department of Transport. London

Edwards, N.I. and Jones, D.A. (1998) Ownership and use of assistive devices amongst older people in the community. *Age and Ageing* **27(4)**, 463–468.

Hoffman, T. and Worrall, L. (2004) Designing effective written health education materials: Consideration for health professionals. *Disability and Rehabilitation* **26(19)**, 1166–1173.

Gardezi, F., Wilson, K.G., Man-Son-Hing, M., Marshall, S.C., Molnar, F.J., Dobbs, B.M. et al. (2006). Qualitative research on older drivers. *Clinical Gerontologist* **30(1)**, 5–22.

Gilhooly, M., Hamilton, K., O'Neill, G.J., Webster, N. and Pike, F. (2003) *Transport and Ageing. Extending Quality of Life via Public and Private Transport*. Economic Social Research Council Growing Older Programme.

Gitlin, L.N. (1995) Why older people accept or reject assistive technology. *Journal of the American Society of Aging* **1(19)**, 41–47.

Gitlin, L.N., Winter, L., Dennis, M.P., Corcoran, M., Schinfeld, S. and Hauck, W.W. (2006) A randomized trial of a multicomponent home intervention to reduce functional difficulties in older adults. *Journal of the American Geriatrics Society* **54(5)**, 809–816.

Goodacre, K., McCreadie, C., Flanigan, S. and Lansley, P. (2008) Enabling older people to stay at home: The costs of substituting and supplementing care with assistive technology. *British Journal of Occupational Therapy* **71(4)**, 130–140.

Griffin, J., McKenna, K. and Tooth, L. (2003) Written health educational materials: Making them more effective. *Australian Occupational Therapy Journal* **50(3)**, 170–177.

Ham, R., Aldersea, P. and Porter, D. (1998) *Wheelchair Users and Postural Seating: A clinical approach*. London: Churchill Livingstone.

Hannon, C, and Bradwell, P. (2007) *Web I'm 64: Ageing, the internet and digital inclusion*. London: Demos.

Hawley, C. (2010) The attitudes of health professionals to giving advice on fitness to drive Department for Transport Road Safety Report 91. London: Department of Transport. Available at: http://assets. dft.gov.uk/publications/pgr-roadsafety-research-rsrr-theme6-report91-pdf/report91.pdf

Help Age International (2012) Older people in emergencies – identifying and reducing risks. Help Age International. Available at: www.helpage.org/download/4fd728a1b410b

Hislop, C. (2010) Improving access to information: A key requirement for reducing social exclusion. *Working with Older People* **14(4)**, 38–43.

Johnson, A., Sandford, J. and Tyndall, J. (2003) Written and verbal information versus verbal information only for patients being discharged from acute hospital settings to home. *Cochrane Database 4*, CD003716.

Korner-Bitensky, N., Menon, A., von Zweck, C., Van Benthem, K. (2010) Occupational therapists' capacity-building needs related to older driver screening, assessment, and intervention: A Canada-wide survey. *The American Journal of Occupational Therapy* **64(2)**, 316–324.

Iezzoni, L.I., McCarthy, E.P., Davis, R.B. and Siebens, H. (2001) Mobility difficulties are not only a problem of old age. *Journal of General Internal Medicine* **16(4)**, 235–243.

Mackenzie, M. (2007) Telecare Factsheet: Ethics and assessment, Edinburgh: Scottish Government.

Mann, W.C., Ottenbacher, K.J., Frass, L., Tomita, M. and Granger, C.V. (1999) Effectiveness of assistive technology and environmental interventions in maintaining independence and reducing home care costs for the frail elderly. A randomised controlled trial. *Archives of Family Medicine* **8(3)** 210–217.

Martin, J.K., Martin, L.G., Stumbo, N.J. and Morrill, J.H. (2012) The impact of consumer involvement on satisfaction with and use of assistive technology. *Disability & Rehabilitation: Assistive Technology* **6(3)**, 225–242.

Marshall, L.A. and Williams, D. (2006) Health information: Does quality count for the consumers? *Librarianship and Information Science* **38(3)**, 141–156.

Money, A. McIntyre, A., Atwal, A., Spiliotopoulou, G., Elliman, T. and French, T (2011) Bringing the home into the hospital: Assisting the pre-discharge home visit process using 3D Home Visualization software. *Universal access in human-computer interaction; Applications and services*, **6768**, 416–426.

Mountain, G. (2000) *Occupational Therapy in Social Services Departments: A review of the literature.* London: College of Occupational Therapists.

National Health Service (2007) *Toolkit for Producing Patient Information.* London: National Health Service.

The National Wheelchair Managers Forum (2010) Healthcare Standards for NHS-Commissioned Wheelchairs. London: NHS. Available at: Serviceshttp://www.wheelchairmanagers.nhs.uk/pubs.html

Office for National Statistics (2002) *Living in Britain.* Results from the 2001 General Household Survey. London: Office for National Statistics.

Office for National Statistics (2010) UK National Statistics. Available at: http://www.statistics.gov.uk/hub/index.html

Office for National Statistics (2011) Statistical Bulletin. Older People's Day. Office for National Statistics. Available at: http://www.ons.gov.uk/ons/dcp171778_235000.pdf

Petersson, I., Lilja, M. and Borell, L. (2012) To feel safe in everyday life at home – a study of older adults after home modifications. *Ageing and Society* **32(5)**, 791–811.

Phillips, B. and Zhao, H. (1993) Predictors of assistive technology abandonment. *Assistive Technology* **5(1)**, 36–45.

Riley, J., Whitcombe, S. and Vincent, C. (2008) *Occupational Therapy in Adult Social Care in England.* London: Department of Health.

Sanford, J.A., Griffiths, P.C., Richardson, P., Hargraves, K.,Butterfield, T. and Hoenig, H. (2006) The effects of in-home rehabilitation on task self-efficacy in mobility-impaired adults: A randomized clinical trial. *Journal of the American Geriatrics Society* **54(11)**, 1641–1648.

Scherer, M.J. and Galvin, J.C. (1996) An outcomes perspective of quality pathways to most appropriate technology. In: Galvin, M.J. (ed.) *Evaluating, Selecting and Using Appropriate Assistive Technology.* Gaithersburg: Aspen Publishers, Inc, pp. 1–26.

Schneidert, M., Hurst, R., Miller, J. and Ustun, B. (2003) The role of environment in the International Classification of Functioning, Disability and Health (ICF). *Disability and Rehabilitation* **25(11–12)**, 588–595.

Schultheis, M.T. and Rizzo, A.A. (2001) The application of virtual reality technology in rehabilitation. *Rehabilitation Psychology* **46(3)**, 296–311.

Simpson, J.M., Darwin, C. and Marsh, N. (2003) What are older people prepared to do to avoid falling? A qualitative study in London. *British Journal of Community Nursing* **8(4)**, 152–159.

Stansfield, S., Butkiewicz, T., Suma, E. and Kane, M. (2005) Interactive virtual client for teaching occupational therapy evaluative processes. In: Proceedings of the 7th International ACM SIGACCESS Conference on Computers and Accessibility

Stav, W., Weidley, L.S. and Love, A. (2011) Barriers to developing and sustaining driving and community mobility programs. *American Journal of Occupational Therapy* **65(4)**, 38–45.

Unsworth, C. (2007) Development and current status of occupational therapy driver assessment and rehabilitation in Victoria, Australia. *Australian Occupational Therapy Journal* **54(2)**, 153–156.

Vrkljan, B.H. and Anaby, V.A. (2011) What vehicle features are considered important when buying an automobile? An examination of driver preferences by age and gender. *Canadian Journal of Occupational Therapy* **42(1)**, 61–65.

Weiderhold, B.K. (2006) The potential of virtual reality to improve healthcare. Available at: http:// iactor.eu/downloads/WP%20The%20Potential%20for%20VR%20to%20Improve%20 Healthcare.pdf

Weiss, P.L., Rand, D., Katz, N. and Kizony, R. (2004) Video capture virtual reality as a flexible and effective rehabilitation tool. *Journal of Neuroengineering and Rehabilitation* **1(1)**, 12.

Wey, S. (2007) The Ethical Use of Assistive Technology for People with Dementia. Trent Dementia Services Development Centre. Available at: http://www.atdementia.org.uk/editorial.asp?page_ id=47

White, D.K., Jette, A.M., Felson, D.T., Lavalley, M.P., Lewis, C.E., Torner, J.C., Nevitt, M.C. and Keysor, J.J. (2010) Are features of the neighborhood environment associated with disability in older adults? *Disability and Rehabilitation* **32(8)**, 639–645.

Whitehead, B., Howie, L. and Lovell, R.K. (2006) Older people's experience of driver licence cancellation: A phenomenological study. *Australian Occupational Therapy Journal* **53(3)**, 173–180.

Wielandt, T. and Strong, J. (2000) Compliance with prescribed adaptive equipment: A literature review. *British Journal of Occupational Therapy* **63(2)**, 65–75.

Wilson, D.J., Mitchell, J.M., Kemp, B.J., Adkins, R.H. and Mann, W. (2009) Effects of assistive technology on functional decline in people aging with a disability. *Assistive Technology* **21(4)**, 208–217.

Winchcombe, M. and Ballinger, C. (2005) *A Competence Framework for Trusted Assessors.* London: Assist UK.

World Health Organization (2001) *The International Classification of Functioning Disability and Health.* Geneva: World Health Organization.

Zhang, L., Abreu, B.C., Seale, G.S., Masel, B., Christiansen, C.H. and Ottenbacher, K.J. (2003) A virtual reality environment for evaluation of a daily living skill in brain injury rehabilitation: Reliability and validity. *Archives of Physical Medicine and Rehabilitation* **84(8)**, 1118–1124.

Index

Occupational Therapy and Older People, Second Edition. Edited by Anita Atwal and Anne McIntyre.
© 2013 Blackwell Publishing Ltd. Published 2013 by Blackwell Publishing Ltd.

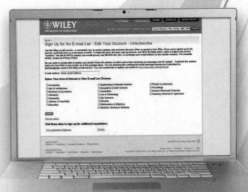
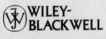